Pediatric Pulmonology

Pediatric Pulmonology

Editor: Lillie McGuire

AMERICAN
MEDICAL PUBLISHERS
www.americanmedicalpublishers.com

AMERICAN
MEDICAL PUBLISHERS
www.americanmedicalpublishers.com

Cataloging-in-Publication Data

Pediatric pulmonology / edited by Lillie McGuire.
p. cm.
Includes bibliographical references and index.
ISBN 978-1-63927-428-4
1. Pediatric respiratory diseases. 2. Lungs--Diseases. 3. Children--Diseases. I. McGuire, Lillie.
RJ431 .P43 2022
618.922--dc23

American Medical Publishers,
41 Flatbush Avenue,
1st Floor, New York,
NY 11217, USA

ISBN 978-1-63927-428-4 (Hardback)

Contents

Preface

Over the recent decade, advancements and applications have progressed exponentially. This has led to the increased interest in this field and projects are being conducted to enhance knowledge. The main objective of this book is to present some of the critical challenges and provide insights into possible solutions. This book will answer the varied questions that arise in the field and also provide an increased scope for furthering studies.

Pediatric pulmonology is a specialized field concerned with the treatment of children with respiratory conditions. Respiratory infections contribute to the high rates of mortality in children under the age of five in many parts of the world. The common respiratory issues in children include asthma, bronchitis, pneumonia and wheezing, while some less common conditions are cystic fibrosis, apnea, assisted breathing, etc. Flexible fiberoptic bronchoscopy and pulmonary function testing are certain diagnostic methods in pediatric pulmonology. The use of molecular diagnostics for respiratory illnesses and minimally invasive procedures, have advanced the diagnostic and treatment outcomes in pediatric pulmonology. This book is compiled in such a manner, that it will provide an in-depth knowledge about the theory and practice of pediatric pulmonology. From theories to research to practical applications, case studies related to all contemporary topics of relevance to this field have been included herein. This book will provide comprehensive knowledge to readers.

I hope that this book, with its visionary approach, will be a valuable addition and will promote interest among readers. Each of the authors has provided their extraordinary competence in their specific fields by providing different perspectives as they come from diverse nations and regions. I thank them for their contributions.

Editor

1

Acute respiratory distress syndrome in a child with severe epileptic disorder treated successfully by extracorporeal membrane oxygenation

Nobuyuki Nosaka[1,2], Shingo Ichiba[1,3*], Kohei Tsukahara[1], Emily Knaup[1], Kumiko Hayashi[1], Shingo Kasahara[4], Yoshinori Kobayashi[5], Makio Oka[5], Katsuhiro Kobayashi[5], Harumi Yoshinaga[5] and Yoshihito Ujike[1]

Abstract

Background: Extracorporeal membrane oxygenation (ECMO) is now a candidate therapy for children with acute respiratory failure.

Case presentation: We report our experience of using central ECMO therapy for acute respiratory distress syndrome followed by seizure in a 15-month-old girl with a severe epileptic disorder. Her respiratory distress was refractory to standard medical treatment and mechanical ventilatory support. Her condition was complicated by development of a pneumothorax. The patient was successfully weaned off ECMO and discharged without deterioration of her neurological status.

Conclusion: The successful outcome in this case resulted from the central ECMO, which enabled "lung rest" and adequate cerebral blood flow. In skilled ECMO facilities, early implementation of ECMO would give some advantages to patients such as the one presented here. Given the invasiveness and the ease of the procedure, introduction of dual-lumen catheters adequately sized for pediatric patients in Japan is required.

Keywords: Acute respiratory distress syndrome (ARDS), Extracorporeal membrane oxygenation (ECMO), Severe epileptic disorder, Pediatrics

Background

Extracorporeal membrane oxygenation (ECMO) is now a candidate therapy for patients with acute respiratory failure [1-4] based on several reports of ECMO treatment for acute respiratory failure associated with influenza A H1N1 infection in both adult and pediatric patients [5-10]. Implementation of ECMO for pediatric respiratory failure has almost doubled since 2000. Approximately 350 patients have been treated annually over the past 3 years worldwide, with a 56% survival rate [11]. We report our experience of using ECMO for acute respiratory distress syndrome (ARDS) followed by seizure in a 15-month-old girl with a severe epileptic disorder. Her respiratory distress was refractory to standard medical treatment and mechanical ventilatory support and complicated by development of a pneumothorax. The patient was successfully weaned from ECMO and discharged home without deterioration in her neurological status.

Case presentation

A 15-month-old girl (10.1 kg, 80 cm) presented to our emergency department because of status epilepticus. She had been diagnosed as having Dravet syndrome [12] with *SCN1A* mutation at the age of 10 months and had received antiepileptic therapy with stiripentol, valproic acid, and clobazam. Psychomotor retardation had been detected at the age of 11 months. She had continued to

* Correspondence: ecmoshingo@gmail.com
[1]Advanced Emergency and Critical Care Medical Center, Okayama University Hospital, Okayama, Japan
[3]Department of Community and Emergency Medicine, Okayama University Graduate School of Medicine, Dentistry and Pharmaceutical Sciences, Okayama, Japan
Full list of author information is available at the end of the article

be subject to repeated convulsions, which were managed by as-needed rectal diazepam.

She was having a partial seizure on arrival at hospital, which was aborted with intravenous midazolam. She was intubated for airway protection and transferred to our emergency intensive care unit. Sulbactam/ampicillin (300 mg/kg/day) was administered for suspected aspiration pneumonia. Once her body temperature had been controlled, she was free of seizures and did not require increased doses of antiepileptic drugs.

Her respiratory function deteriorated, however, and she developed ARDS the day after her admission. Her partial pressure of O_2 (PaO_2)/fraction of inspired O_2 (FIO_2) (P/F) ratio was 207. She was placed on synchronized intermittent mandatory ventilation. The ventilator settings had to be gradually increased during the next 4 days from 18/5 cmH_2O to 20/10 cmH_2O with an increase in FIO_2 from 0.40 to 0.80. On day 6, the ventilator settings were changed to high-frequency oscillation ventilation (HFOV) because her P/F ratio and oxygenation index (OI) had worsened to 84 and 19, respectively. Having achieved complete muscle relaxation, the HFOV settings were adjusted (mean airway pressure 32 cm H_2O, FIO_2 0.65, stroke volume 60 mL, frequency 10 Hz), after which the P/F ratio and OI improved to 196 and 15.2, respectively.

Her respiratory status stabilized on HFOV. However, on day 8 her oxygenation suddenly deteriorated to a P/F ratio of 54 and OI of 55 because of development of a right pneumothorax (a complication of HFOV), which required urgent placement of a chest tube. Despite a deaeration procedure, her pulmonary function deteriorated to an OI of 78.9. A decision was made to introduce venovenous ECMO therapy. A 14 Fr return cannula was successfully inserted percutaneously into the left internal jugular vein. However, an attempt to place a 17 Fr drainage cannula into the right internal jugular vein percutaneously failed because of an error in guidewire handling and formation of a hematoma on her neck.

In this emergency situation, the therapeutic strategy was aggressively changed to venoarterial ECMO. With the help of a cardiac surgeon, a 21 Fr drainage cannula and 12 Fr return cannula were placed in the right atrium and ascending aorta, respectively, via mid-sternotomy. The ECMO flow was initially set at 1 L/min with rotational frequency of the centrifugal pump. After introduction of 70% O_2 via ECMO, her arterial blood gas values dramatically improved (PaO_2 404 mmHg), and the FIO_2 from mechanical ventilation was reduced to 30% with a lower tidal volume and lower airway pressure (positive end-expiratory pressure 8 cmH_2O, inspiration time 1.5–1.8 seconds, frequency 5/min). Because of continuous oozing from the thoracotomy site and hematoma formation in the right thoracic cavity, substantial volumes of blood were transfused during ECMO management (red blood cell concentrate 3250 mL; fresh frozen plasma 920 mL; platelets 1350 mL). As the patient was already fluid-overloaded because of her severe hypoxic and inflammatory status prior to introducing ECMO, continuous renal replacement therapy was introduced after stabilization on ECMO to control her fluid balance precisely. To reduce the risk of bleeding, nafamostat mesilate was used as an anticoagulant, with a targeted activated clotting time of 150–160 s. The ECMO circuit used had a heparin coating.

On day 12 (fourth day of ECMO), mediastinal lavage and removal of hematoma from the right thoracic cavity was performed through re-thoracotomy with no complications. On day 13 (fifth day of ECMO), 600 mg of surfactant was administered mainly into the right upper and middle lobar branches, with direct bronchoscopic observation. According to her lung compliance measured by the ventilator (Evita Infinity V500, Dräger, Lübeck, Germany) and serial chest X-ray films, there was gradual improvement, especially after the surfactant therapy (Figure 1). During ECMO support, central venous oxygen saturation was stable at around 70%.

Stable hemodynamics having been achieved after 7 days of ECMO support, the patient was successfully weaned from ECMO on day 15. Continuous renal replacement therapy was discontinued simultaneously. Tracheal extubation was performed on day 26. She was discharged from our intensive care unit on day 34 and discharged home on day 79 without deterioration in her neurological status.

Support from multiple departments facilitated rapid introduction of central ECMO and stabilization of the patient, which contributed greatly to successful treatment of this pediatric patient with ARDS [2]. There may be counterarguments against using central respiratory ECMO, but it enabled provision of complete "lung rest," attenuating ventilator-induced lung injury [13,14], as did aggressive treatment with the surfactant. Because of the patient's abnormal vessel course and small vessel size, which are associated with Dravet syndrome, there was no adequately sized double-lumen cannula for this patient that was available in Japan. The use of bilateral jugular vein cannulation in ECMO has some risk of increasing the intracranial venous pressure and development of superior vena cava syndrome. Also, if we had chosen to cannulate the jugular veins bilaterally in this patient, it may have caused deterioration in her neurodevelopmental status. Therefore, we believe that central ECMO was a reasonable choice for this patient.

We decided to implement ECMO after detecting a pneumothorax, which is one of the complications of HFOV. Whether the timing of ECMO introduction was optimal in this patient is open to debate. Our respiratory management strategy for pediatric ARDS patients is based on the OI as follows: With OI ≥20, implement HFOV; with OI ≥30, implement ECMO. Two large randomized

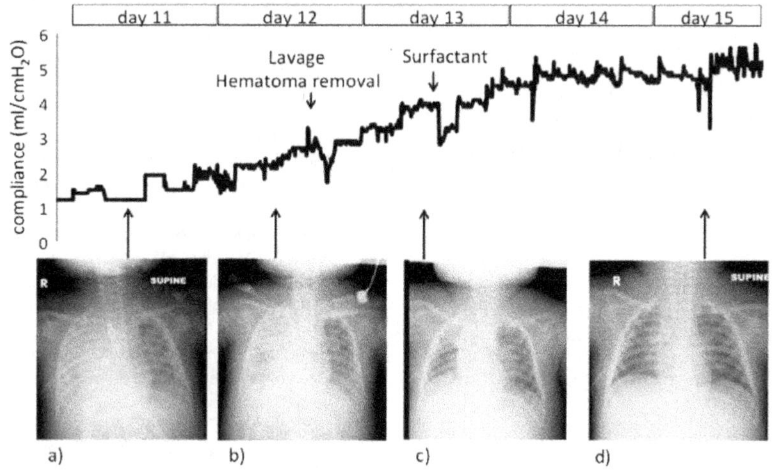

Figure 1 Lung compliance and chest radiographs. The line graph shows improvement in lung compliance as calculated by the mechanical ventilator. Lung compliance was temporarily compromised with interventions such as lavage or surfactant administration; however, it subsequently recovered to adequate levels. Parallel with recovery of lung compliance, the radiolucency of the lung gradually improved. **a)** Day 11. **b)** Day 12 before lavage and hematoma removal. **c)** Day 13 before surfactant administration. **d)** Day 15.

controlled trials comparing HFOV with conventional lung-protective ventilation were published in 2013: the Oscillation for Acute Respiratory Distress Syndrome Treated Early (OSCILLATE) trial [15] and the Oscillation in ARDS (OSCAR) trial [16]. These trials suggested that, in adults with early moderate-to-severe ARDS, HFOV conferred no benefit and may have been harmful [17]. Historically, HFOV is preferred for lung protective therapy in small children. However the pathophysiology of acute respiratory failure in neonates is known to differ from that of older infants and children. Thus, HFOV may also be harmful to children. With sufficient understanding of the characteristics of both HFOV and ECMO, lowering the criteria for implementation of ECMO might improve patients' safety and outcomes.

Easier, less invasive implementation of ECMO should provide great advantages for pediatric patients with severe ARDS. The current technique in Japan involves implementing venovenous ECMO using bilateral jugular veins or venoarterial ECMO using an internal jugular vein and a common carotid artery. The internal diameter of the catheter is crucial to facilitating sufficient drainage of venous blood [18]. However, the available catheters with sufficiently large diameters (larger than 15 Fr) in Japan may be too long for pediatric patients. This makes aspects of the cannulation procedure (e.g., handling of the guidewire) more difficult, as we experienced in this patient. Recently, dual-lumen catheters have gained popularity in western countries for administering pediatric ECMO [19]. Currently, these devices are unavailable in Japan. However, given the invasiveness and the ease of the procedure, introduction of dual-lumen catheters for pediatric patients is urgently required in our country.

ECMO enabled safe administration of surfactant into targeted lung lobar branches with bronchoscopic guidance. ECMO provides a safe setting for procedures that are risky during ventilation. Several researchers have reported that surfactant is effective in patients with ARDS, especially children [20,21]. Based on our observations of improvement in lung compliance, we believe that surfactant contributed to our patient's recovery. However, further research to verify the effect of surfactant in ARDS patients is needed. It would be desirable to accumulate a series of pediatric ARDS patients who have been treated with surfactant and in whom relevant variables, including lung compliance, have been measured.

Severe neurological disorders have been thought to contraindicate the use of ECMO [22]. According to the most recent Extracorporeal Life Support Organization guidelines, however, most contraindications are relative. Hence, the risk of a procedure should be balanced against its potential benefits [18]. Pneumonia is one of the most frequent causes of death in epileptic patients, including those with Dravet syndrome [23-25]. The development of ECMO has increased the range of means of managing such patients. However, ECMO remains an expensive treatment with a high risk of complications. The indications should be carefully scrutinized, case by case. From this perspective, the possibility of implementing ECMO should be considered at an early stage to ensure sufficient time to discuss its applicability.

Conclusions

We implemented central venoarterial ECMO for respiratory failure in a pediatric patient with a severe epileptic disorder in an emergency situation. Central respiratory

ECMO could be a reasonable choice for small pediatric patients with severe ARDS. With enough understanding of the characteristics of ECMO, its early implementation might improve outcomes. Our results suggest that the introduction of dual-lumen catheters for pediatric patients to Japan could lead to safer, less invasive implementation of ECMO.

Abbreviations

ARDS: Acute respiratory distress syndrome; ECMO: Extracorporeal membrane oxygenation; FIO_2: Fraction of inspired O_2; HFOV: High-frequency oscillation ventilation; OI: Oxygenation index; PaO_2: Partial pressure of oxygen; P/F: Pressure of O_2/fraction of inspired O_2.

Competing interests

The authors declare that they have no competing interests.

Authors' contributions

NN drafted the manuscript. NN, SI, EK, KT, KH, SK, YK, MO, KK, and HY contributed to treating the patient. SI and YU revised and edited the manuscript. All authors have read and approved the final manuscript.

Acknowledgment

The authors thank Edanz (http://www.edanzediting.co.jp) for the English language review.

Author details

[1]Advanced Emergency and Critical Care Medical Center, Okayama University Hospital, Okayama, Japan. [2]Department of Pediatrics, Okayama University Graduate School of Medicine, Dentistry and Pharmaceutical Sciences, Okayama, Japan. [3]Department of Community and Emergency Medicine, Okayama University Graduate School of Medicine, Dentistry and Pharmaceutical Sciences, Okayama, Japan. [4]Department of Cardiovascular Surgery, Okayama University Graduate School of Medicine, Dentistry and Pharmaceutical Sciences, Okayama, Japan. [5]Department of Child Neurology, Okayama University Graduate School of Medicine, Dentistry and Pharmaceutical Sciences, Okayama, Japan.

References

1. Peek GJ, Sosnowski AW. Extra-corporeal membrane oxygenation for paediatric respiratory failure. Br Med Bull. 1997;53:745–56.
2. Peris A, Cianchi G, Biondi S, Bonizzoli M, Pasquini A, Bonacchi M, et al. Extracorporeal life support for management of refractory cardiac or respiratory failure: initial experience in a tertiary centre. Scand J Trauma Resusc Emerg Med. 2010;21:18–28.
3. Maslach-Hubbard A, Bratton SL. Extracorporeal membrane oxygenation for pediatric respiratory failure: History, development and current status. World J Crit Care Med. 2013;4:29–39.
4. Extracorporeal Life Support Organization (ELSO): Guidelines for Pediatric Respiratory Failure. Ver. 1.3, November 2013. [https://www.elso.org/Portals/0/IGD/Archive/FileManager/929122ae88cusersshyerdocumentselsoguidelinesgeneralalleclsversion1.3.pdf]
5. Buckley E, Sidebotham D, McGeorge A, Roberts S, Allen SJ, Beca J. Extracorporeal membrane oxygenation for cardiorespiratory failure in four patients with pandemic H1N1 2009 influenza virus and secondary bacterial infection. Br J Anaesth. 2010;104:326–9.
6. Noah MA, Peek GJ, Finney SJ, Griffiths MJ, Harrison DA, Grieve R, et al. Referral to an extracorporeal membrane oxygenation center and mortality among patients with severe 2009 influenza A(H1N1). JAMA. 2011;306:1659–68.
7. Australia and New Zealand Extracorporeal Membrane Oxygenation (ANZ ECMO) Influenza Investigators, Davies A, Jones D, Bailey M, Beca J, Bellomo R, et al. Extracorporeal Membrane Oxygenation for 2009 Influenza A(H1N1) Acute Respiratory Distress Syndrome. JAMA. 2009;302:1888–95.
8. Turner DA, Rehder KJ, Peterson-Carmichael SL, Ozment CP, Al-Hegelan MS, Williford WL, et al. Extracorporeal membrane oxygenation for severe refractory respiratory failure secondary to 2009 H1N1 influenza A. Respir Care. 2011;56:941–6.
9. Freed DH, Henzler D, White CW, Fowler R, Zarychanski R, Hutchison J, et al. Extracorporeal lung support for patients who had severe respiratory failure secondary to influenza A (H1N1) 2009 infection in Canada. Can J Anaesth. 2010;57:240–7.
10. Tokuhira N, Shime N, Inoue M, Kawasaki T, Sakurai Y, Kurosaka N, et al. Mechanically ventilated children with 2009 pandemic influenza A/H1N1: results from the National Pediatric Intensive Care Registry in Japan. Pediatr Crit Care Med. 2012;13:e294–8.
11. Paden ML, Conrad SA, Rycus PT, Thiagarajan RR, ELSO Registry. Extracorporeal Life Support Organization Registry Report 2012. ASAIO J. 2013;59:202–10.
12. Akiyama M, Kobayashi K, Ohtsuka Y. Dravet syndrome: a genetic epileptic disorder. Acta Med Okayama. 2012;66:369–76.
13. Fan E, Villar J, Slutsky AS. Novel approaches to minimize ventilator-induced lung injury. BMC Med. 2013;28:85.
14. The Acute Respiratory Distress Syndrome Network. Ventilation with lower tidal volumes as compared with traditional tidal volumes for acute lung injury and the acute respiratory distress syndrome. N Engl J Med. 2000;342:1301–8.
15. Ferguson ND, Cook DJ, Guyatt GH, Mehta S, Hand L, Austin P, et al. High-frequency oscillation in early acute respiratory distress syndrome. N Engl J Med. 2013;368:795–805.
16. Young D, Lamb SE, Shah S, MacKenzie I, Tunnicliffe W, Lall R, et al. High-frequency oscillation for acute respiratory distress syndrome. N Engl J Med. 2013;368:806–13.
17. Goffi A, Ferguson ND. High-frequency oscillatory ventilation for early acute respiratory distress syndrome in adults. Curr Opin Crit Care. 2014;20:77–85.
18. Extracorporeal Life Support Organization (ELSO) General Guidelines for all ECLS Cases. [https://www.elso.org/Portals/0/IGD/Archive/FileManager/929122ae88cusersshyerdocumentselsoguidelinesgeneralalleclsversion1.3.pdf]
19. Fallon SC, Shekerdemian LS, Olutoye OO, Cass DL, Zamora IJ, Nguyen T, et al. Initial experience with single-vessel cannulation for venovenous extracorporeal membrane oxygenation in pediatric respiratory failure. Pediatr Crit Care Med. 2013;14:366–73.
20. Kula R, Maca J, Sklienka P, Tichy J, Szturz P, Jahoda J, et al. Exogenous surfactant as a component of complex non-ECMO therapy of ARDS caused by influenza A virus (2009 H1N1). Bratisl Lek Listy. 2011;112:218–22.
21. Willson DF, Notter RH. The future of exogenous surfactant therapy. Respir Care. 2011;56:1369–86.
22. Extracorporeal Life Support Organization (ELSO) Guidelines for Pediatric Respiratory Failure. Ver. 1.1, April 2009. [http://www.elso.med.umich.edu/wordforms/elso%20pt%20specific%20guidelines.pdf]
23. Terra VC, Scorza FA, Arida RM, Fernandes RM, Wichert-Ana L, Machado HR, et al. Mortality in children with severe epilepsy: 10 years of follow-up. Arq Neuropsiquiatr. 2011;69:766–9.
24. Lhatoo SD, Sander JW. Cause-specific mortality in epilepsy. Epilepsia. 2005;46 Suppl 11:36–9.
25. Forsgren L, Hauser WA, Olafsson E, Sander JW, Sillanpää M, Tomson T. Mortality of epilepsy in developed countries: a review. Epilepsia. 2005;46(11):18–27.

2

Lung function in very preterm infants with patent ductus arteriosus under conservative management

Hsiu-Lin Chen[1,3], Rei-Cheng Yang[2,3], Wei-Te Lee[3], Pei-Lun Lee[3], Jong-Hau Hsu[2,3], Jiunn-Ren Wu[2,3] and Zen-Kong Dai[2,3*]

Abstract

Background: Persistent patent ductus arteriosus (PDA) during hospitalization is thought to be associated with adverse pulmonary outcomes in very preterm infants. This observational study aimed to compare the lung function in very preterm infants with and without PDA at discharge.

Methods: Very preterm infants, admitted to our neonatal intensive unit, who required respiratory support soon after birth and had undergone a lung function test at discharge, were enrolled. Infants with a need for positive-pressure support (either an invasive ventilator, or nasal continuous positive airway pressure without oxygen) or supplemental oxygen at a postmenstrual age of 36 weeks were defined as having bronchopulmonary dysplasia (BPD). Echocardiography was performed weekly for each of the very preterm infants with PDA to confirm closure of the PDA. The data were collected retrospectively.

Results: Fifty-two very preterm infants received lung function tests before discharge during the study period, 28 of whom had PDA and received conservative management, and 20 who did not. The other 4 infants who were given active treatment for PDA were excluded. Gestational age was significantly smaller in the PDA group than in the no-PDA group (27.1 ± 2.0 vs. 28.6 ± 1.6 weeks, $p = 0.009$). Birth weight did not differ significantly in those with and those without PDA (0.98 ± 0.26 vs. 1.12 ± 0.26 kg, $p = 0.074$). Significantly more infants with PDA had BPD ($p = 0.002$) and required respiratory support for a longer period ($p = 0.001$) than those without PDA. However, functional residual capacity (ml/kg) at discharge was comparable between the two groups after adjusting for gestational age and postmenstrual age at testing (21.6 ± 8.4 vs. 21.5 ± 6.7 ml/kg, $p = 0.894$). Other lung function test parameters were also comparable.

Conclusion: Under a definition of BPD (including infants needing CPAP but without oxygen) other than the conventional definition, the very preterm infants in our study who received conservative management for PDA had a higher percentage of BPD than the infants without PDA. The parameters of the lung function test and lung clearance index were comparable between these two groups at discharge.

Keywords: Bronchopulmonary dysplasia, Lung function, Patent ductus arteriosus, Very preterm infants

* Correspondence: zenkong@kmu.edu.tw
[2]School of Medicine, College of Medicine, Kaohsiung Medical University, Kaohsiung, Taiwan
[3]Department of Pediatrics, Kaohsiung Medical University Hospital, No.100 , Tzyou 1st RoadSan Ming District, Kaohsiung 807, Taiwan
Full list of author information is available at the end of the article

Background

Very preterm birth results in neonatal morbidity, primarily due to the functional immaturity of multiple organ systems, such as respiratory distress syndrome, patent ductus arteriosus (PDA), intraventricular hemorrhage, necrotizing enterocolitis, retinopathy of prematurity, and the development of bronchopulmonary dysplasia (BPD) [1, 2].

PDA is a common problem in very preterm infants. Persistent PDA is thought to be associated with adverse outcomes such as necrotizing enterocolitis, intraventricular hemorrhage, BPD, and death in very preterm infants [3, 4]. Large systemic to pulmonary (left to right) ductal shunts may result in an increase in pulmonary circulation, which may lead to pulmonary edema, worsened lung mechanics, decreased lung compliance, and deterioration in gas exchange with hypercapnia and hypoxemia [5, 6]. However, the treatment of persistent PDA in very preterm infants remains controversial [7]. Active management of persistent PDA includes both pharmaceutical and surgical interventions. Because an increasing number of reports have focused on the adverse effects of pharmacotherapy (indomethacin, ibuprofen) [8, 9] and surgical ligation [10], physicians increasingly use conservative management in very preterm infants with PDA.

Currently, in the neonatal intensive care unit of Kaohsiung Medical University Hospital, neonatologists also prefer to treat very preterm infants with PDA conservatively. We hypothesized that persistence of PDA in very preterm infants treated with conservative management may result in worsened lung mechanics and changes in the development of lung function. Therefore, in this observational study, we aimed to compare the morbidity and lung function of very preterm infants with persistent PDA under conservative management and those without PDA at discharge.

Methods

Subjects

This was a clinical observational study. Very preterm infants (birth weight <1500 g and gestational age <32 weeks) admitted to the neonatal intensive care unit of Kaohsiung Medical University Hospital in Taiwan who required respiratory support soon after birth and had undergone a lung function test at discharge were enrolled between January 2011 to December 2013. Patients with major birth defects or chromosomal abnormalities were excluded. The clinical data collected included gestational age, birth weight, gender, antenatal use of steroids, severity of respiratory distress syndrome as determined by chest X-ray at admission, postnatal use of exogenous surfactants, and mode and duration of respiratory support. Infants with a need for positive-pressure support (including invasive ventilator, nasal continuous positive airway pressure (CPAP), with any FiO_2) or supplemental oxygen, at a postmenstrual age (PMA) of 36 weeks were defined as having BPD. We did not use the conventional definition of BPD, i.e., need for oxygen at a PMA of 36 weeks. In our neonatal intensive care unit, cyclic nasal CPAP under room air is the method of choice for weaning from respiratory support, and room air CPAP is stopped when the patients achieve a stable respiratory condition; therefore, patients would not receive only supplemental oxygen in our clinical setting. The conventional definition of BPD is therefore not applicable in such situations.

Diagnosis of PDA in very preterm infants

In our neonatal intensive care unit, the pediatric cardiologist performs once-weekly echocardiography at the bedside for very preterm infants, and preterm infants in our neonatal intensive care unit are thus echocardiographically assessed once during their first week of life. The echocardiographic criteria for PDA included visualization of the ductus or an increased left atrial to aortic root ratio of more than 1.2, and a left to right shunt of ductal flow seen under color Doppler ultrasound [11–13]. Echocardiography was performed weekly for each of the very preterm infants with PDA to confirm closure of the PDA. The diameter of the duct was also measured and recorded.

The conservative management for the very preterm infants with PDA included fluid restriction (daily fluid up to 130 $ml{\cdot}kg^{-1}{\cdot}day^{-1}$ beyond day 3), diuretic agents if necessary (furosemide, or trichlormethiazide), appropriate respiratory support (supplemental oxygen, CPAP, or invasive mechanical ventilator), and assessment of symptoms and signs of congestive heart failure. All of the enrolled infants received care according to the established and standard protocols for care of very preterm infants used in our neonatal intensive care unit, including the ventilatory strategy, nutritional policy, infection control, and criteria for blood transfusion.

Lung function test

The enrolled infants underwent lung function tests once when they were ready for discharge, i.e., when the infants were in a clinically stable condition. The tests were performed using an infant lung function testing system (EXHALYZER® D, ECO MEDICS AG, Duernten, Switzerland), using multiple-breath washout and ultrasonic transit-time measurements [14]. During the examination, pulse rate and oxygen saturation were monitored continuously by a pulse oximeter. Measurements were performed by the same respiratory therapist, using an infant face mask according to the manufacturer's instructions, with the infants in the supine position during unsedated sleep. Functional residual capacity (FRC), tidal volume (TV), respiratory rate, time to peak tidal expiratory flow (T_{PTEF}), total expiratory time (T_E), and indices of ventilation inhomogeneity (lung clearance index, first and second moment ratios) were measured during normal tidal breathing using a tracer gas (4 % SF6) and the multiple-breath washout technique.

Statistical analysis

The characteristics and parameters of the lung function test of the very preterm infants with and without PDA were compared using the Mann–Whitney U test for numerical data and the chi-square test for categorical data. Multivariate analysis, including gestational age and PMA at testing, was performed to adjust for the gestational differences between the groups. Correlations between the maximum size of PDA and the parameters of the lung function test were assessed using the Pearson correlation test. The required sample size was estimated to be 48 for detecting a difference of 5 ml/kg in FRC between the two groups, with a standard deviation of 6, at an alpha level of 0.05 [15]; thus, 24 individuals would be required per group, which was close to the actual size of the groups. All statistical analyses were performed using JMP® statistical software version 10.0.0 (SAS Institute Inc., Cary, NC). A two-tailed p-value of less than 0.05 was considered to be statistically significant.

Ethical approval

This study was approved by the Institutional Review Board (IRB) of the Kaohsiung Medical University Hospital, and the IRB number is KMUH-IRB-990282. The informed consent was obtained from all parents.

Results

Fifty-two very preterm infants underwent lung function tests before discharge between January 2011 and December 2013, 32 of whom had PDA. Three of these infants who were treated with surgical ligation and one who received three doses of enteral indomethacin were excluded. Of the remaining 48 infants, 28 had PDA (the PDA group) and 20 did not (the no-PDA group). All of the 28 very preterm infants with PDA underwent conservative management (Fig. 1). The gestational age was significantly lower in the PDA group than in the no-PDA group ($p = 0.009$). Birth weight was not different significantly between those with and those without PDA ($p = 0.074$; Table 1).

The rate of intubation at birth was higher in the PDA group, and the duration of invasive ventilation and respiratory support was longer in the PDA group than in the no-PDA group (Table 1). There were no significant differences in gender, antenatal steroid use, severity of respiratory distress syndrome at admission, use of exogenous surfactants, and complications, including oxygen dependence at 28 days of age, retinopathy of prematurity, necrotizing enterocolitis, and intraventricular hemorrhage, between the two groups. However, 75 % of the infants with PDA had BPD, which was significantly higher than that in the infants without PDA (30 %) ($p = 0.002$).

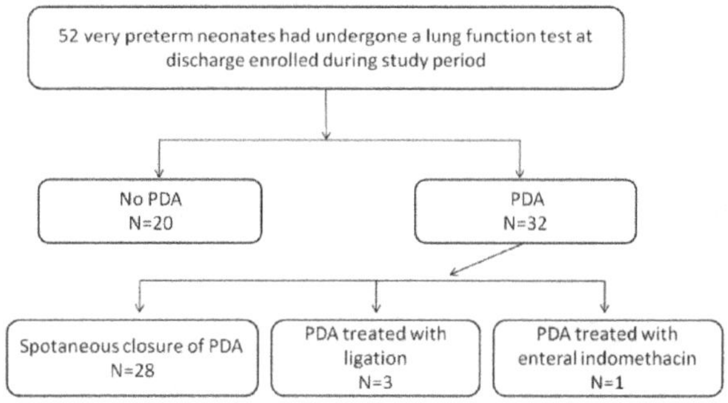

Fig. 1 Flow chart of the study infants with data on lung function tests for the study period

Twenty-seven individuals in the PDA group (96.4 %) demonstrated spontaneous closure during hospitalization, but PDA persisted after discharge in the remaining infant. The maximum size of PDA during hospitalization was 3.2 ± 1.1 mm (range: 1.8–4.6 mm) in the PDA group. Spontaneous PDA closure occurred at 50 ± 27.8 days (range: 13–155 days) postnatally, with a mean PMA of 34.6 ± 4.1 weeks (range: 29.3–51.6 weeks). A cumulative distribution function plot showed that the cumulative probability of spontaneous closure of PDA was 0.7 at a PMA of 35 weeks, and more than 0.9 at a PMA of 38 weeks (Fig. 2). All of the enrolled infants were

Table 1 The clinical characteristics of the study infants

	PDA[a] ($n = 28$)	No-PDA ($n = 20$)	*P*-value
Birth weight, kg	0.98 ± 0.26	1.12 ± 0.26	0.074
Gestational age, weeks	27.1 ± 2.0	28.6 ± 1.6	0.009
Male, *n* (%)	14 (50)	11 (55)	0.733
Antenatal steroid use, *n* (%)	15 (53.6)	12 (60)	0.658
Intubation after birth, *n* (%)	20 (71.4)	8 (40)	0.029
RDS, Grade 3 or 4, *n* (%)	14 (50)	6 (30)	0.166
Exogenous surfactant use, *n* (%)	8 (28.6)	2 (10)	0.118
Days of invasive ventilation	22.2 ± 28.1	1.6 ± 2.3	0.008
Total days of respiratory support	66.8 ± 25.6	40.8 ± 21.8	0.001
O2 dependence at 28 days, *n* (%)	25 (89.3)	14 (70)	0.092
BPD, *n* (%)	21 (75)	6 (30)	0.002
ROP, ≥ stage 3, *n* (%)	7 (25)	2 (10)	0.189
NEC, *n* (%)	0 (0)	2 (10)	0.087
IVH, any grade, *n* (%)	11 (39.3)	5 (25)	0.301
Pneumothorax, *n* (%)	4 (14.3)	0 (0)	0.136

[a]PDA with conservative treatment

All continuous data are presented as mean ± SD

RDS respiratory distress syndrome; *BPD* bronchopulmonary dysplasia; *ROP* retinopathy of prematurity; *NEC* necrotizing enterocolitis; *IVH* intraventricular hemorrhage

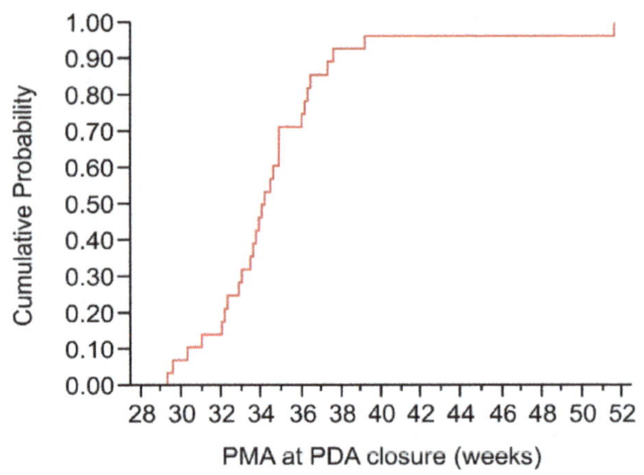

Fig. 2 Cumulative distribution function plot showing the cumulative probability of spontaneous closure of PDA at postmenstrual ages (PMA)

discharged home without oxygen supply or respiratory support.

The results of the lung function tests by multiple-breath washout are shown for both groups in Table 2. Due to the difference in maturity between the two groups when lung function was measured, we further conducted multivariate analysis to adjust for the gestational differences between the groups. After adjusting for gestational age and PMA at testing, there was no statistically significant difference in FRC (ml/kg) at discharge between the two groups (21.6 ± 8.4 ml/kg with PDA vs. 21.5 ± 6.7 ml/kg without PDA, $p = 0.894$). The other parameters of the lung function tests, including TV, respiratory rate, T_{PTEF}, T_E, and indices of ventilation inhomogeneity, were also comparable between both groups after adjustment (Table 2). An adjustment for PMA alone or postnatal age was also performed, and again there were no significant differences in FRC or other parameters of the lung function tests between the two groups (data not shown).

Because detrimental effects are thought to be directly related to the magnitude of the PDA shunt, we further performed correlation analysis between the maximum size of the PDA and parameters of the lung function tests in the PDA group, but found no significant correlations.

Table 2 Comparison of pulmonary function parameters in the two groups

	PDA[a] (*n* = 28)	No-PDA (*n* = 20)	*P* value
Postnatal age at testing, days	91.8 ± 30.7	69.2 ± 23.1	0.012[b]
PMA at testing, weeks	40.4 ± 2.8	38.8 ± 3.0	0.063[b]
Body weight at testing, kg	2.71 ± 0.58	2.65 ± 0.59	0.385[b]
Body length at testing, cm	46.7 ± 4.9	46.5 ± 4.1	0.690[b]
FRC (ml)	57.1 ± 19.5	56.4 ± 19.0	0.580[c]
FRC (ml/kg)	21.6 ± 8.4	21.5 ± 6.7	0.894[c]
FRC (ml/cm)	1.23 ± 0.44	1.20 ± 0.33	0.866[c]
Vt (ml)	23.3 ± 4.9	23.4 ± 4.6	0.430[c]
Vt (ml/kg)	8.8 ± 2.4	9.0 ± 1.5	0.432[c]
MV (ml/kg/min)	1359.9 ± 693.5	1358.3 ± 536.0	0.778[c]
RR (/min)	78.1 ± 20.2	80.2 ± 15.0	0.637[c]
T_I (s)	0.39 ± 0.10	0.36 ± 0.08	0.151[c]
T_{PTEF} (s)	0.16 ± 0.06	0.20 ± 0.15	0.390[c]
T_{PTEF}/T_E (%)	41.1 ± 16.4	46.0 ± 18.4	0.759[c]
LCI	15.4 ± 4.4	16.2 ± 3.4	0.745[c]
M1/M0	5.0 ± 2.2	5.1 ± 1.7	0.529[c]
M2/M0	41.1 ± 16.4	46.0 ± 18.4	0.887[c]

[a]PDA with conservative treatment
[b]compared using the Mann–Whitney *U*-test
[c]*P* value: after adjustment with GA, and PMA at testing
All continuous data are presented as mean ± SD
FRC functional residual capacity; *Vt* tidal volume; T_I inspiratory time; T_{PTEF} time to peak tidal expiratory flow; T_{PTEF}/T_E the ratio of time to peak tidal expiratory flow over total expiratory time; *LCI* lung clearance index; *M1/M0* and *M2/M0*, first and second moment ratios

Discussion

Our results showed that lung volume and indices of ventilation inhomogeneity in very preterm infants receiving conservative management for PDA were comparable to those of very preterm infants without PDA at discharge, although the infants with PDA had a higher percentage of BPD than those without PDA.

PDA is a common condition in very preterm infants; however, the management of PDA in very preterm infants is still a controversial issue. Bose and Laughon stated that the patency of the ductus arteriosus may be a physiological phenomenon in very preterm infants [16]. The EPICure study [17] reported that approximately 65 % of preterm infants born at a gestational age of less than 28 weeks who survive to discharge have persistent PDA. Regarding the natural course and rate of spontaneous closure of ductus arteriosus in very preterm infants, previous studies [18, 19] reported a spontaneous PDA closure rate of 66–94 % after conservative management in very preterm infants born at a gestational age of less than 30 weeks. In this observational study, the spontaneous closure rate of PDA in the infants receiving conservative management was 96.4 %, which was compatible with the high rate of spontaneous closure of PDA in very preterm infants. We also found that there is a direct relationship between PMA and the spontaneous closure of PDA in very preterm infants (Fig. 2). Thus, maturity is important for spontaneous closure of ductus arteriosus.

Persistent ductal patency is thought to be associated with adverse outcomes, such as hemodynamic derangements and several major complications, including necrotizing enterocolitis, intraventricular hemorrhage, BPD, and death in premature infants [3, 4]. With concerns over adverse effects of aggressive treatment of PDA, conservative management is increasingly considered to be an option [18]. Jhaveri et al. reported that the rates of BPD, retinopathy of prematurity, neurological injury, and death are similar between infants receiving conservative management and those undergoing early PDA ligation [20]. In this study, we showed there were no significant differences in major complications between infants with PDA who underwent conservative management and those without PDA. However, the rate of BPD (including infants needing CPAP, but without oxygen, at a PMA of 36 weeks) was higher in the infants with PDA than in those without PDA (75 % vs. 30 %, $p = 0.002$). Since, in our neonatal intensive care unit, we apply room air CPAP (i.e., oxygen equals 21 % when using CPAP) for most very preterm infants with acceptable oxygen saturation (88–94 %) [21], the definition we use for BPD is different from the diagnostic criteria developed by the National Institute of Child Health and Human Development Workshop on BPD in 2001 [22], in which BPD is defined as treatment with oxygen of more than 21 % at a PMA of 36 weeks, plus a total oxygen duration of more than 28 days for infants born at less than 32 weeks' gestation. The use of oxygen therapy as a single criterion for defining BPD has limitations in clinical situations [5]. We considered that lung function is impaired when infants require positive-pressure ventilation or CPAP, even though oxygen requirement equals 21 % at a PMA of 36 weeks.

In this study, we were concerned about whether pulmonary sequelae differed between very preterm infants with and those without PDA. With PDA, large systemic to pulmonary (left to right) ductal shunts result in an increase in pulmonary flow and pulmonary remodeling in preterm infants. As a result, these infants need prolonged respiratory support to maintain adequate ventilation, which then increases the likelihood of respiratory morbidity [6, 23]. Bancalari et al. reported a strong association between the presence and duration of PDA, and an increased risk of developing BPD in premature infants [6]. However, the association between PDA and BPD may be distorted by confounding factors, such as gestational age and other co-morbidities [24]. A recent study by Laughon et al. reported that the role of PDA as an independent risk factor for BPD was less marked [25]. Therefore, the lung functions in very preterm infants with persistent PDA under conservative management should be addressed when they are ready to be discharged.

FRC is frequently used for monitoring lung disease during infancy, and FRC has been found to be reduced in infants with BPD in some studies [26–29]. However, we found that FRC was not lower in the patients with PDA compared to those without, although there was a higher rate of BPD in infants with PDA under conservative management. Furthermore, some authors have suggested that normalized FRC in infants with BPD may result from both hyperinflation and/or gas trapping due to airway obstruction [30]. The amount of time to reach peak tidal expiratory flow to total expiratory time (T_{PTEF}/T_E ratio), which is recognized to be a tool for evaluating airway obstructions [31], has been reported to be lower in infants with airway obstruction and lower compliance [32, 33]. Our patients may not have had airway obstructions severe enough to reveal a significant difference in the T_{PTEF}/T_E ratio between those with and without PDA, because there was no difference in T_{PTEF}/T_E ratio between the two groups.

Increased lung clearance index and moment ratio values imply reduced ventilation efficiency in infants [28, 34, 35]. We did not find any differences in lung clearance index or moment ratio values between the PDA and no-PDA groups, suggesting that the very preterm infants with prolonged PDA did not have greater ventilation inhomogeneity than those without PDA.

The major limitation of this study was that the lung function tests used can detect changes in volume-dependent pulmonary mechanics and airway function, but not specific changes in the lung periphery. New BPD infants are characterized by an arrest in lung development, with simplification of the lung periphery. The simplification of the lung periphery includes arrested alveolar growth, with fewer, larger, and simplified alveoli, and fewer and dysmorphic arteries [36]. In future, methods for evaluating changes in the lung periphery, such as volumetric capnography [36], should be considered. The other limitations of this observational study are that we did not include infants with PDA under active management, due to the small number of such patients during the study period, and because the sample size overall was small. The potential strength of this study is that we examined lung function, after the PDA had closed spontaneously, to determine whether there were residual effects on lung function due to its earlier occurrence.

Conclusions

In our study, very preterm infants who received conservative management for PDA had a higher percentage of BPD, defined as infants needing CPAP, but without oxygen, than infants without PDA. The parameters of the lung function test and lung clearance index were comparable between these two groups at discharge. Long-term follow up of pulmonary outcomes in later life is necessary.

Abbreviations

BPD: bronchopulmonary dysplasia; PMA: postmenstrual age; CPAP: continuous positive airway pressure; FRC: functional residual capacity; IVH: intraventricular hemorrhage; LCI: lung clearance index; M1/M0 and M2/

M0: first and second moment ratios; NEC: necrotizing enterocolitis; RDS: respiratory distress syndrome; ROP: retinopathy of prematurity; T_I: inspiratory time; T_{PTEF}: time to peak tidal expiratory flow; T_{PTEF}/T_E: the ratio of time to peak tidal expiratory flow over total expiratory time; Vt: tidal volume.

Competing interests

The authors declare that they have no competing interests.

Authors' contributions

Conception and design of study: H.L. Chen, R.C. Yang. Acquisition of data: W.T. Lee, P.L. Lee, J.H. Hsu, J.R. Wu. Analysis and/or interpretation of data: H.L. Chen, Z.K. Dai. Drafting the manuscript: H.L. Chen. Revising the manuscript critically for important intellectual content: R.C. Yang, Z.K. Dai. All authors read and approved the final manuscript.

Acknowledgments

This study was supported by a grant from the Kaohsiung Medical University (KMU-Q100008). The authors greatly appreciate the Statistical Analysis Laboratory, Department of Medical Research, Kaohsiung Medical University Hospital, Kaohsiung Medical University for assisting with statistical analysis. The authors also thank the nursing staff of the neonatal intensive care unit, Kaohsiung Medical University Hospital, for patient enrollment.

Author details

[1]Department of Respiratory Therapy, College of Medicine, Kaohsiung Medical University, Kaohsiung, Taiwan. [2]School of Medicine, College of Medicine, Kaohsiung Medical University, Kaohsiung, Taiwan. [3]Department of Pediatrics, Kaohsiung Medical University Hospital, No.100 , Tzyou 1st RoadSan Ming District, Kaohsiung 807, Taiwan.

References

1. Stoll BJ, Hansen NI, Bell EF, Shankaran S, Laptook AR, Walsh MC, et al. Neonatal outcomes of extremely preterm infants from the NICHD Neonatal Research Network. Pediatrics. 2010;126(3):443–56.
2. Kusuda S, Fujimura M, Uchiyama A, Totsu S, Matsunami K. Trends in morbidity and mortality among very-low-birth-weight infants from 2003 to 2008 in Japan. Pediatr Res. 2012;72(5):531–8.
3. Sellmer A, Bjerre JV, Schmidt MR, McNamara PJ, Hjortdal VE, Host B, et al. Morbidity and mortality in preterm neonates with patent ductus arteriosus on day 3. Arch Dis Child Fetal Neonatal Ed. 2013;98(6):F505–10.
4. Noori S, McCoy M, Friedlich P, Bright B, Gottipati V, Seri I, et al. Failure of ductus arteriosus closure is associated with increased mortality in preterm infants. Pediatrics. 2009;123(1):e138–44.
5. Bancalari E, Claure N, Sosenko IR. Bronchopulmonary dysplasia: changes in pathogenesis, epidemiology and definition. Semin Neonatol. 2003;8(1):63–71.
6. Bancalari E, Claure N, Gonzalez A. Patent ductus arteriosus and respiratory outcome in premature infants. Biol Neonate. 2005;88(3):192–201.
7. Benitz WE. Patent ductus arteriosus: to treat or not to treat? Arch Dis Child Fetal Neonatal Ed. 2012;97(2):F80–2.
8. Pezzati M, Vangi V, Biagiotti R, Bertini G, Cianciulli D, Rubaltelli FF. Effects of indomethacin and ibuprofen on mesenteric and renal blood flow in preterm infants with patent ductus arteriosus. J Pediatr. 1999;135(6):733–8.
9. Vieux R, Desandes R, Boubred F, Semama D, Guillemin F, Buchweiller MC, et al. Ibuprofen in very preterm infants impairs renal function for the first month of life. Pediatr Nephrol. 2010;25(2):267–74.
10. Moin F, Kennedy KA, Moya FR. Risk factors predicting vasopressor use after patent ductus arteriosus ligation. Am J Perinatol. 2003;20(6):313–20.
11. Sperandio M, Beedgen B, Feneberg R, Huppertz C, Brussau J, Poschl J, et al. Effectiveness and side effects of an escalating, stepwise approach to indomethacin treatment for symptomatic patent ductus arteriosus in premature infants below 33 weeks of gestation. Pediatrics. 2005;116(6):1361–6.
12. Hsu JH, Yang SN, Chen HL, Tseng HI, Dai ZK, Wu JR. B-type natriuretic peptide predicts responses to indomethacin in premature neonates with patent ductus arteriosus. J Pediatr. 2010;157(1):79–84.
13. Van Overmeire B, Follens I, Hartmann S, Creten WL, Van Acker KJ. Treatment of patent ductus arteriosus with ibuprofen. Arch Dis Child Fetal Neonatal Ed. 1997;76(3):F179–84.
14. Schibler A, Hall GL, Businger F, Reinmann B, Wildhaber JH, Cernelc M, et al. Measurement of lung volume and ventilation distribution with an ultrasonic flow meter in healthy infants. Eur Respir J. 2002;20(4):912–8.
15. Hulskamp G, Lum S, Stocks J, Wade A, Hoo AF, Costeloe K, et al. Association of prematurity, lung disease and body size with lung volume and ventilation inhomogeneity in unsedated neonates: a multicentre study. Thorax. 2009;64(3):240–5.
16. Bose CL, Laughon MM. Patent ductus arteriosus: lack of evidence for common treatments. Arch Dis Child Fetal Neonatal Ed. 2007;92(6):F498–502.
17. Costeloe K, Hennessy E, Gibson AT, Marlow N, Wilkinson AR. The EPICure study: outcomes to discharge from hospital for infants born at the threshold of viability. Pediatrics. 2000;106(4):659–71.
18. Vanhaesebrouck S, Zonnenberg I, Vandervoort P, Bruneel E, Van Hoestenberghe MR, Theyskens C. Conservative treatment for patent ductus arteriosus in the preterm. Arch Dis Child Fetal Neonatal Ed. 2007;92(4):F244–7.
19. Herrman K, Bose C, Lewis K, Laughon M. Spontaneous closure of the patent ductus arteriosus in very low birth weight infants following discharge from the neonatal unit. Arch Dis Child Fetal Neonatal Ed. 2009;94(1):F48–50.
20. Jhaveri N, Moon-Grady A, Clyman RI. Early surgical ligation versus a conservative approach for management of patent ductus arteriosus that fails to close after indomethacin treatment. J Pediatr. 2010;157(3):381–7. 387 e381.
21. Sola A, Golombek SG, Montes Bueno MT, Lemus-Varela L, Zuluaga C, Dominguez F, et al. Safe oxygen saturation targeting and monitoring in preterm infants: can we avoid hypoxia and hyperoxia? Acta Paediatr. 2014;103(10):1009–18.
22. Jobe AH, Bancalari E. Bronchopulmonary dysplasia. Am J Respir Crit Care Med. 2001;163(7):1723–9.
23. Van Marter LJ, Pagano M, Allred EN, Leviton A, Kuban KC. Rate of bronchopulmonary dysplasia as a function of neonatal intensive care practices. J Pediatr. 1992;120(6):938–46.
24. Trembath A, Laughon MM. Predictors of bronchopulmonary dysplasia. Clin Perinatol. 2012;39(3):585–601.
25. Laughon MM, Langer JC, Bose CL, Smith PB, Ambalavanan N, Kennedy KA, et al. Prediction of bronchopulmonary dysplasia by postnatal age in extremely premature infants. Am J Respir Crit Care Med. 2011;183(12):1715–22.
26. Latzin P, Roth S, Thamrin C, Hutten GJ, Pramana I, Kuehni CE, et al. Lung volume, breathing pattern and ventilation inhomogeneity in preterm and term infants. PLoS One. 2009;4(2), e4635.
27. Schmalisch G, Wilitzki S, Roehr CC, Proquitte H, Buhrer C. Development of lung function in very low birth weight infants with or without bronchopulmonary dysplasia: longitudinal assessment during the first 15 months of corrected age. BMC Pediatr. 2012;12:37.
28. Hjalmarson O, Sandberg KL. Lung function at term reflects severity of bronchopulmonary dysplasia. J Pediatr. 2005;146(1):86–90.
29. May C, Kennedy C, Milner AD, Rafferty GF, Peacock JL, Greenough A. Lung function abnormalities in infants developing bronchopulmonary dysplasia. Arch Dis Child. 2011;96(11):1014–9.
30. Hulskamp G, Pillow JJ, Dinger J, Stocks J. Lung function tests in neonates and infants with chronic lung disease of infancy: functional residual capacity. Pediatr Pulmonol. 2006;41(1):1–22.
31. Davis SD. Neonatal and pediatric respiratory diagnostics. Respir Care. 2003;48(4):367–84. discussion 384–365.
32. Hoo AF, Henschen M, Dezateux C, Costeloe K, Stocks J. Respiratory function among preterm infants whose mothers smoked during pregnancy. Am J Respir Crit Care Med. 1998;158(3):700–5.
33. Dezateux CA, Stocks J, Dundas I, Jackson EA, Fletcher ME. The relationship between tPTEF:tE and specific airway conductance in infancy. Pediatr Pulmonol. 1994;18(5):299–307.
34. Pillow JJ, Frerichs I, Stocks J. Lung function tests in neonates and infants with chronic lung disease: global and regional ventilation inhomogeneity. Pediatr Pulmonol. 2006;41(2):105–21.
35. Shao H, Sandberg K, Hjalmarson O. Impaired gas mixing and low lung volume in preterm infants with mild chronic lung disease. Pediatr Res. 1998;43(4 Pt 1):536–41.
36. Fouzas S, Häcki C, Latzin P, Proietti E, Schulzke S, Frey U, et al. Volumetric capnography in infants with bronchopulmonary dysplasia. J Pediatr. 2014;164(2):283–8. e281-283.

3

Characteristics and severity of asthma in children with and without atopic conditions

Ali Arabkhazaeli[1], Susanne J. H. Vijverberg[1], Francine C. van Erp[2], Jan A. M. Raaijmakers[1], Cornelis K. van der Ent[2] and Anke H. Maitland van der Zee[1*]

Abstract

Background: Childhood allergic diseases have a major impact on a child's quality of life, as well as that of their parents. We studied the coexistence of reported allergies in children who use asthma medication. Additionally, we tested the hypothesis that asthma severity is greater among children with certain combinations of co-morbid allergic conditions.

Methods: For this cross-sectional study, 703 children (ages 4 to 12 years) from the PACMAN cohort study were selected. All of the children were regular users of asthma medication. The study population was divided into nine subgroups according to parental-reported allergies of the child (hay fever, eczema, food allergy or combinations of these). In order to assess whether these subgroups differed clinically, the groups were compared for child characteristics (age, gender, family history of asthma), asthma exacerbations in the past year (oral corticosteroids (OCS) use; asthma-related emergency department (ED) visits), asthma control, fractional exhaled nitric oxide level (FeNO), and antihistaminic usage.

Results: In our study, 79.0 % of the parents reported that their child suffered from at least one atopic condition (hay fever, food allergy and eczema), and one quarter of the parents (25.6 %) reported that their child suffered from all three atopic conditions. Having more than one atopic condition was associated with an increased risk of OCS use (OR = 3.3, 95 % CI = 1.6 – 6.6), ED visits (OR = 2.3, 95 % CI = 1.2 – 4.6) in the past year and inadequate short term asthma control (OR = 1.9, 95 % CI = 1.3 – 2.8).

Conclusions: Children who use asthma medication often also have other allergic conditions. Parental reported allergies were associated with a higher risk of more severe asthma (more asthma complaints and more asthma exacerbations).

Keywords: Allergy, Asthma, Atopic condition, Eczema, Exacerbation, FeNO, Food allergy, Hay fever

Background

Childhood allergic diseases have a major impact on a child's quality of life, as well as that of their parents [1]. Therefore, it is important to have a better understanding of the risk factors associated with the development of asthma in children, as well as the factors associated with more severe asthma. The term "allergy" refers to a hypersensitivity reaction initiated by immunologic mechanisms, and although all people are continuously exposed to different allergens, only a limited group of individuals experience adverse immunologic mechanisms [2]. Persistent asthma is often treated with inhaled corticosteroids (ICS) in combination with short acting beta agonists (SABA) as needed, or sometimes in more severe cases, long acting beta agonists and/or leukotriene antagonists [3]. When asthma is controlled, there should only be occasional recurrence of symptoms, and severe asthma exacerbations should be rare [4]. One of the risk factors for asthma severity that has been

* Correspondence: a.h.maitland@uu.nl
[1]Division of Pharmacoepidemiology & Clinical Pharmacology, Utrecht Institute for Pharmaceutical Sciences (UIPS), Faculty of Science, Utrecht University, P.O. Box 80082David de Wied Building, Universiteitsweg 99, Utrecht 3508 TB, The Netherlands
Full list of author information is available at the end of the article

identified is atopy [5, 6]. Atopic individuals are prone to developing allergic symptoms. Asthma, food allergies, eczema, and hay fever are common childhood atopic conditions with an increasing prevalence in the western world [7].

In general, eczema peaks in the child's first years of life as an "entry point" for subsequent allergic disease, and consequently the prevalence of asthma and allergic rhinitis increases over time as sensitization develops [8].

Several studies have investigated the coexistence of food allergies and asthma, hay fever and asthma, or eczema and asthma [8–11]. However, most of these studies have only assessed the relationship between two conditions. They did not assess the effect of a combination of allergies, and they only focused on atopic patients. In this study, we examined the coexistence of allergies and the use of allergy related medication in a large cohort of children who use asthma medication and were recruited through community pharmacies. As a result of the inclusion of the participants from the community pharmacies, this cohort covered the whole spectrum of children with mild to severe asthma. Furthermore, we assessed the differences in the measurement of asthma severity among children with and without different allergies and combinations thereof.

Methods

Study population

At the time of this analysis, 744 children (ages 4 to 12 years) were included in the ongoing PACMAN (Pharmacogenetics of Asthma medication in Children: Medication with Anti-inflammatory effects) cohort study. Complete data on allergies was available for 703 children. The children were regular users (≥3 prescriptions in the last two years and ≥ 1 prescription in the last 6 months) of asthma medications (R03 on the ATC (Anatomical Therapeutic Chemical) coding system) and were recruited through community pharmacies in the Netherlands. The children and their parents were invited to their regular pharmacy for a study visit [12]. The design and rationale of the PACMAN study has been described elsewhere [12]. Data were collected with the help of pharmacists belonging to the Utrecht Pharmacy Practice Network for Education and Research (UPPER), and the work was conducted in compliance with the requirements of the UPPER institutional review board of the Department of Pharmacoepidemiology and Clinical Pharmacology, Utrecht University. The PACMAN study has been approved by the Medical Ethics Committee of the University Medical Centre Utrecht. Written, informed consent for all participants in the study was obtained from either the participants themselves, or, where participants were minors, a parent or guardian [12].

Data collection

The parents completed a questionnaire during the pharmacy visit. The questionnaire contained questions regarding general health, asthma and respiratory symptoms, allergy symptoms, medication use, adherence to medication (Medication Adherence Rating Scale (MARS) questionnaire [13]), socio-demographic factors, and asthma symptoms. In addition, the child's fractional exhaled nitric oxide level (FeNO) was measured with a handheld analyzer (Niox Mino, Aerocrine, Solna, Sweden).

To measure co-morbid atopic conditions, parents were asked: Has your child ever had a food allergy (FA) (itching, rash/hives, vomiting, diarrhea, runny nose, sneezing, stuffiness and cough)? Has your child ever had eczema? Has your child ever had hay fever (HF)?

The use of oral corticosteroids (OCS) and the amount of emergency department (ED) visits were used to measure asthma severity. Furthermore, the Dutch version of the 6-item Asthma Control Questionnaire (ACQ) was applied to assess current asthma control. ACQ ≥ 1.5 was used as a cut-off value indicating poorly controlled asthma [14].

Statistical analyses

The study was a cross-sectional analysis in the baseline measurements of the PACMAN cohort study. The study population was stratified into nine subgroups according to the allergies that the parents had reported. The first three groups reported HF, FA, or eczema irrespective of whether or not they had also reported one or more of the other studied allergies. Then all possible combinations of

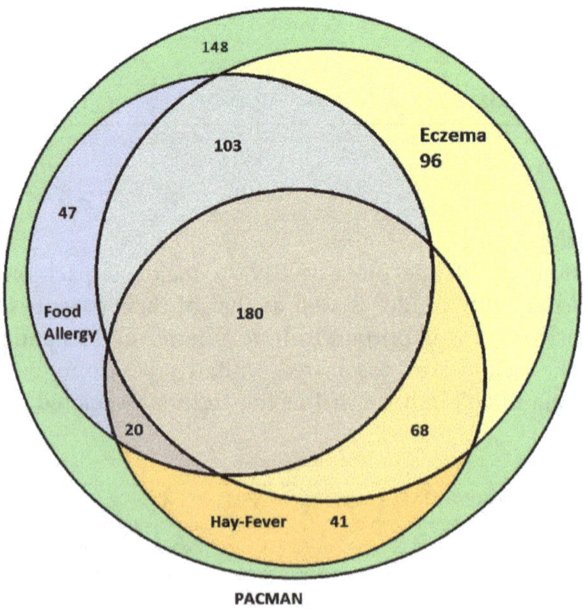

Fig. 1 The co-existence of allergies in the study population

Table 1 Characteristics and antihistamines usage

The population in the Venn diagram [a]		Number (Percentage)	Mean Age ± SD (P Value)[b]	Median FeNO (P Value)[c] [IQR]
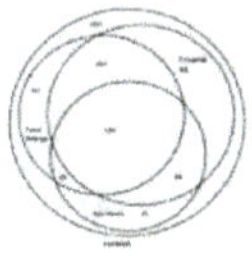	Study Population	703	8.4 ± 2.4	13.0 [7.0 – 27.0]
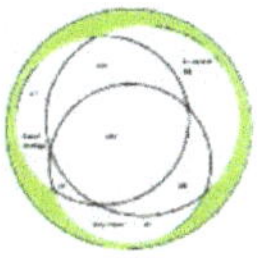	Without history of allergies	148 (21.1 %)	8.1 ± 2.4 (.104)	11.0(.084) [6.0 – 27.0]
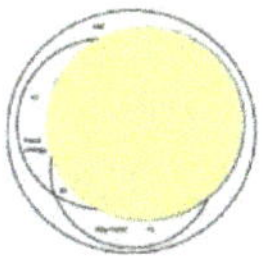	Eczema	447 (63.6 %)	8.5 ± 2.5 (.485)	13.0 (.222) [8.0 – 26.0]
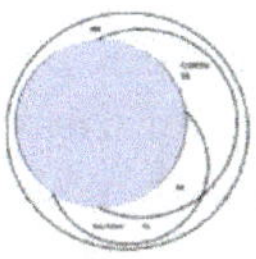	Food allergy	350 (49.8 %)	8.4 ± 2.5 (.695)	13.0 (.294) [8.0 – 27.0]
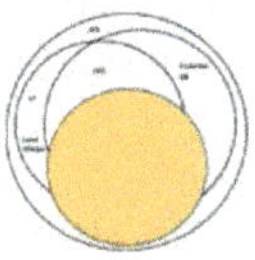	Hay fever	309 (44.0 %)	8.9[d] ± 2.3 (.000)	15.0[d] (.005) [8.0 – 29.8]
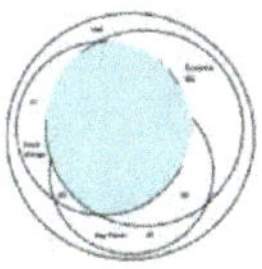	Food allergy + Eczema	283 (40.3 %)	8.5 ± 2.5 (.646)	14.0(.072) [8.3 – 27.8]
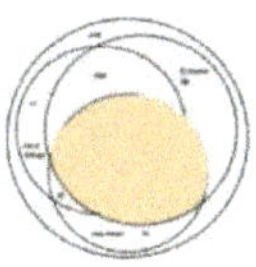	Eczema + Hay fever	248 (35.3 %)	8.8[d] ± 2.4 (.002)	15.0[d] (.036) [8.5 – 27.5]
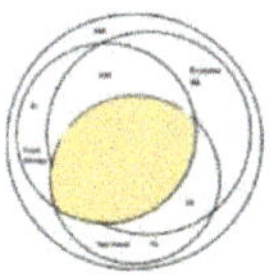	Food allergy + Hay fever	200 (28.5 %)	8.7[d] ± 2.4 (.035)	15.0 (.153) [8.0 – 28.0]

Table 1 Characteristics and antihistamines usage *(Continued)*

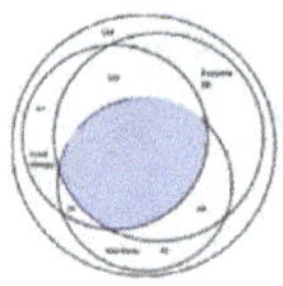	Food allergy + Eczema + Hay fever	180 (25.6 %)	8.8[d] ± 2.4 (.035)	15.0 (.099) [9.0 – 27.0]
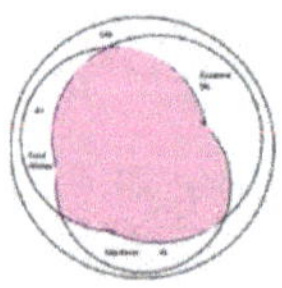	At least two allergies	371 (52.8 %)	8.6 ± 2.4 (.109)	14.0[d] (.029) [8.0 – 28.0]

[a]For a larger diagram see Fig. 1
[b]With independent samples T-test
[c]With Mann–Whitney test
[d]P Value < 0.05

allergies were defined (FA + eczema, eczema + HF, FA + HF, FA + eczema + HF) (see Fig. 1 and Table 1).

The characteristics and asthma severity measures of these groups (age, gender, family history of asthma, breast feeding, FeNO, use of allergy medications, OSC usage, ED visits and ACQ) were compared between the groups of children with and without specific combination of atopic conditions (colored area in the first column of Table 1 and the rest of PACMAN population).

We used the independent samples T-test and the Chi-Square test where appropriate. As the distribution of FeNO was not normal, according to the Kolomogorov-Smirnov and the Shapiro-Wilk test, the Mann–Whitney test was used to compare median FeNO between different groups. Logistic regression was applied for multivariate analyses. Age, gender and use of antihistamines were considered potential confounding factors. The potential confounding factors were included in the multivariate model. The Odds Ratios (OR) for OCS use, ED visits and ACQ were adjusted for age and gender and reported with 95% confidence intervals CI). Adjusting the OR for the use of antihistamines and adherence to therapy did not change the results (Table 4).

Results

Co-existence of allergies

In the study population, 79.0% (555/703) of the parents reported that their children had suffered from at least one of the assessed allergies. Eczema was the most common condition (63.6 %). Almost half of the study population reported a history of food allergy (49.8 %), and hay fever was reported by 44.0 %. 25.6 % (180/703) of the participants reported symptoms of all three allergies (food allergy, eczema and hay fever), while 21.1 % did not report any of these symptoms. (See Fig. 1 and Table 1).

Baseline characteristics

Characteristics of the study population are shown in Table 2.

The trends of the main allergic groups' age distributions are shown in Fig. 2. For hay fever an ascending trend is visible (Fig. 2). The mean age of the study population was 8.4 years. However, the mean age of the subgroup of children that reported having hay fever (irrespective of whether they had other allergies) was significantly higher (8.9 years, $p < 0.001$) (Table 1). Also, the occurrence of hay fever increased from almost 20 % in the 4-year-olds to more than 50 % in the 12-year-olds

Table 2 Characteristics of study population

Study population (*n* = 703)	
General characteristics	
Male gender, %	62.0
Age, mean ± SD	8.4 ± 2.5
Clinical characteristics	
Parental-reported Eczema, %	63.6
Parental-reported Food Allergy, %	49.8
Parental-reported Hay fever, %	44.0
Asthma family history (One or more parents with history of asthma), %	48.0
Antihistamine usage, %	30.6
ICS usage, %	87.8
SABA usage, %	84.8
LABA usage, %	23.5
LTRA usage, %	8.8
Breast fed, %	74.9
Median FeNO (IQR)	13.0 (7.0 – 27.0)
OCS usage in the past year, %	7.0
Asthma-related ED visit in the past year, %	6.3

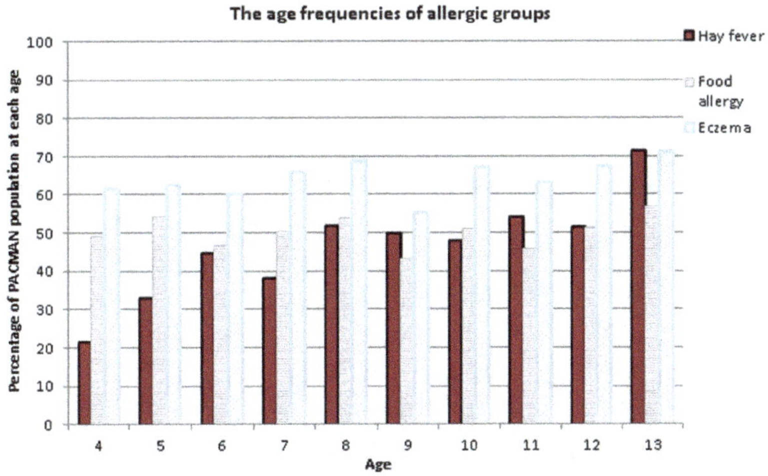

Fig. 2 The age frequencies of allergic groups in the study population

(Fig. 2). The frequency of children with a positive asthma family history (father or mother) in the total studied PACMAN population was 48.0 %. In the subgroup of children who reported having had hay fever, there was an even higher risk of a family history of asthma (55 %) compared to the children who did not report having had hay fever (45.0 %) (OR = 1.7 95 % CI = 1.2 – 2.3). Furthermore, in the subgroup of children with a reported food allergy, there was a trend towards a higher risk of a family history of asthma (51.2 % to 48.8 %, OR = 1.3 95 % CI = 1.0 - 1.8) (Table 3). The median of FeNO in the study population was 13.0 (Interquartile Range (IQR) = 7.0 – 27.0). The children who reported having had hay fever had a significantly higher FeNO (median = 15.0, IQR = 8.0 – 29.8, $p < 0.01$) (Table 1). Gender or having been breastfed did not significantly differ between allergic subgroups.

Oral antihistaminic drug usage

Oral antihistaminic drugs were used by almost 30 % of the study population. The top three oral antihistaminic drugs (Loratadine, Cetirizine and Fenistil) were equally distributed among all the allergy subgroups.

Asthma outcomes

Severity of asthma was assessed by OCS usage, ED visits and ACQ using both univariate and multivariate analyses. 9.1 % of the children who reported eczema symptoms used OCS (Table 4). This was significantly higher when compared to the use of OCS in the non-eczema population (3.2 %) (OR = 3.0, 95 % CI = 1.4 – 6.6). The use of OCS for the subgroup that had symptoms of food allergy was 9.6 %; this was also statistically significantly different compared to 4.3 % of the non-food allergy population (OR = 2.3, 95 % CI = 1.2 – 4.4). There was a

Table 3 Differences in asthma family history in the allergic subgroups

Group	Asthma family history % (P Value)		Odds Ratio (95 % CI)
	Present	Not present	
Study population	48.0		
Without history of allergies	44.0 (.230)	56.0	0.8 (0.5 – 1.2)
Eczema	48.5 (.741)	51.5	1.1 (0.8 – 1.4)
Food allergy	51.2 (.096)	48.8	1.3 (1.0 - 1.8)
Hay fever	55.0[a] (.001)	45.0	1.7[a] (1.2 – 2.3)
Food allergy + Eczema	51.5 (.137)	48.5	1.3 (0.9 – 1.7)
Eczema + Hay fever	54.8[a] (.009)	45.2	1.5[a] (1.1 – 2.1)
Food allergy + Hay fever	57.7[a] (.001)	42.3	1.7[a] (1.2 – 2.4)
Food allergy + Eczema + Hay fever	57.5[a] (.004)	42.5	1.7[a] (1.2 – 2.4)
At least two allergies	51.3 (.070)	48.7	1.3 (1.0 – 1.8)

[a]P Value < 0.05 with chi-square test

Table 4 Differences in outcomes of each subgroups in whole study population

	OCS usage % (P Value)	Univariate analysis OR (95 % CI)	Multivariate analysis [b] OR (95 % CI)	E.D visit in past year % (P Value)	Univariate analysis OR (95 % CI)	Multivariate analysis [b] OR (95 % CI)	Poorly controlled refer to ACQ-6 % (P Value)	Univariate analysis OR (95 % CI)	Multivariate analysis [b] OR (95 % CI)
Study population	7.0			6.3			18.2		
Without history of allergies	4.1 (0.12)	0.5 (0.2–1.2)	0.5 (0.2–1.2)	4.1 (.215)	0.6 (0.2–1.4)	0.5 (0.2–1.3)	14.3 (.118)	0.7 (0.4–1.1)	0.7 (0.4–1.1)
Eczema	9.1[a] (.003)	3.0[a] (1.4–6.6)	3.0[a] (1.4–6.6)	8.1[a] (.010)	2.7[a] (1.2–5.9)	2.7[a] (1.2–6.0)	20.4 (.053)	1.5 (1.0–2.3)	1.5[a] (1.0–2.4)
Food allergy	9.6[a] (.007)	2.3[a] (1.2–4.4)	2.3[a] (1.2–4.4)	8.0 (.068)	1.8 (1.0–3.4)	1.8 (0.9–3.4)	21.3[a] (.039)	1.5[a] (1.0–2.2)	1.5[a] (1.0–2.2)
Hay fever	8.0 (0.36)	1.3 (0.7–2.4)	1.4 (0.8–2.5)	6.0 (.765)	0.9 (0.5–1.7)	1.1 (0.6–2.1)	22.7[a] (.007)	1.7[a] (1.2–2.5)	1.8[a] (1.2–2.7)
Food allergy + Eczema	11.6[a] (.000)	3.2[a] (1.7–6.0)	3.3[a] (1.8–6.1)	9.6[a] (.005)	2.4[a] (1.3–4.6)	2.5[a] (1.3–4.7)	22.1[a] (.028)	1.5[a] (1.0–2.3)	1.6[a] (1.1–2.3)
Eczema + Hay fever	9.5 (.056)	1.8 (1.0–3.2)	1.8[a] (1.0–3.3)	7.1 (.557)	1.2 (0.6–2.3)	1.4 (0.7–2.7)	24.5[a] (.002)	1.9[a] (1.3–2.8)	1.9[a] (1.3–2.9)
Food allergy + Hay fever	9.2 (0.14)	1.6 (0.9–2.9)	1.6 (0.9–3.0)	6.7 (.776)	1.1 (0.6–2.2)	1.2 (0.6–2.5)	25.4[a] (.002)	1.9[a] (1.3–2.8)	1.9[a] (1.3–2.9)
Food allergy + Eczema + Hay fever	10.3[a] (.045)	1.9[a] (1.0–3.4)	1.9 (1.0–3.6)	7.5 (.467)	1.3 (0.7–2.5)	1.5 (0.7–2.9)	25.3[a] (.005)	1.8[a] (1.2–2.7)	1.9[a] (1.2–2.8)
At least two allergies	10.1[a] (.001)	3.2[a] (1.6–6.4)	3.3[a] (1.6–6.6)	8.4[a] (.020)	2.2[a] (1.1–4.3)	2.3[a] (1.2–4.6)	22.4[a] (.003)	1.9[a] (1.2-2.8)	1.9[a] (1.3–2.8)

The referent group for all these odds ratios is the entire study population

[a]*P* Value < 0.05 with logistic regression test

[b]Adjusted for age and gender

trend towards a higher risk for the use of OCS in all allergy subgroups. However, the group of children who did not report a history of allergic conditions did not have an increased risk for the use of OCS (Table 4).

Emergency department visits during the past year were significantly higher (8.1 %, OR = 2.7, 95 % CI = 1.2 – 6.0) in the population who had a history of eczema as compared to the rest of the population (3.2 %) (Table 4).

The Asthma Control Questionnaire (ACQ) was assessed in all the defined groups, and 18.2 % of the total study population suffered from poorly controlled asthma. The frequencies of poorly controlled asthmatics in all allergic subgroups were significantly higher ($p < 0.05$) as compared to the non-allergic population. They were 21.3 %, 20.4 % and 22.1 % in the populations with a history of eczema, food allergy or both, respectively. The frequencies of poorly controlled patients were even higher in all the subgroups that reported hay fever (22.7 % - 25.4 %) or more than one allergy (22.4 %) compared to the rest of study population (Table 4).

Discussion

In this large pharmacy-based study of children with a reported use of asthma medication, we found that the prevalence of children that reported symptoms of one or more allergy syndromes was high, and patients that reported more atopic conditions had a greater odds of more severe asthma.

In general, children with asthma and co-morbid allergic conditions were more often poorly controlled compared to their non-allergic peers. Furthermore, usage of OCS and asthma-related ED visits were more common in children who reported more than one atopic condition, which was approximately half of the study population. This indicates that the presence of a more complicated allergic phenotype significantly influences the severity of asthma [15].

To our knowledge, there is limited research that has studied the association of allergic comorbidities and asthma severity [16]. However several longitudinal studies have shown that approximately half of eczema patients will develop asthma, particularly patients with severe eczema [8]. A study by Roberts et al. showed that children with food allergies are around 6 times more likely to suffer from severe asthma later in life than children who did not have food allergies. Similarly, Priftis et al. showed that approximately 40 % of children who were diagnosed with an egg and/or fish allergy in the first three years of their life reported current asthma symptoms at school age [17, 18]. Moreover, hay fever has been described as a major risk factor for asthma [19, 20]. In the current study, eczema was the most frequently reported allergy among the three allergies (food allergy, eczema and hay fever), reported by 63 % of the population (Table 2). A remarkably high percentage of the parents (25.6 %) reported that their children had experienced all three allergies (Fig. 1). The prevalence of food allergy in the current study was also very high (49.8 %). Earlier studies showed that the prevalence of food allergy varied between 3 % and 35 % [7]. Likewise a Dutch study reported a prevalence of (current) self-reported food allergy around 7.2 % among school children in the Netherlands [21]. The high prevalence in our study may have been influenced by the fact that we asked whether the child had ever experienced symptoms. Some children might have only experienced symptoms in early childhood, and this may have caused a larger prevalence than the prevalence of current food allergy symptoms. Nevertheless, we do realize that self-reporting might lead to an overestimation. Unfortunately, data regarding provocation testing to confirm an actual diagnosis of food allergy were not available. However, it has been shown that results from screening questionnaires, comparable to the one we used in this study, were in concordance with results from specific IgE measurements and information obtained from patient records [22, 23].

When we assessed the effect of age on the development of allergic disease, we noticed that the occurrence of hay fever increased with age in our study population (Fig. 2). Moreover, the mean age of the hay fever group (8.9 ± 2.5) was significantly higher than the mean age in the overall study population (Table 2). The same trend was reported by Spergel et al. where the incidence of hay fever increased over time during childhood. This might be caused by sensitization developed through other allergic conditions [8]. Ghouri et al. showed an increase in the prevalence of hay fever during childhood in England as well [24]. On the other hand, age trends in the occurrence of the eczema were not observed. Spergel et al. reported age incidence of eczema peaks in the first years of life [8]. It might, therefore, be that our population was too old to observe this trend. The median FeNO level was significantly higher in the hay fever group. This is in alignment with other studies that confirm high FeNO levels in hay fever sufferers [25, 26].

Our study was limited by the lack of physicians' diagnoses on allergic diseases or objective immunological test results. We used a questionnaire to obtain information about the history of allergic conditions. Other studies (such as ISAAC [27]) have also used questionnaire data. We realize, however, that this questionnaire data might differ from objective tests, and the occurrence of allergic diseases might therefore have been overestimated due to the use of parental-reported data. However, the strength of our study is in the selection of a large set of asthmatic children through community pharmacies. Our population represents a cross-section of the everyday pediatric asthma population that varies in the severity of the disease, health care utilization and asthma control.

Conclusions

In conclusion, our study suggests that children with asthma and co-morbid atopic conditions are at risk for more exacerbations and less well-controlled asthma in comparison to children who did not report allergies. The children who were reported to have had more than one allergic co-morbidity were especially at risk of having less well controlled asthma and more severe exacerbations. This may have clinical implications, such as more unscheduled health care visits and hospitalizations, as these patients may experience more severe asthma. These children should be carefully monitored and might benefit from asthma/allergy specialist care at an earlier stage.

Abbreviations

ACQ: Asthma Control Questionnaire; ATC: Anatomical Therapeutic Chemical; CI: confidence interval; ED: emergency department; FA: food allergy; FeNO: fractional exhaled nitric oxide level; HF: hay fever; ICS: Inhaled Corticosteroids; IQR: Interquartile Range; MARS: Medication Adherence Rating Scale; OCS: oral corticosteroids; OR: Odds Ratios; PACMAN: Pharmacogenetics of Asthma medication in Children: Medication with Anti-inflammatory effects; SABA: short acting beta agonists; UPPER: Utrecht Pharmacy Practice Network for Education and Research.

Competing interests

Francine C. van Erp declares that she has no competing interests. Susanne J.H. Vijverberg had been paid by an unrestricted grant from GlaxoSmithKline (GSK). Jan A. M. Raaijmakers is a part-time professor at the Utrecht University and he was Vice-president External Scientific Collaborations for GSK in Europe, and holds stock in GSK. Anke-Hilse Maitland-van der Zee received an unrestricted grant from GSK. Cornelis K. van der Ent received unrestricted grants from GSK and Grunenthal. Furthermore, the Department of Pharmacoepidemiology and Clinical Pharmacology, Utrecht Institute for Pharmaceutical Sciences, employing authors Ali Arabkhazaeli, Susanne J.H. Vijverberg, Jan A.M. Raaijmakers, and Anke-Hilse Maitland-van der Zee, has received unrestricted research funding from the Netherlands Organisation for Health Research and Development (ZonMW), the Dutch Health Care Insurance Board (CVZ), the Royal Dutch Pharmacists Association (KNMP), the private-public funded Top Institute Pharma (http://www.tipharma.nl website, includes co-funding from universities, government, and industry), the EU Innovative Medicines Initiative (IMI), EU 7th Framework Program (FP7), the Dutch Medicines Evaluation Board, the Dutch Ministry of Health and industry (including GSK, Pfizer, and others).

Authors' contributions

AA carried out the study design, analysis and interpretation of data, and drafted the manuscript. SV carried out the acquisition of data, participated in interpretation and helped to draft the manuscript. FE participated in interpretation. JR participated in study design and interpretation. CKE participated in study design and interpretation. AM contributed to conception and design of the study, and participated in its design and coordination and helped to draft the manuscript. All authors read and approved the final manuscript.

Acknowledgements

The authors wish to thank the children and the parents of the PACMAN cohort study, as well as UPPER and the participating pharmacies for their cooperation. Furthermore, we acknowledge the field workers for their valuable efforts. Susanne J.H. Vijverberg had been paid by an unrestricted grant from GlaxoSmithKline (GSK). Jan A. M. Raaijmakers is a part-time professor at the Utrecht University and he was Vice-president External Scientific Collaborations for GSK in Europe, and holds stock in GSK. Anke-Hilse Maitland-van der Zee received an unrestricted grant from GSK. Cornelis K. van der Ent received unrestricted grants from GSK and Grunenthal. Furthermore, the Department of Pharmacoepidemiology and Clinical Pharmacology, Utrecht Institute for Pharmaceutical Sciences, employing authors Ali Arabkhazaeli, Susanne J.H. Vijverberg, Jan A.M. Raaijmakers, and Anke-Hilse Maitland-van der Zee, has received unrestricted research funding from the Netherlands Organisation for Health Research and Development (ZonMW), the Dutch Health Care Insurance Board (CVZ), the Royal Dutch Pharmacists Association (KNMP), the private-public funded Top Institute Pharma (http://www.tipharma.nl website, includes co-funding from universities, government, and industry), the EU Innovative Medicines Initiative (IMI), EU 7th Framework Program (FP7), the Dutch Medicines Evaluation Board, the Dutch Ministry of Health and industry (including GSK, Pfizer, and others).

Author details

[1]Division of Pharmacoepidemiology & Clinical Pharmacology, Utrecht Institute for Pharmaceutical Sciences (UIPS), Faculty of Science, Utrecht University, P.O. Box 80082David de Wied Building, Universiteitsweg 99, Utrecht 3508 TB, The Netherlands. [2]Department of Pediatric Respiratory Medicine, Wilhelmina Children's Hospital, University Medical Centre Utrecht, Lundlaan 6, Utrecht 3584 EA, The Netherlands.

References

1. Covaciu C, Bergstrom A, Lind T, Svartengren M, Kull I. Childhood allergies affect health-related quality of life. J Asthma. 2013;50(5):522–8.
2. Nauta AJ, Engels F, Knippels LM, Garssen J, Nijkamp FP, Redegeld FA. Mechanisms of allergy and asthma. Eur J Pharmacol. 2008;585(2–3):354–60.
3. Barnes J. Chapter 254. Asthma. In: Longo D, Fauci A, Kasper D, Hauser S, Jameson J, Loscalzo J, editors. Harrison's Principles of Internal Medicine. 18th ed. New York: McGraw-Hill; 2012.
4. Bateman ED, Hurd SS, Barnes PJ, Bousquet J, Drazen JM, FitzGerald M, et al. Global strategy for asthma management and prevention: GINA executive summary. Eur Respir J. 2008;31(1):143–78.
5. Hon KL, Wang SS, Leung TF. The atopic march: from skin to the airways. Iran J Allergy Asthma Immunol. 2012;11(1):73–7.
6. Schwindt CD, Bacchus H, Leu SY, Tjoa T, Klebanova Y, Delfino RJ. Characterization of the asthmatic population of St. Vincent and the Grenadines: asthma severity levels and atopic sensitization. J Asthma. 2010;47(8):871–7.
7. Kewalramani A, Bollinger ME. The impact of food allergy on asthma. J Asthma Allergy. 2010;3:65–74.
8. Spergel JM, Paller AS. Atopic dermatitis and the atopic march. J Allergy Clin Immunol. 2003;112(6 Suppl):S118–27.
9. Branum AM, Lukacs SL. Food allergy among children in the United States. Pediatrics. 2009;124(6):1549–55.
10. Eichenfield LF, Hanifin JM, Beck LA, Lemanske Jr RF, Sampson HA, Weiss ST, et al. Atopic dermatitis and asthma: parallels in the evolution of treatment. Pediatrics. 2003;111(3):608–16.
11. Morgan WJ, Crain EF, Gruchalla RS, O'Connor GT, Kattan M, Evans III R, et al. Results of a home-based environmental intervention among urban children with asthma. N Engl J Med. 2004;351(11):1068–80.
12. Koster ES, Raaijmakers JA, Koppelman GH, Postma DS, van der Ent CK, Koenderman L, et al. Pharmacogenetics of anti-inflammatory treatment in children with asthma: rationale and design of the PACMAN cohort. Pharmacogenomics. 2009;10(8):1351–61.
13. Menckeberg T, Bouvy M, Bracke M. Adherence to inhaled corticosteroids and patient perception: towards a better understanding and individualised care. Utrecht: Utrecht University; 2008.
14. Juniper EF, Bousquet J, Abetz L, Bateman ED, GOAL Committee. Identifying 'well-controlled' and 'not well-controlled' asthma using the Asthma Control Questionnaire. Respir Med. 2006;100(4):616–21.
15. Schwindt CD, Tjoa T, Floro JN, McLaren C, Delfino RJ. Association of atopy to asthma severity and medication use in children. J Asthma. 2006;43(6):439–46.
16. Just J, Gouvis-Echraghi R, Rouve S, Wanin S, Moreau D, Annesi-Maesano I. Two novel, severe asthma phenotypes identified during childhood using a clustering approach. Eur Respir J. 2012;40(1):55–60.
17. Roberts G, Patel N, Levi-Schaffer F, Habibi P, Lack G. Food allergy as a risk factor for life-threatening asthma in childhood: a case-controlled study. J Allergy Clin Immunol. 2003;112(1):168–74.

18. Priftis KN, Mermiri D, Papadopoulou A, Papadopoulos M, Fretzayas A, Lagona E. Asthma symptoms and bronchial reactivity in school children sensitized to food allergens in infancy. J Asthma. 2008;45(7):590–5.
19. Pawankar R, Bunnag C, Chen Y, Fukuda T, Kim YY, Le LT, et al. Allergic rhinitis and its impact on asthma update (ARIA 2008)–western and Asian-Pacific perspective. Asian Pac J Allergy Immunol. 2009;27(4):237–43.
20. Lin J, Su N, Liu G, Yin K, Zhou X, Shen H, et al. The impact of concomitant allergic rhinitis on asthma control: a cross-sectional nationwide survey in China. J Asthma. 2014;51(1):34–43.
21. Brugman E, Meulmeester JF, Spee-van der Wekke A, Beuker RJ, Radder JJ, Verloove-Vanhorick SP, et al. Prevalence of self-reported food hypersensitivity among school children in The Netherlands. Eur J Clin Nutr. 1998;52(8):577–81.
22. Lakwijk N, Van Strien RT, Doekes G, Brunekreef B, Gerritsen J. Validation of a screening questionnaire for atopy with serum IgE tests in a population of pregnant Dutch women. Clin Exp Allergy. 1998;28(4):454–8.
23. Tuokkola J, Kaila M, Pietinen P, Simell O, Knip M, Virtanen SM. Agreement between parental reports and patient records in food allergies among infants and young children in Finland. J Eval Clin Pract. 2008;14(6):984–9.
24. Ghouri N, Hippisley-Cox J, Newton J, Sheikh A. Trends in the epidemiology and prescribing of medication for allergic rhinitis in England. J R Soc Med. 2008;101(9):466–72.
25. Gratziou C, Lignos M, Dassiou M, Roussos C. Influence of atopy on exhaled nitric oxide in patients with stable asthma and rhinitis. Eur Respir J. 1999;14(4):897–901.
26. Buchvald F, Baraldi E, Carraro S, Gaston B, De Jongste J, Pijnenburg MW, et al. Measurements of exhaled nitric oxide in healthy subjects age 4 to 17 years. J Allergy Clin Immunol. 2005;115(6):1130–6.
27. ISAAC Methodology. [http://isaac.auckland.ac.nz/story/methods/methods.php]

4

Parental knowledge, attitudes and practices regarding antibiotic use for acute upper respiratory tract infections in children

Sa'ed H. Zyoud[1,2,3*], Adham Abu Taha[4], Khulood F. Araj[5], Islam A. Abahri[5], Ansam F. Sawalha[4], Waleed M. Sweileh[4], Rahmat Awang[3] and Samah W. Al-Jabi[2]

Abstract

Background: In primary health care centres, upper respiratory tract infections (URTIs) in children are commonly encountered by physicians. Viruses cause most URTIs, but parents' attitudes often represent an important reason for antibiotic abuse, which leads to the development and spread of antimicrobial resistance. The goal of this study was to examine parents' knowledge, attitudes, and practices (KAP) about antibiotic use for children with URTIs in Palestine.

Methods: A cross-sectional study was performed in primary health care centres in Nablus city from 1 June to 31 October 2012. A questionnaire was developed and administered to determine parents' KAP regarding antibiotic use for their children with URTIs.

Results: Three hundred and eighty-five parents completed the questionnaire. A total of 79.7 % of the parents were attentive to the truth that antibiotic misuse is responsible for bacterial resistance. Only 18.9 % of parents thought that antibiotics did not have any harmful side effects. Fifty nine per cent of parents did not agree that URTIs are mostly viral in origin and are self-limited. Almost 73 % of parents choose antibiotics as a treatment for URTIs, while earache (68 %) and fever (64 %) were the most common reasons for which parents expected antibiotics. However, more than 38 % of the parents never asked the paediatrician to prescribe antibiotics, and only 6 % congratulated their paediatricians for not prescribing antibiotics.

Conclusions: Although there is a trusted relationship between parents and paediatricians, Palestinian parents have insufficient knowledge related to antibiotic use for URTIs in children, which results in inappropriate attitudes and practices. Educational interventions for both parents and physicians will reduce unnecessary antibiotic use and resistance.

Keywords: Upper respiratory tract infections, Parents, Children, Antibiotic

* Correspondence: saedzyoud@yahoo.com
[1]Poison Control and Drug Information Center (PCDIC), College of Medicine and Health Sciences, An-Najah National University, Nablus 44839, Palestine
[2]Department of Clinical and Community Pharmacy, College of Medicine and Health Sciences, An-Najah National University, Nablus 44839, Palestine
Full list of author information is available at the end of the article

Background

In primary health care centres, upper respiratory tract infections (URTIs) in children are commonly encountered by physicians [1–4]. These infections are considered the main cause of absenteeism from schools by children or from work by parents [5]. Furthermore, such infections in children bear a lot of economic burden on parents and healthcare system [5].

The World Health Organization, in its late report released in April 2014, revealed that antibiotic resistance is a serious and growing global problem [6]. Several studies reported the relationship between antibiotic use and the development of resistance [7–9]. Countries consuming the highest amounts of antibiotics have the highest rates of resistance [10]. Despite the fact that the majority of URTIs are viral in origin [11], antibiotic prescribing for URTIs is a common practice in paediatrics [12–14]. It is probable that 20–50 % of all antimicrobial use is medically inappropriate [15, 16]. Inappropriate prescribing of antibiotics is the most important reason behind the development of antibiotic resistance [17, 18].

The main contributors to the development of resistance in children are paediatricians and parents. Parental beliefs and expectations are important factors in determining whether an antibiotic is prescribed. When parents panic about acute illnesses, it leads to more frequent paediatric physician visits for URTIs and, subsequently, unnecessary antibiotic use [19–22]. Therefore, numerous reports have evaluated the factors related to antibiotic overuse. These factors consist of knowledge, attitudes and beliefs regarding antibiotic use [23–25], behaviours [26, 27], patient treatment satisfaction, patient-doctor communication, and patient experiences with antibiotics [25–28]. Proper public knowledge and attitude toward antibiotics is an important factor in rational antibiotic use and therefore minimizing development of antibiotic resistance [29]. Unfortunately, the pressure imposed on physicians to meet patients' expectations is a major contributing factor for physicians to prescribe antibiotics for viral URTI [24, 30]. Therefore, parental knowledge, attitude and practice toward antibiotic use in URTI in their children is of great value [24, 31].

Many studies were conducted in Palestine regarding antibiotic misuse and purchasing antibiotics without a prescription [32, 33]. These studies evaluated the extent of storage and wastage of antibacterial agents in Palestinian households [34], self-medication with antibiotics [35], and patterns of parenteral antimicrobial prescription among paediatric hospitalised patients [36]. Neither of these studies, nor other studies conducted in Palestine, assessed parents' knowledge, attitudes, and practices (KAP) regarding antibiotic use in URTIs in children. Thus, this study is the first of its kind in Palestine to evaluate parental KAP regarding antibiotic use in paediatrics. This study could provide baseline data for developing strategies for local health authorities' educational purposes.

Methods

Study area and study design

A cross-sectional survey was performed in Primary Health Care (PHC) centres in selected areas in Nablus governorate. The study was carried out from June, 1st to the end of October in 2012. The PHC centre's selection was based on geographic clustering sampling to obtain a representative sample of parents. Previously published studies about knowledge and attitudes toward antibiotics have been mostly carried out among physicians in primary healthcare centres [4, 37, 38]. For the purpose of this study, four primary health care centres were chosen. These centres have the followings in common which made them suitable as a study area [39, 40]: (1) they provide a full package of primary health care services; (2) they serve a large number of patients; and (3) they cover the three types of communities within this region (rural, urban, and Palestinian refugee camps). To the best of our knowledge, limited such studies were conducted on consumers such as parents [24, 31].

Study population

The population of the study was the parents of children attending PHC centres aged between 18 and 50 years.

Sampling procedure and sample size calculation

Sample size was calculated using a Raosoft sample size calculator. The calculation was based on 50 % response distribution, 5 % margin of error and 95 % confidence interval [41]. The assumption that the response rate is 50 % was based on the idea that both responses and response rates were completely unknown since there are no previously published similar studies from Palestine. The calculated sample size was 377. To ensure accuracy, the sample size was increased to 400 to account for any missing data or non-response rate. Ultimately, parents were selected using a convenience sampling method because it saves time, cost, and ease of accessibility to the researchers [42].

Questionnaire development

A self-administered questionnaire was developed in Arabic after reviewing related studies [24, 31, 43]. Most of the developed questions were extracted from previously published validated studies in Greece and were tailored to suit the local situation and assure its applicability [31, 44]. The questionnaire is comprised of four main sections: demographic data related to participants; and knowledge, attitude, and practice concerning the use of antibiotics. Some items were added, and the questionnaire was modified to be used in the Palestinian setting. Content validity of the questionnaire was assured by a group of experts in the field of paediatrics, infectious diseases, clinical pharmacy and biostatisticians. A pilot study was conducted among 30 participants in order to check the clarity and readability of the questionnaire. The final version of the questionnaire was refined and corrected based on feedback from the participants.

The final questionnaire consisted of four sections (A, B, C, and D). Section A contained demographic data, including age, gender, education levels, residency, income, number of children, health insurance status and whether the child had a chronic disease such as asthma. Section B was adopted from Panagakou et al., [31] and included items concerning parental knowledge of antibiotics. Parents were requested to mark antibiotic names out of six frequently used medications in the Nablus district and to answer questions related to general antibiotic use, adverse effects and their use in viral infections. Furthermore, Section B explored sources of information regarding the use of antibiotics. Section "C" included items concerning parental attitudes toward antibiotics. Parents were asked for possible treatment options for paediatric URTI management. In addition, parents were asked specifically about the most serious symptoms that would have to be present in order for them to visit the paediatricians' office. Other questions asked if parents thought that antibiotics were useful in relieving a variety of symptoms. Furthermore, parents were asked to indicate their expectations for antibiotic use corresponding to URTI symptoms and to designate the reasons for antibiotic use without medical advice. Finally, Section D illustrated parents' answers to questions linked to the medical practice. Parents were asked to indicate if their paediatrician spends adequate time elucidating the illness and suggesting antibiotic treatment for a child's illness, and if he/she is affected by their demand to prescribe antibiotics for their child. Parents were asked to answer the statements on a 5-point Likert scale ("strongly agree", "agree", "uncertain", "disagree", "strongly disagree" or "never", "sometimes", "often", "most of the time", "always"). A detailed description is provided in Additional file 1 about questions regarding knowledge, attitudes and practices of antibiotic use as an Arabic version.

Ethical approval

The study was approved by the Palestinian Ministry of Health, and the institutional review board (IRB) of An-Najah National University (approval number 23-Apr 2012 on April 13, 2012) and verbal consent was obtained from survey participants. An written consent was waived according to the regulation of IRB.

Statistical analysis

Data were entered and assessed with the Statistical Package for the Social Sciences (SPSS), version 16.0 for Windows. The analysis of answers for questions involved descriptive quantitative statistics, e.g., frequency and percentage for categorical variables and means ± standard deviation (SD) or medians (lower-upper quartiles) for numerical variables. The figures were created using Microsoft® Office Excel 2007.

Results

Three hundred and eighty five questionnaires were collected back out of 400 that were initially distributed, giving a response rate of 96.2 %. The majority of respondents (62.6 %) were mothers with a mean age of 31.6 years (SD ± 7), and 74 % of parents considered their income as moderate. Approximately two-thirds of parents lived in the city. Nearly 43 % of participants

Table 1 Socio-demographic characteristics of the population studied ($n = 385$)

Variable	Frequency (%), or mean ± SD, or median [interquartile] $N = 385$
Gender	
Male	144 (37.4)
Female	241 (62.6)
Age ± SD (year)	31.6 ± 7
Median number of children aged less than six years	2 [1–2]
Median number of children aged more than six years	0 [0–2]
Health insurance	
Governmental insurance	142 (36.9)
Private insurance	127 (33.0)
Do not have insurance	116 (30.1)
Participant's educational level	
Elementary school (primary)	79 (20.5)
High school (secondary school)	149 (36.4)
University	166 (43.1)
Income level of the family per month[a]	
Low (less than 500 JD)	67 (17.4)
Average (500–1000 JD)	285 (74)
High (more than 3000 JD)	33 (8.6)
Residency	
City	239 (62.1)
Rural	101 (26.2)
Palestinian refugee camps	45 (11.7)
Child with chronic disease	41 (10.6)

[a]1 Jordanian Dinar (JD) equals 1.41 US Dollar

had a university degree. The socio-demographic characteristics of respondents are shown in Table 1.

Knowledge

Most parents (61.6 %) stated that their physician was the main source of information regarding antibiotics, followed by their pharmacist (34.3 %); other sources, such as television, newspapers, and family members/friends accounted only for 2.8 % of parents' sources of information. However, 1.3 % of parents stated they never received any information from any of these sources.

When parents were asked to discriminate between antibiotic products and other drugs, including analgesics, cough preparations and expectorants, and antipyretics, most parents (55.6 %) were able to identify that amoxicillin was an antibiotic, while only 8.1 and 3.1 % were able to identify that amoxicillin-clavulanic acid and cefuroxime, respectively, were antibiotics. Moreover, 24.2, 4.7 and 4.1 % of parents identified ibuprofen,

Table 2 Parental knowledge regarding antibiotic use in children with URTIs ($N = 385$). Questions adopted from Panagakou et al. [31]

Variable	Item	Frequency	Percentage %
Antibiotics can be used for any feverish child	Strongly agree	76	19.7
	Agree	153	39.7
	Disagree	110	28.6
	Strongly disagree	40	10.4
	Uncertain	6	1.6
Children with flu like symptoms get better faster when antibiotics are used	Strongly agree	69	17.9
	Agree	201	52.2
	Disagree	95	24.7
	Strongly disagree	15	3.9
	Uncertain	5	1.3
Most URTIs are viral in origin and are self-limited; thus, there is no need for antibiotic use	Strongly agree	43	11.2
	Agree	114	29.9
	Disagree	173	44.9
	Strongly disagree	37	9.6
	Uncertain	18	4.7
Antibiotics do not have any side effects	Strongly agree	19	4.9
	Agree	54	14.0
	Disagree	163	42.3
	Strongly disagree	138	35.8
	Uncertain	11	2.9
Inappropriate use of antibiotics reduces their efficacy and drives bacterial resistance	Strongly agree	126	32.7
	Agree	181	47
	Disagree	53	13.8
	Strongly disagree	15	3.9
	Uncertain	10	2.6
Antibiotic use can prevent complications from URTIs	Strongly agree	68	17.7
	Agree	223	57.9
	Disagree	63	16.4
	Strongly disagree	12	3.1
	Uncertain	19	4.6
Scientists can produce new antibiotics for resistant bacteria	Strongly agree	96	24.4
	Agree	180	46.8
	Disagree	27	7.0
	Strongly disagree	18	4.7
	Uncertain	64	16.6

paracetamol, and cough preparations, respectively, as antibiotics.

Table 2 demonstrate the responses to questions related to knowledge. A total of 79.7 % of parents were attentive to the truth that antibiotic misuse is responsible for bacterial resistance, but 70.1 % would still give antibiotics to their child because they thought this would lead to a faster recovery. 59 % of parents did not agree that URTIs are mostly viral in origin and are self-limited without the need for antibiotic use. Only 18.9 % of parents thought that antibiotics did not cause any harmful side effects, while 78.1 % were certain that antibiotics might cause many harmful adverse effects (Fig. 1). Moreover, 71.7 % of parents thought that new stronger antibiotics are always emerging.

Attitude and expectation

When parents were given possible treatment options for the management of paediatric URTIs, more than two-thirds (73.2 %) of participants chose antibiotic therapy, and 66 % of parents choose analgesics and antipyretics as a possible treatment options for URTIs, while only 15.3 % of participants choose inhalers as a possible therapy (Fig. 2). In addition, when parents were asked specifically about the most serious symptoms that would have to be present in order for them to visit the paediatricians office (including fever, runny nose, cough, sore throat, ear pain, and change in behaviour) in the case of URTIs, 78.4 and 44.7 % of symptoms were fever and ear pain, respectively, often accompanied by other symptoms.

Few parents would ask their paediatrician for antibiotics for nasal drainage (22 %) or dry throat (11 %), while the majority of parents would want their paediatrician to recommend an antibiotic if their child had an earache (68 %), fever (64 %), cold (52 %), cough (34 %), or was vomiting (30 %). Figure 3 shows parental expectations for antibiotic use corresponding to URTI symptoms. There are many reasons for parents to administer antibiotics to their children without having received previous medical advice. In particular, 24.7 % of parents used antibiotics as self-medication due to economic hardships or lack of time, while 50.6 % would give antibiotics to their child because they believed that symptoms (e.g., earache, fever, cold, cough) were not dangerous as much as necessary to see the paediatrician.

Figure 4 indicates parental attitudes for antibiotic use in URTIs. The majority of parents (72.7 %) agreed that antibiotics are extensively used without proper indications and affirmed that they would not change paediatricians if they did not easily prescribe antibiotics (76 %); however, 27 % declared that they would change paediatricians because they easily prescribed antibiotics. About 63.5 % of parents agreed that it was better to keep away from the use of antibiotics to their child for simple or uncomplicated URTIs.

Practice

Figure 5 illustrates parents' responses to questions related to practice. More than 38 % of parents declared that they never asked their paediatrician to prescribe antibiotics, while only 6 % of parents congratulated paediatricians for not prescribing antibiotics. However, about 41.1 % of parents would ask the paediatrician whether antibiotic administration was necessary. About 28.3 % of parents thought that their paediatrician prescribed antibiotics based on their request, and, more notably, 76.6 % declared they exactly follow paediatricians' directions.

Discussion

The current study aimed to analyse knowledge and attitudes concerning antibiotic use and practices in the management of childhood URTIs in a large sample of

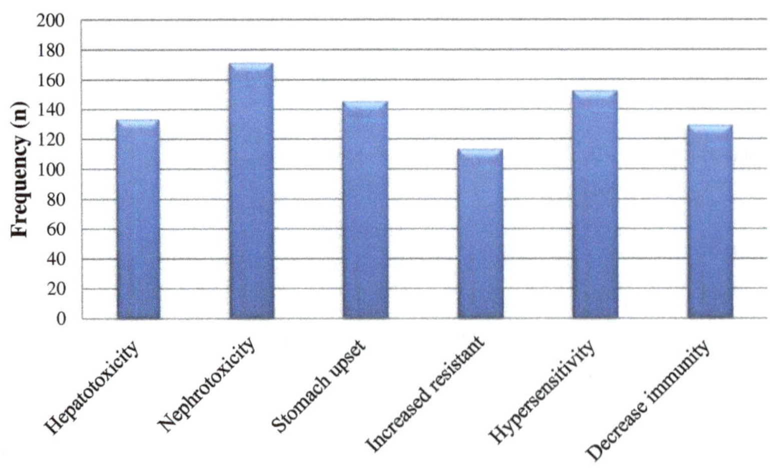

Fig. 1 Parents' knowledge regarding harmful adverse effects of antibiotics

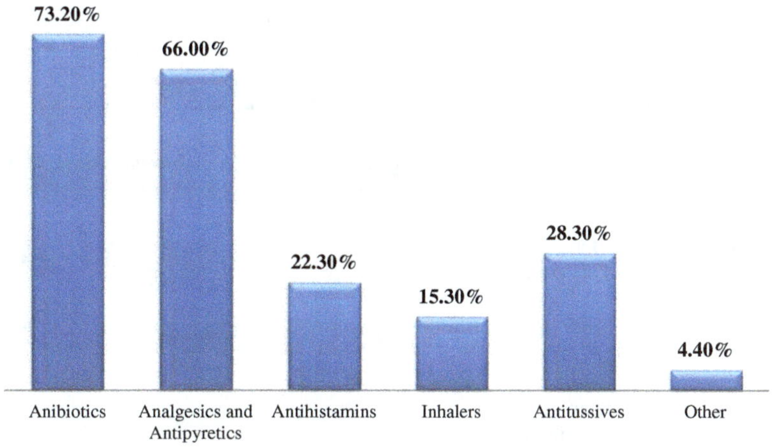

Fig. 2 Parental expected treatment for paediatric URTIs

parents. The issue of the current study is novel in the Palestinian population. It is considered a part of social science that often lags behind.

Our study demonstrated that Palestinian parents and paediatricians have a trusting relationship; the great majority of parents have confidence in the information and prescriptions supplied to them by paediatricians, and only a few parents would change paediatricians if they over- or under-prescribed antibiotics in the case of URTIs in children. Furthermore, 76.6 % stated that they precisely follow paediatricians' recommendations, and almost two-thirds of parents indicated their paediatricians as the main source of information about use or misuse of antibiotics. Xiang et al. [45] identified media (e.g., television) as the main source of such information about use or misuse of antibiotics, despite the fact that similar KAP studies reported paediatricians as the preferred source of information [43].

Most of the Palestinian parents were attentive to the truth that antibiotic misuse is responsible for bacterial resistance, although 59 % of them did not agree that URTIs are mostly viral in origin and are self-limited without the need for antibiotic use, which is in contrast to Greek parents, of which 80 % believed that URTIs are mostly self-limited [31]. It is inaccurate to suppose that 59 % of the parents preferred only antibiotic treatment because most of them also favoured other medications indicated for symptom relief such as analgesics, antipyretic, antihistamines, inhalers, and cough preparations.

Our results demonstrated that fever symptoms accompanied with URTIs were the most common reason for a paediatric visit in which parents would expect to receive

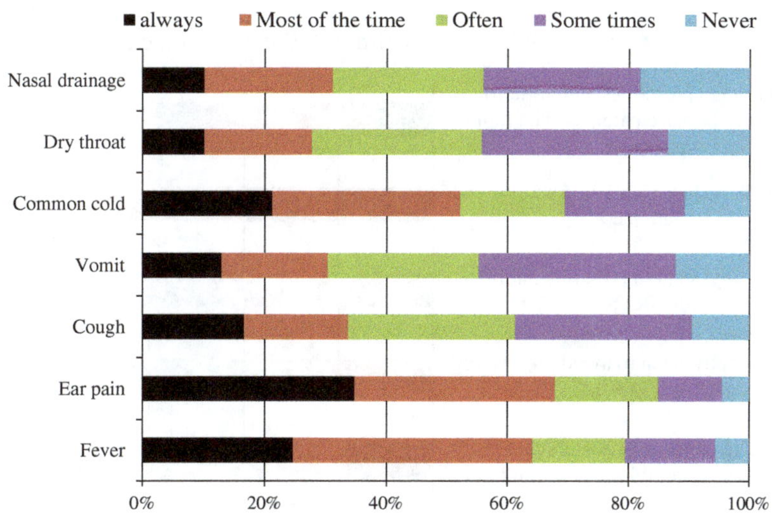

Fig. 3 Parental expectations for antibiotic use corresponding to upper respiratory tract infection symptoms. Questions adopted from Panagakou et al. [31]

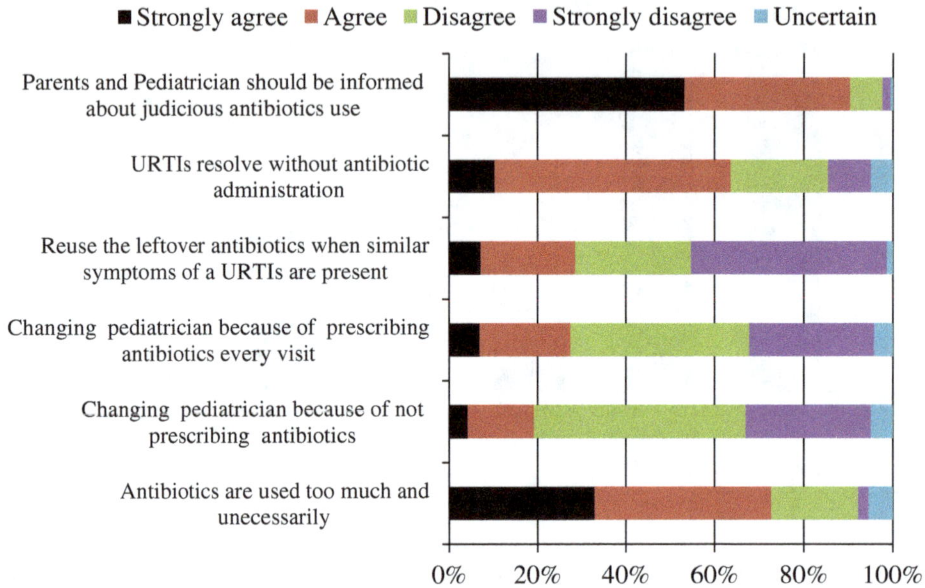

Fig. 4 Percentage of parents' responses to questions related to attitude. Questions adopted from Panagakou et al. [31]

antibiotics. Similarly, a cross-sectional KAP study involving 421 parents in Malaysia showed that 76 % of parents believed that antibiotics were helpful in the treatment of fever [24].

The use of "leftover" and "shared" antibiotics by parents to their child are common situations in the Palestinian and Malaysian communities; 27.6 % of Palestinian parents reused the leftover and shared antibiotics between their children, while 15 % of Malaysian parents reused leftovers and 24 % shared antibiotics. Parents believed that their child complained of the same illnesses because they had similar symptoms, therefore they would give the leftover antibiotics and shared it with others, and only bring their children to paediatrician if there was no improvement [24]. Interestingly, almost 51 % of parents choose antibiotics as the first choice of treatment for URTIs despite 78 % of them understanding that antibiotic use is associated with harmful and adverse effects on body systems, especially nephrotoxicity and hepatotoxicity.

Furthermore, 72.7 % of parents in the current study believed that antibiotics were used too much and unnecessarily. Comparable findings were found in previous similar studies such as Panagakou et al. [31] (78 %) and Rouusounides et al. [43] (81 %). This could be

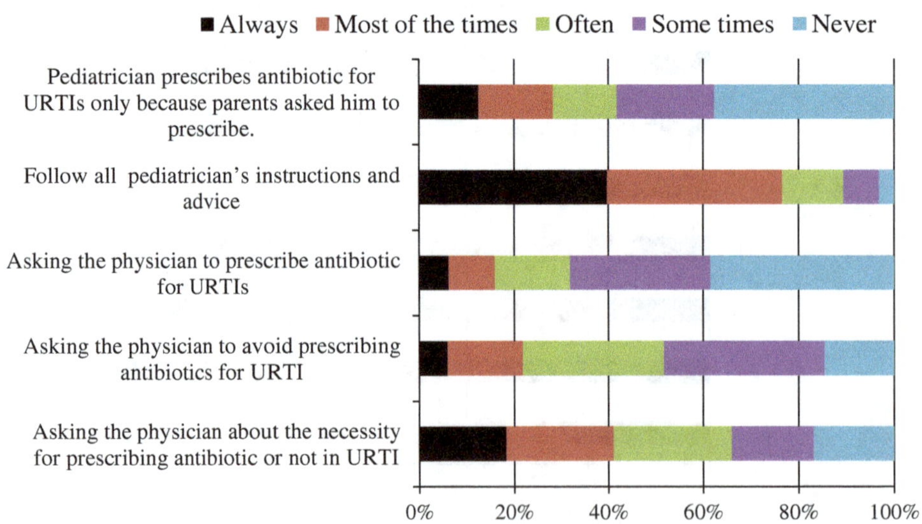

Fig. 5 Percentage of parents' responses to questions related to practice. Questions adopted from Panagakou et al. [31]

somewhat contributed to by paediatricians' behaviours and their antibiotic prescribing practices in Palestine [35, 36, 46, 47], which is one of the developing countries in the Middle East that has a high antimicrobial resistance rate [32, 48, 49]. There were several factors that may have induced inappropriate antibiotic prescription, including diagnostic uncertainty, socio-cultural and economic pressures, lack of knowledge, and fear of litigation [50, 51]. A more recent study demonstrated that many general practitioners had a moderate level of knowledge concerning the management of URTIs [4].

Strengths and limitations of the study

This is the first study that was conducted to assess parental KAP on antibiotic use in URTIs in Palestine. In addition, the study response rate of 96.1 % is considered reasonable for a community survey. Nevertheless, there were some limitations of this study. These limitations were associated with using a convenience sample, which might not be representative of the whole community in Palestine. Furthermore, the data were collected from parents attending PHC centres which limit the generalizability of the results to other types of health care services such as private sectors. While efforts were made to obtain representative samples, the over representation of PHC and higher educational level in the study sample might indicate a possible selection bias. Another limitation is that parents were asked several questions about their experience and antibiotic use in the past, which may lead to recall bias. Lastly, small sample size of the subgroups made comparative analyses to be problematic. For example, comparison between those living in refugee camps and city residents would have been helpful in identifying the most appropriate groups to target with educational programmes.

Conclusions and recommendations

In conclusion, we found that Palestinian parents' lack of knowledge on antibiotic use for paediatric URTIs resulted in inappropriate attitudes and practices. On the other hand, there is a trusted relationship between parents and paediatricians, and there is confidence in the information and prescriptions provided to them from doctors: only a few parents would change their paediatrician according to antibiotic prescription patterns. However, parents also believed that inappropriate use of antibiotics reduces their efficacy and drives resistance. Unfortunately, a large number of parents did not agree that URTIs are mostly viral of origin; parents' also self-limited antibiotic use, and three-fourths expected antibiotics to be a choice for paediatric URTI treatment. Educational interventions for both parents and physicians will reduce unnecessary antibiotic use and resistance. Strengthening and application of pharmacy regulations related to the over-the-counter sale of antibiotics is needed in community pharmacies.

Abbreviations

URTIs: Upper respiratory tract infections; KAP: Knowledge, attitudes, and practices; PHC: Primary health care; SD: Standard deviation; IRB: Institutional review board.

Competing interests

The authors declare that they have no competing interests.

Authors' contributions

SZ led study design, data collection, statistical analysis, interpreted the data, and drafting of manuscript; AA, SA, AS, WS and RA involved in study concept and design, and revised the article for important intellectual content; and KA, and IA carried out the data collection, results tabulation, statistical analysis, and wrote part of the article. All authors read and approved the final manuscript and agreed on its submission.

Acknowledgements

The research team would like to thank all participants who agreed to complete the survey. Furthermore, the authors would like to express many thanks and gratitude to An-Najah National University and the Palestinian Ministry of Health for their help and ethical approval to conduct this study.

Author details

[1]Poison Control and Drug Information Center (PCDIC), College of Medicine and Health Sciences, An-Najah National University, Nablus 44839, Palestine. [2]Department of Clinical and Community Pharmacy, College of Medicine and Health Sciences, An-Najah National University, Nablus 44839, Palestine. [3]WHO Collaborating Centre for Drug Information, National Poison Centre, Universiti Sains Malaysia (USM), Penang 11800, Malaysia. [4]Department of Pharmacology and Toxicology, College of Medicine and Health Sciences, An-Najah National University, Nablus 44839, Palestine. [5]PharmD Program, College of Medicine and Health Sciences, An-Najah National University, Nablus, Palestine.

References

1. Yang L, Liu C, Wang L, Yin X, Zhang X. Public reporting improves antibiotic prescribing for upper respiratory tract infections in primary care: a matched-pair cluster-randomized trial in China. Health Res Policy Syst. 2014;12:61.
2. Eckel N, Sarganas G, Wolf IK, Knopf H. Pharmacoepidemiology of common colds and upper respiratory tract infections in children and adolescents in Germany. BMC Pharmacol Toxicol. 2014;15:44.
3. Zeng L, Zhang L, Hu Z, Ehle EA, Chen Y, Liu L, et al. Systematic review of evidence-based guidelines on medication therapy for upper respiratory tract infection in children with AGREE instrument. PLoS One. 2014;9(2):e87711.
4. Hassali MA, Kamil TK, Md Yusof FA, Alrasheedy AA, Yusoff ZM, Saleem F, et al. General practitioners' knowledge, attitude and prescribing of antibiotics for upper respiratory tract infections in Selangor, Malaysia: findings and implications. Expert Rev Anti Infect Ther. 2015;13(4):511–20.
5. West JV. Acute upper airway infections. Br Med Bull. 2002;61:215–30.
6. WHO. Antimicrobial resistance: global report on surveillance 2014 [http://apps.who.int/iris/bitstream/10665/112642/1/9789241564748_eng.pdf?ua=1].
7. Turnidge J, Christiansen K. Antibiotic use and resistance–proving the obvious. Lancet. 2005;365(9459):548–9.
8. Levy SB, Marshall B. Antibacterial resistance worldwide: causes, challenges and responses. Nat Med. 2004;10(12 Suppl):S122–9.

9. Shibl AM, Memish Z, Osoba A. Antibiotic resistance in developing countries. J Chemother. 2001;13 Suppl 1:40–4.
10. Ferech M, Coenen S, Malhotra-Kumar S, Dvorakova K, Hendrickx E, Suetens C, et al. European Surveillance of Antimicrobial Consumption (ESAC): outpatient antibiotic use in Europe. J Antimicrob Chemother. 2006;58(2):401–7.
11. Harnden A, Perera R, Brueggemann AB, Mayon-White R, Crook DW, Thomson A, et al. Respiratory infections for which general practitioners consider prescribing an antibiotic: a prospective study. Arch Dis Child. 2007;92(7):594–7.
12. Goossens H, Ferech M, Vander Stichele R, Elseviers M, Group EP. Outpatient antibiotic use in Europe and association with resistance: a cross-national database study. Lancet. 2005;365(9459):579–87.
13. Watson RL, Dowell SF, Jayaraman M, Keyserling H, Kolczak M, Schwartz B. Antimicrobial use for pediatric upper respiratory infections: reported practice, actual practice, and parent beliefs. Pediatrics. 1999;104(6):1251–7.
14. McCaig LF, Besser RE, Hughes JM. Trends in antimicrobial prescribing rates for children and adolescents. JAMA. 2002;287(23):3096–102.
15. Guven GS, Uzun O. Principles of good use of antibiotics in hospitals. J Hosp Infect. 2003;53(2):91–6. quiz 149.
16. Cizman M. The use and resistance to antibiotics in the community. Int J Antimicrob Agents. 2003;21(4):297–307.
17. Nasrin D, Collignon PJ, Roberts L, Wilson EJ, Pilotto LS, Douglas RM. Effect of beta lactam antibiotic use in children on pneumococcal resistance to penicillin: prospective cohort study. BMJ. 2002;324(7328):28–30.
18. Yagupsky P. Selection of antibiotic-resistant pathogens in the community. Pediatr Infect Dis J. 2006;25(10):974–6.
19. Paluck E, Katzenstein D, Frankish CJ, Herbert CP, Milner R, Speert D, et al. Prescribing practices and attitudes toward giving children antibiotics. Can Fam Physician. 2001;47:521–7.
20. Stivers T. Participating in decisions about treatment: overt parent pressure for antibiotic medication in pediatric encounters. Soc Sci Med. 2002;54(7):1111–30.
21. Mangione-Smith R, McGlynn EA, Elliott MN, McDonald L, Franz CE, Kravitz RL. Parent expectations for antibiotics, physician-parent communication, and satisfaction. Arch Pediatr Adolesc Med. 2001;155(7):800–6.
22. Pechere JC. Patients' interviews and misuse of antibiotics. Clin Infect Dis. 2001;33 Suppl 3:S170–3.
23. Awad AI, Eltayeb IB. Self-medication practices with antibiotics and antimalarials among Sudanese undergraduate university students. Ann Pharmacother. 2007;41(7):1249–55.
24. Chan GC, Tang SF. Parental knowledge, attitudes and antibiotic use for acute upper respiratory tract infection in children attending a primary healthcare clinic in Malaysia. Singapore Med J. 2006;47(4):266–70.
25. Mitsi G, Jelastopulu E, Basiaris H, Skoutelis A, Gogos C. Patterns of antibiotic use among adults and parents in the community: a questionnaire-based survey in a Greek urban population. Int J Antimicrob Agents. 2005;25(5):439–43.
26. Al-Azzam SI, Al-Husein BA, Alzoubi F, Masadeh MM, Al-Horani MA. Self-medication with antibiotics in Jordanian population. Int J Occup Med Environ Health. 2007;20(4):373–80.
27. Sarahroodi S, Arzi A, Sawalha A, Ashtarinezhad A. Antibiotics self-medication among southern iranian university students. Int J Pharmacol. 2010;6(1):48–52.
28. Crossley J, Eiser C, Davies HA. Children and their parents assessing the doctor-patient interaction: a rating system for doctors' communication skills. Med Educ. 2005;39(8):820–8.
29. Awad AI, Aboud EA. Knowledge, attitude and practice towards antibiotic use among the public in Kuwait. PLoS One. 2015;10(2):e0117910.
30. Belongia EA, Naimi TS, Gale CM, Besser RE. Antibiotic use and upper respiratory infections: a survey of knowledge, attitudes, and experience in Wisconsin and Minnesota. Prev Med. 2002;34(3):346–52.
31. Panagakou SG, Spyridis N, Papaevangelou V, Theodoridou KM, Goutziana GP, Theodoridou MN, et al. Antibiotic use for upper respiratory tract infections in children: a cross-sectional survey of knowledge, attitudes, and practices (KAP) of parents in Greece. BMC Pediatr. 2011;11:60.
32. Hajjaj MZA-A. Utilization of antibiotics in Nablus City-Palestine pharmaco-epidemiological study. Nablus: National University; 2005.
33. Sawalha AF, Sweileh WM, Zyoud SH, Al-Jabi SW, Shamseh FFB, Odah AA. Analysis of prescriptions dispensed at community pharmacies in Nablus, Palestine. East Mediterr Health J. 2010;16(7):788–92.
34. Sawalha A. Extent of storage and wastage of antibacterial agents in Palestinian households. Pharm World Sci. 2010;32(4):530–5.
35. Sawalha AF. Self-medication with antibiotics: A study in Palestine. Int J Risk Saf Med. 2008;20(4):213–22.
36. Sawalha A, Al-Bishtawi G, Al-Khayyat L, Sweileh W, Al-Ramahi R, Jaradat N. Pattern of parenteral antimicrobial prescription among pediatric patients in Al-watani governmental hospital in Palestine. An-Najah Univ J Res. 2006;20:191–206.
37. Sahin H, Arsu G, Koseli D, Buke C. Evaluation of primary health care physicians' knowledge on rational antibiotic use. Mikrobiyol Bul. 2008;42(2):343–8.
38. Md Rezal RS, Hassali MA, Alrasheedy AA, Saleem F, Md Yusof FA, Godman B. Physicians' knowledge, perceptions and behaviour towards antibiotic prescribing: a systematic review of the literature. Expert Rev Anti Infect Ther. 2015;13(5):665–80.
39. Zyoud SH, Al-Jabi SW, Nabulsi MM, Tubaila MF, Sweileh WM, Awang R, et al. The validity and reliability of the parent fever management scale: A study from Palestine. Matern Child Health J. 2015;19(8):1890–7.
40. Zyoud SH, Al-Jabi SW, Sweileh WM, Nabulsi MM, Tubaila MF, Awang R, et al. Beliefs and practices regarding childhood fever among parents: A cross-sectional study from Palestine. BMC Pediatr. 2013;13:66.
41. Raosoft Inc. Sample size calculator [http://www.raosoft.com/samplesize.html].
42. van der Deijl M, Etman A, Kamphuis CB, van Lenthe FJ. Participation levels of physical activity programs for community-dwelling older adults: a systematic review. BMC Public Health. 2014;14:1301.
43. Rousounidis A, Papaevangelou V, Hadjipanayis A, Panagakou S, Theodoridou M, Syrogiannopoulos G, et al. Descriptive study on parents' knowledge, attitudes and practices on antibiotic use and misuse in children with upper respiratory tract infections in Cyprus. Int J Environ Res Public Health. 2011;8(8):3246–62.
44. Panagakou SG, Theodoridou MN, Papaevangelou V, Papastergiou P, Syrogiannopoulos GA, Goutziana GP, et al. Development and assessment of a questionnaire for a descriptive cross-sectional study concerning parents' knowledge, attitudes and practises in antibiotic use in Greece. BMC Infect Dis. 2009;9:52.
45. Xiang N, Shi Y, Wu J, Zhang S, Ye M, Peng Z, et al. Knowledge, attitudes and practices (KAP) relating to avian influenza in urban and rural areas of China. BMC Infect Dis. 2010;10:34.
46. Abu-Taha AS, Sweileh WM. Antibiotic resistance of bacterial strains isolated from patients with community-acquired urinary tract infections: An exploratory study in Palestine. Curr Clin Pharmacol. 2011;6(4):304–7.
47. Al-Dawodi R, Farraj MA, Essawi T. Antimicrobial resistance in non-typhi Salmonella enterica isolated from humans and poultry in Palestine. J Infect Dev Ctries. 2012;6(2):132–6.
48. Shibl A, Daniels J, Sievers J, the SOAR in AME Study Group. Antimicrobial resistance among Streptococcus pneumoniae and Haemophilus influenzae from Africa and the Middle East: 2002- 2003 winter season, Clin Microbiol Infect. 2004;10(Suppl 3):111.
49. de Andrade SS, Gales AC, Sader HS. Antimicrobial resistance in Gram-negative bacteria from developing countries. In: DeJSosa A, Byarugaba DK, Amábile-Cuevas CF, Hsueh PR, Kariuki S, Okeke IN, editors. Antimicrobial resistance in developing countries. New York, Dordrecht, Heidelberg, London: Springer; 2010. p. 249–66.
50. Moro ML, Marchi M, Gagliotti C, Di Mario S, Resi D. Why do paediatricians prescribe antibiotics? Results of an Italian regional project. BMC Pediatr. 2009;9:69.
51. Pichichero ME. Understanding antibiotic overuse for respiratory tract infections in children. Pediatrics. 1999;104(6):1384–8.

5

A randomized controlled trial of hospital versus home based therapy with oral amoxicillin for severe pneumonia in children aged 3 – 59 months: The IndiaCLEN Severe Pneumonia Oral Therapy (ISPOT) Study

Archana B. Patel[1], Akash Bang[2*], Meenu Singh[3], Leena Dhande[1], Luke Ravi Chelliah[4], Ashraf Malik[5], Sandhya Khadse[6] and ISPOT Study Group

Abstract

Background: Pneumonia is the leading cause of child mortality under five years of age worldwide. For pneumonia with chest indrawing in children aged 3–59 months, injectable penicillin and hospitalization was the recommended treatment. This increased the health care cost and exposure to nosocomial infections. We compared the clinical and cost outcomes of a seven day treatment with oral amoxicillin with the first 48 h of treatment given in the hospital (hospital group) or at home (home group).

Methods: We conducted an open-label, multi-center, two-arm randomized clinical trial at six tertiary hospitals in India. Children aged 3 to 59 months with chest indrawing pneumonia were randomized to home or hospital group. Clinical outcomes, treatment adherence, and patient safety were monitored through home visits on day 3, 5, 8, and 14 with an additional visit for the home group at 24 h. Clinical outcomes included treatment failure rates up to 7 days (primary outcome) and between 8–14 days (secondary outcome) using the intention to treat and per protocol analyses. Cost outcomes included direct medical, direct non-medical and indirect costs for a random 17 % subsample using the micro-costing technique.

Results: 1118 children were enrolled and randomized to home ($n = 554$) or hospital group ($n = 564$). Both groups had similar baseline characteristics. Overall treatment failure rate was 11.5 % (per protocol analysis). The hospital group was significantly more likely to fail treatment than the home group in the intention to treat analysis. Predictors with increased risk of treatment failure at any time were age 3–11 months, receiving antibiotics within 48 h prior to enrolment and use of high polluting fuel. Death rates at 7 or 14 days did not differ significantly. (Difference −0.0 %; 95 % CI −0.5 to 0.5). The median total treatment cost was Rs. 399 for the home group versus Rs. 602 for the hospital group ($p < 0.001$), for the same effect of 5 % failure rate at the end of 7 days of treatment in the random subsample.

(Continued on next page)

* Correspondence: drakashbang@gmail.com
[2]Mahatma Gandhi Institute of Medical Sciences, Sewagram, Maharashtra, India
Full list of author information is available at the end of the article

(Continued from previous page)

Conclusions: Home based oral amoxicillin treatment was equivalent to hospital treatment for first 48 h in selected children of chest indrawing pneumonia and was cheaper. Consistent with the recent WHO simplified guidelines, management with home based oral amoxicillin for select children with only fast breathing and chest-indrawing can be a cost effective intervention.

Keywords: Severe pneumonia, Lower chest indrawing, Hospitalization, Oral amoxicillin, Cost effective, Randomized trial

Background

Pneumonia is the single largest killer of children under the age of five worldwide [1]. The disease kills over two million children under the age of five every year— nearly one fourth (400,000) of these deaths occur in India alone [2]. About half of pneumonia cases in India are caused by bacteria and could be treated with antibiotics. However, only 13 % of Indian children under the age of five with suspected pneumonia receive antibiotics [3].

The 2008 WHO guidelines for treatment of non-severe pneumonia (cough, fever and fast breathing) recommend health workers to provide oral antibiotics for three days at home but urgent referral for hospitalization for parenteral (injectable) antibiotics and other supportive therapy after administration of first dose of antibiotics, if the child has severe pneumonia (cough, fever, fast breathing and lower chest indrawing) or very severe disease (pneumonia with the presence of WHO defined danger signs) [4]. Often inability to access a referral facility deprives these children from getting appropriate care. For many families, seeking treatment for their children at a health care facility is often logistically and financially burdensome thus denying them early administration of antibiotics within 48 h that can potentially improve their outcomes. Additionally transport to a distant facility can entail serious delays in effective treatment. Many children with severe pneumonia referred for admission to a hospital could die in transit or reach too sick to be saved [5]. In addition, when hospitalized, the children with severe pneumonia are vulnerable to nosocomial infections in crowded hospital wards and are also at risk of needle-borne infections due to parenteral therapy. Two important studies have addressed such barriers to the recommended treatment of severe pneumonia. The first study was intended to determine whether oral antibiotics are equivalent to injectable antibiotics when both are given in the hospital. This was an open label equivalency study called APPIS (Amoxicillin Penicillin Pneumonia International Study), which was a large multicentre randomized controlled trial comparing injectable penicillin versus oral amoxicillin given for 7 days to children in the hospital [6]. The second study was called "NO-SHOTS" (New Outpatient Short-Course Home Oral Therapy for Severe Pneumonia Study) and was a randomized, open-label equivalency trial done at seven study sites in Pakistan and compared initial hospitalization and parenteral ampicillin for 48 h followed by 3 days of oral amoxicillin at home, to 5 days of home-based treatment with oral amoxicillin [7]. NO-SHOTS showed that home treatment with high-dose oral amoxicillin is equivalent to hospital based treatment with parenteral ampicillin in selected children aged 3–59 months with WHO defined severe pneumonia [7]. Later, another study- the MASS study (Multicenter Amoxicillin Severe pneumonia Study) showed that clinical treatment failure and adverse event rates among children with severe pneumonia treated at home with oral amoxicillin did not substantially differ across geographic areas (Bangladesh, Ghana, Vietnam and Egypt) and hence home-based therapy of severe pneumonia could possibly be applied to a wide variety of settings [8]. Thus oral amoxicillin at home has proven clinically efficacious in various settings across the world for treatment of selected children with WHO defined severe pneumonia. The Lancet Series on Childhood Pneumonia and Diarrhoea has reported that case management is one of the three most effective interventions to reduce pneumonia deaths in children but also noted that the cost effectiveness of these interventions in national health systems needs urgent assessment [9]. So the cost savings or cost-effectiveness of home-based oral antibiotic treatment for WHO defined severe pneumonia in childhood would be important to inform public policy and has not been previously evaluated.

Therefore our objective was to assess the efficacy and cost-effectiveness of a 7-day home-based course of oral amoxicillin as compared to oral amoxicillin administered for the first 48 h in the hospital followed by 5 days of home-administration.

Methods

We conducted an open labelled multi-center prospective two-arm randomized clinical trial at 6 referral hospitals in India (Chandigarh, Chennai, Nagpur, Pune, Sewagram and Aligarh) to evaluate the difference of rates of treatment failures of a 7-day course of oral amoxicillin when administered at home as compared to a 7-day course of oral amoxicillin administered for the first 48 h in the hospital followed by 5 days of home-administration to treat WHO defined severe pneumonia in children aged 3–59 months. In addition to the clinical outcomes, the costs of treating severe pneumonia, the differences in costs of treatment in the two study groups and the cost-effectiveness of the two alternative treatment strategy was also assessed in this trial.

The study was approved by the institutional ethics committees of: Indira Gandhi Government Medical College, Nagpur; Post Graduate Institute of Medical Sciences, Chandigarh; Government General Hospital, Chennai; B.J. Medical College, Pune; Mahatma Gandhi Institute of Medical Sciences, Sevagram, Wardha; Jawaharlal Nehru Medical College, Aligarh; the Research Ethics Review Committee, World Health Organization; and the INCLEN Institutional Review Board through the India Clinical Epidemiology Network (IndiaCLEN, dated 18th Nov 2006).

Eligibility

Children aged 3–59 months with cough/difficulty in breathing of less than 2 weeks duration, lower chest indrawing (LCI), unresponsive to nebulisation, who did not have any of the exclusion criteria (Table 1) and whose parents gave a written informed consent for their participation were enrolled in the study by trained research staff. All included children were administered the first dose of amoxicillin, sent for chest radiology and then reassessed after radiology. Children were randomized to either treatment arms if there was no clinical deterioration or radiographic signs of consolidation, effusion or pneumothorax (using the the WHO manual for standardization of interpretation of chest radiographs for the diagnosis of pneumonia in children) [10].

Randomization

Random numbers were computer generated, by using variable length permuted blocks at the coordinating site using STATA 10 program. A separate list was generated for each site and the individual patient assignments were placed in a series of sealed opaque envelopes that were opened for serially eligible patients. The eligible study participants were randomly allocated to either the hospital group in which syrup amoxicillin (50 mg/kg/d in two divided doses) was administered in hospital for initial two days by hospital staff followed by administration at home for five days by the care-giver, or, to the home group in which the first dose of amoxicillin was administered in hospital and subsequent doses were administered by the care-giver at home for seven days.

Table 1 Exclusion Criteria

1. Known or clinically recognizable chronic conditions
2. History of > 2 weeks of cough /difficulty in breathing
3. Past history of more than 3 wheezing episodes or physician diagnosed asthma
4. LCI that responds to trial of nebulization
5. Respiratory rate (RR) >70 breaths per minute in calm child
6. Known HIV positive child or HIV status of mother known to be positive and status of child not known/defined.
7. Hospitalization for > 48 h in the last two weeks
8. Measles in the last month
9. Clinically severe malnutrition (weight for length < −3 SD or kwashiorkor) (refer to WHO growth chart)
10. Rickets
11. Central cyanosis
12. Kerosene poisoning within last 48 h
13. Oxygen saturation (pulse oximetry) <88 % on room air
14. Abnormally sleepy or difficult to wake
15. Inability to drink
16. Stridor in calm child
17. Convulsions during this illness
18. Known any antibiotic therapy for 48 h or more immediately prior to admission
19. Other diseases requiring antibiotic therapy, e.g. Meningitis, tuberculosis, dysentery, etc.
20. Persistent vomiting (>3 episodes of vomiting within 1 h)
21. Grunting
22. Known prior anaphylactic reaction to penicillin or amoxycillin
23. Severe dehydration according to WHO guidelines
24. Severe pallor
25. Suspected surgical pathology
26. Living out of the follow-up area of the study (30 kms)
27. Subject previously included in the same trial or already included in another ongoing trial anywhere
28. Presence of radiological consolidation / effusion / pneumothorax

Data collection

Clinical and demographic data was collected at baseline along with throat swab and nasopharyngeal aspirate. Both groups were followed up through home visits on day 3, 5, 8 & 14 and home group had an additional home visit at 24 h. During these follow-up home visits, data regarding outcomes were collected. This included clinical deterioration of disease any time after enrolment, change of antibiotics, hospitalization, serious adverse events considered related to amoxicillin, left against medical advice (LAMA), voluntary withdrawal of consent, or loss to follow up.

Clinical outcomes

Treatment failure was defined as presence of any one of the following conditions - clinical deterioration of disease any time after enrolment that required change of antibiotics, hospitalization (any time for the children in the home managed group or clinical decision to extend the hospitalization longer than 48 h in the hospitalized group), an occurrence of a serious adverse event related to amoxicillin, left against medical advice (LAMA), voluntary withdrawal of consent from the study, or loss to follow up. Clinical deterioration was defined as appearance of signs of very severe disease such as persistent vomiting (vomiting repeated three times within an hour due to any reason), central cyanosis, grunt, stridor, abnormal sleepiness or difficulty to wake, inability to drink, SpO2 < 85 %, convulsions, or death [6]. Antibiotics would be changed if there was clinical deterioration, developing a co-morbid condition, or, persisting fever > 98.6 °F with lower chest indrawing even after 3rd day, or, fever alone at day 5, or, lower chest indrawing alone (non responsive to three doses of nebulisation with bronchodilator) at day 5 (as reported by the mother), or, persistence of fast breathing after day 7 which is unresponsive to three doses of nebulization with bronchodilator. Rigorous training and retraining of the research physicians using standard operating procedures was used to minimize the biases that may arise due to lack of uniformity in assessing clinical signs between treatment groups and across sites. Strong quality monitoring processes were also established. An additional file describes the relevant standard operating procedures in details [see Additional file 1].

Cost outcomes

Cost data were collected for 17.2 % patients starting from before enrolment till day 14 or till the patient recovered whichever was earlier. Three distinct types of forms were used at enrolment, daily in the hospital and at each visit respectively. The cost data were also collected for those patients who left against medical advice. The forms included information about the service provider and the type of service. We disregarded fixed costs that were common for the two strategies. The protocol driven costs, such as investigations required for the study but not otherwise conducted routinely, were excluded from calculation of these costs. The variable costs i.e. direct medical, direct non-medical and indirect costs of the two treatment arms were measured using micro-costing technique [11].

Direct medical costs included costs of medical resources utilized by the patient at the out-patient and during hospital stay as calculated from the patient's perspective eg cost of medications, physician and nurses services and other paramedical services, bed cost, and the laboratory investigations.

Direct non-medical costs included the cost of travelling to the hospital for the patient and the family, cost of food to the family and patient during hospitalization and other incidental cost to the family attributed to the illness.

Indirect costs were measured by the lost wages for employed parents or guardians attending to the participant.

The median differences in costs and the predictors of total cost were analyzed as cost data was not normally distributed. The incremental cost-effectiveness of the two treatment strategies was also assessed.

Sample size

Sample size estimates were based to detect equivalence and on the hypothesis that children who were treated with oral amoxicillin at home would experience a failure rate of 15 %, and, would be within 5 % of those treated for first 48 h in hospital. The estimated sample size was 1,234 i.e. 617 per group. The sample size was calculated for the clinical trial but provided 90 % power for a two-tailed alternative hypothesis to calculate a mean difference in costs between the two interventions.

Statistical analysis

Baseline characteristics of the two treatment groups were compared using chi-square tests for categorical variables and ANOVA for continuous variables. We conducted the analysis using both intention to treat (analyzed as randomized) and per protocol analysis (included all clinical causes of treatment failure, but excluded treatment failure due to lost to follow up, LAMA, and voluntary withdrawal from the study). Cox proportional hazards models were used to estimate the relative hazards (RH) of treatment failure in the two groups up to 14 days and to explore associations between the same baseline explanatory covariates (age, feeding status, immunization, antibiotics prior to 48 h, weight for age Z scores, body temperature, respiratory rates, oxygen saturation, auscultatory wheeze, crackles, radiological infiltrates, number of rooms in the house and type of fuel used for cooking) and outcome. We used forward step wise method and identified explanatory candidate variables ($p \leq 0.1$) for inclusion in adjusted models as plausible predictors of treatment failure. The Kaplan-Meier curves for the cumulative probability of treatment success were also plotted for the two groups and the overall difference in their rates of treatment success was examined using the log-rank test. Statistical analysis was conducted using STATA 10 data analysis software.

Economic analysis

The medians of the direct medical, direct non-medical and indirect costs and their inter-quartile ranges were calculated. Group differences in median costs of the treatment strategies were assessed using the median test. Univariate analysis was conducted for the predictors of cost variation, such as data on patient demographic characteristics, clinical history, length of stay and other utilization of resources for treatment of this episode of pneumonia before entry of patients into the trial. Multivariable regression analysis (OLS, with log transformation) was also used to predict total costs across the cost categories using pre-randomization variables, the alternate treatment strategies and other covariates that relate to resource consumption. Differences were considered statistically significant if they had a two-tailed *p* value less than 0.05. The hypothesis, that home treatment is more cost-effective than hospital treatment, was also tested by comparing the cost-effectiveness ratios. The incremental cost-effectiveness was estimated as the difference in the predicted total costs in the numerator and the difference in effects i.e. the number of patients cured (1-treatment failure) or the number of cases of treatment failure avoided in the denominator.

Results

The study was conducted from October 2008 to March 2011. Of the children screened for WHO defined severe pneumonia, 1118 (16.9 %) were enrolled, 554 were assigned to home treatment, and 564 were assigned to hospital treatment, across six sites in India (Fig. 1). The number of children enrolled from different sites were 377 (33.7 %), 328 (29.3 %), 316 (28.3 %), 50 (4.5 %), 37 (3.3 %), and 10 (0.9 %) from Chandigarh, Chennai, Nagpur, Sewagram, Aligarh, and Pune respectively. The

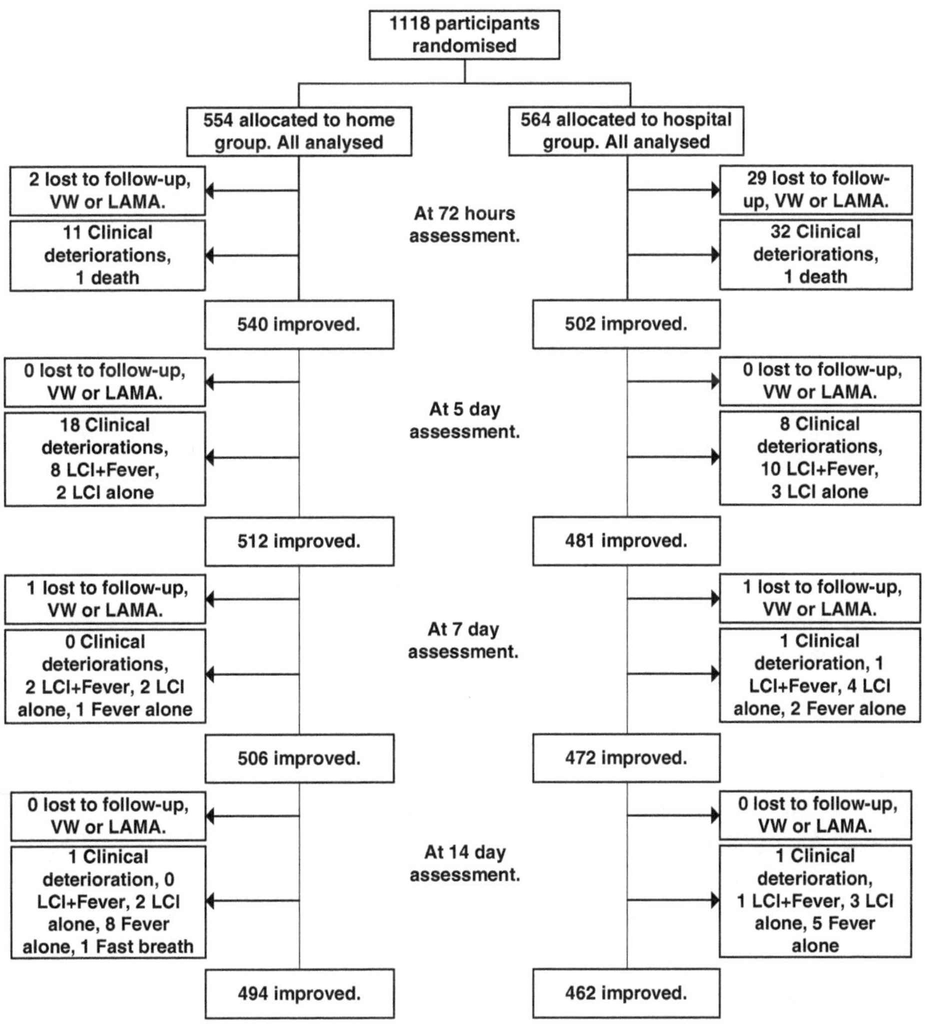

Fig. 1 Trial profile

reasons for excluding 83.1 % of screened children are shown in Table 2. The two intervention groups were not statistically different in their baseline characteristics (Table 3).

Clinical outcomes

The cumulative overall treatment failure (home + hospital) on oral amoxicillin at different time points were 6.8 % at <72 h, 11.2 % at <5 days, 12.5 % at <7 days, and 14.5 % at <14 days by intention to treat and 4 % at <72 h, 8.4 % at <5 days, 9.6 % at <7 days, and 11.5 % at <14 days respectively by per protocol analysis.

The treatment failure rate at 14 days in hospital group was 18.1 % (102/564) as compared to 10.8 % (60/554) in the home group. There were 30 (5.4 %) failures due to clinical deterioration (presence of any one of these conditions - persistent vomiting, central cyanosis, grunt, stridor, abnormally sleepy or difficult to wake, inability to drink, or convulsions) in the home group and 42 (7.4 %) in the hospital group (Fig. 1) which was not significantly different. The failures due to LAMA or voluntary withdrawal were significantly more in hospital group as compared the home group. [5.3 % (30/564) vs 0.5 % (3/554); $p < 0.001$] Kaplan Meier curves for differences between treatment successes in the home

Table 2 Study Screening and Reasons for Exclusion

	Total[#]	
	n	%[a]
Screened	6,634	
Enrolled (%)	1,118	16.9
Inclusion criteria not satisfied		
Not satisfying Age 3–59 months	462	5.1
Had no lower chest indrawing on examination	1489	16.3
Caretaker is not willing to sign informed consent form	4060	44.5
Exclusion criteria, number (%)		
Known or clinically recognizable chronic conditions	224	2.5
History of >2 weeks of cough / difficulty in breathing	195	2.1
Past history of more than 3 wheezing episodes or physician diagnosed asthma	267	2.9
LCI that responds to trial of nebulization	743	8.1
Known HIV positive child. HIV status of mother known to be positive & of child not known/defined	16	0.2
Hospitalization for > 48 h in the last two weeks	127	1.4
Measles in the last month	64	0.7
Clinically severe malnutrition (weight for length < −3 SD or kwashiorkar)	163	1.8
Rickets	21	0.2
Kerosene poisoning within last 48 h.	17	0.2
Antibiotic therapy for 48 h or more immediately prior to admission	431	4.7
Other diseases requiring antibiotic therapy, e.g. Meningitis, tuberculosis, dysentery, etc.	28	0.3
Known prior anaphylactic reaction to penicillin or amoxycillin	8	0.1
Severe dehydration according to WHO guidelines	12	0.1
Severe pallor	19	0.2
Suspected surgical pathology	12	0.1
Living out of the follow-up area of the study (30 kms)	308	3.4
Subject previously included in the same trial or already included in another ongoing trials anywhere.	44	0.5
Presence of danger sign [c] before radiology evaluation	358	3.9
Presence of danger sign after radiology evaluation	9	0.1
Presence of radiological consolidation/ effusion / pneumothorax	45	0.5
Total reasons for exclusion[b]	9122	

[a]Proportion for the presence of exclusion criteria. The denominator is total reasons for exclusion2s

[b]A child could have more than one reason for exclusions

[c]Danger signs are presence of any one clinical condition - abnormally sleepy or difficult to wake, persistent vomiting, inability to drink, grunting, stridor, central cyanosis, convulsions, RR > 70 breaths per minute, Sp02 < 88 % on room air

Table 3 Baseline Characteristics in Home and Hospitalized Children

Baseline characteristic	Home ($N = 554$)		Hospital ($N = 564$)	
	n	%	*n*	%
Sex (Female)	207	37.4	204	36.2
Infants (3–11 months old)	237	42.8	277	49.1
Children (12–23 months old)	164	29.6	138	24.5
Children (24–59 months old)	153	27.6	149	26.4
Breast feeding indicators(3-59months)				
Exclusive breast feeding	361	65.2	373	66.1
Bottle feeding	231	41.7	209	37.1
Timely complementary feeding	431	77.8	443	78.6
Immunization status up-to-date	516	93.1	510	90.4
Report of antibiotics in < 48 h prior to enrollment	56	10.1	59	10.5
Weight-for-age Z score (mean ± sd)	554	−1.5 ± 1.3	564	−1.6 ± 1.3
Weight-for-age Z score (<−2)	197	35.6	205	36.4
Length/ height (cm)(mean ± sd)	548	75.9 ± 11.7	560	74.7 ± 12.1
Temperature (°F)(mean ± sd)	554	99.5 ± 1.5	564	99.6 ± 1.5
Respiratory rate per min (mean ± sd)				
Infants	237	47.3 ± 8.9	277	48.9 ± 8.7
Children	317	43.0 ± 9.1	287	43.9 ± 9.8
Auscultatory wheeze				
Infants	140/237	59.1	176/277	63.5
Children	155/317	48.9	121/287	42.2
Crackles				
Infants	174/237	73.4	211/277	76.2
Children	243/317	76.7	228/287	79.4
Pulse oximetry (mean ± sd)				
Infants	236	96.1 ± 2.9	277	95.9 ± 3.2
Children	317	95.9 ± 3.0	286	95.8 ± 3.1
Any Infiltrates in chest x-ray	322/530	60.8	365/540	67.6
No. of rooms in house (mean ± sd)	554	2.4 ± 1.4	564	2.3 ± 1.4
Fuel used for cooking				
Low polluting fuel	220/553	39.8	249/556	44.8
High polluting fuel	333/553	60.2	307/556	55.2
Any smoker who smokes in the house	121	21.8	129	22.9

and hospital group with log rank tests for the intention to treat (ITT) analysis showed that the hospital group was significantly more likely than home children to fail treatment at any time point. (HR 1.79; 95 % C.I. 1.30, 2.46, $p < 0.01$) (Fig. 2) The per protocol analysis, though tended to show a similar trend (RR 1.32), was statistically non-significant ($p = 0.10$). The Cox Regression model showed that infants (3–11 months) and patients who had antibiotics within 48 h of enrolment had a higher likelihood of failing treatment at any point from enrolment to 14 days (per protocol and intention to treat analysis). Additionally, belonging to the hospital group and residence in homes with high polluting fuels were significantly associated with treatment failure in ITT, because children in the hospital group were more likely to fail treatment at any time than children in the home group (with LAMA accounting for the majority of these failures) (Table 4).

Two children died within the first 72 h, one in the home group, and the other in the hospital group. There were no other serious adverse events. Neither of the deaths were considered to be related to the study treatment with oral amoxicillin.

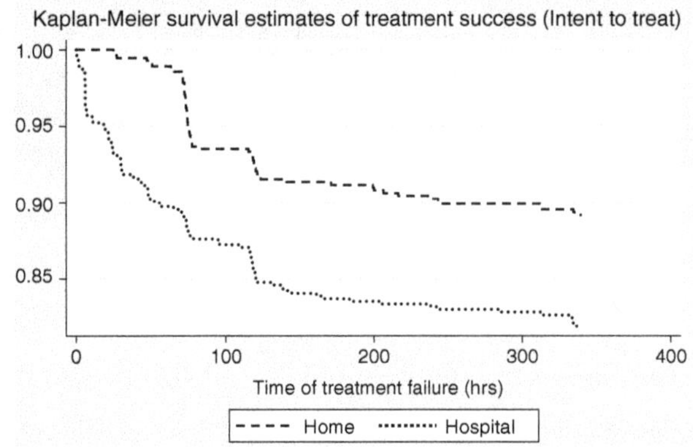

Fig. 2 Kaplan Meier Curves for treatment success rates for intention to treat analysis

Cost outcomes

The average cost of treating a child at a government hospital in India with subsidized rates was Rs. 567 when patients were hospitalized for only two days. The median total cost for treating at home was significantly less than treating at hospital for the first 48 h. (Rs 399 for home vs. Rs 602 for the hospital group, $p < 0.001$) (Table 5) The predictors of total mean costs of treatment are shown in Table 6. The patient characteristics associated with higher costs of treatment were age 3–11 months, higher temperature, lower pulse oximetry readings, and presence of auscultatory wheeze. The boot strap cost estimates of Rs.702 (95 % CI 701, 703) for the hospital group and Rs. 427 (95 % CI 427, 428) for the home group were consistent with those determined by the above regression and were significantly higher for the hospital group ($p < 0.001$). Figure 3 shows the plotting of the boot strap estimates (20,000 re-samples) on the cost effectiveness plane. It indicates that it is cheaper to be treated at home (all points are below zero in the Y co-ordinate of costs) with identical effects (all points are equally distributed on either side of zero in the X co-ordinate of effectiveness).

Discussion

Is oral Amoxicillin effective?

Our study showed that oral amoxicillin, whether administered at hospital or at home for the first 48 h was effective in treating WHO defined severe pneumonia in 93.2 % of eligible patients who were otherwise clinically stable and did not have co-morbid conditions. Although the rates of clinical deterioration were similar over the 14 day follow up, the treatment failure rate was more in the hospital group (18.1 % vs 10.8 %), due to higher rates of LAMA/voluntary withdrawal (5.3 % in hospital group vs 0.5 % in home group), one of the criteria for the

Table 4 Cox Regression Analysis for Treatment Failure Using the Per Protocol and Intention to Treat Analysis up to 14 days

Characteristic	Per-protocol analysis				Intention to treat analysis			
	Hazard ratio	95 % CI		*p*-value	Hazard ratio	95 % CI		*p*-value
Treatment group								
Home	1.00				1.00			
Hospital	1.32	0.93	1.88	0.12	1.61	1.16	2.24	0.00
Age group								
Infants (3–11 months old)	1.00				1.00			
Children (12–59 months old)	0.65	0.45	0.93	0.02	0.69	0.49	0.96	0.03
Exclusive breast feeding								
No	1.00				1.00			
Yes	1.52	0.98	2.36	0.06	1.46	0.99	2.16	0.06
Antibiotics prior to enrollment								
No	1.00				1.00			
Yes	1.79	1.06	3.02	0.03	1.72	1.07	2.76	0.02
Fuel used for cooking								
Low polluting fuel	1.00				1.00			
High polluting fuel	1.43	0.98	2.10	0.06	1.51	1.06	2.15	0.02
Study Site								
Chandigarh	1.00				1.00			
Chennai	0.18	0.09	0.33	0.00	0.41	0.26	0.64	0.00
Nagpur	0.58	0.38	0.91	0.02	0.63	0.42	0.96	0.03
Pune	2.33	0.84	6.48	0.11	2.78	1.11	6.97	0.03

Table 5 Treatment costs in different cost categories in the home and hospital group

Type of costs	Home		Hospital		*P*-value*
	n	(median ± IQR)	*n*	(median ± IQR)	
Cost of outpatient visits					
Direct Medical Cost	94	104 ± 213	97	83 ± 215	0.6
Direct Non Medical cost	94	57.5 ± 68	97	60 ± 85	0.7
Indirect Cost	86	0 ± 0	84	0 ± 0	0.5
Hospital Cost					
Direct Medical Cost	76	130 ± 36	95	166 ± 101	<0.001
Direct Non Medical cost	76	40 ± 37	95	165 ± 130	<0.001
Indirect Cost	76	0 ± 50	95	0 ± 150	0.02
Total Direct Medical Cost	94	208 ± 204	97	215 ± 236	0.09
Total Direct Non Medical cost	94	90 ± 91	97	225 ± 210	<0.001
Total Indirect Cost	94	0 ± 100	97	0 ± 150	0.1
Total Cost	94	399 ± 346	97	602 ± 524	<0.001

**P*-value of median test

composite outcome "treatment failure". This was a conservative estimate of treatment success as there is uncertainty of the clinical outcome and treatment adherence in those who leave the study prematurely. Figure 1 describes frequency of presence of various criteria for treatment failure and of true clinical deterioration. Secondly, children who are hospitalized are closely monitored by skilled research staff for presence of signs of clinical deterioration and are also likely to experience a change in antibiotic (also a criterion for treatment failure) by a treating physician. These could have potentially increased the failure rate in the hospital group. However, clinical deterioration at < 7 days was not significantly different between the groups indicating that it did not cause a potential bias in this study. Selective randomization of sicker children to the hospital was unlikely as the allocation was concealed. The high rate of LAMA in the hospital group (5.1 %) demonstrates that hospitalization is a barrier to children receiving a full course of treatment and perhaps the caregivers prefer to have their children who otherwise do not have co-morbid conditions such as those listed out in the Table 1, treated at home.

The baseline characteristics predictive of treatment failure were known risk factors such as younger age 3–11 months [12, 13], those who received antibiotics less than 48 h prior to enrollment (perhaps clinically sicker children) and use of solid fuels for household cooking, a known risk factor for poor treatment response [14–18]. Also, all other sites had lower failure rates than Chandigarh. This was mostly because of persistence of LCI at 48 h contributed mostly by children of hyperreactive airway disease. National Family Health Survey 2005–06 has reported the northern states to have higher prevalence and symptoms of acute respiratory infections [3]. Chandigarh is in the northern states of India and has colder winters than the remaining sites and reports higher incidence of hyperreactive airway disease. Also, Chandigarh site was a referral tertiary care hospital with larger patient load.

Table 6 Predictors of total mean costs for treating WHO defined severe pneumonia

Variable	β (95 % CI)	*P*-value
Treatment group (Hospital)	239.8 (102.6, 377.0)	0.00
Age group (12–59 months old)	−195.7 (−341.6, −49.9)	0.01
Antibiotics prior to enrollment	−22.7 (−297.5, 252.1)	0.87
Weight for age Z-score	−36.4 (−94.0, 21.2)	0.21
Temperature	28.1 (3.9, 52.2)	0.02
Respiratory rate per min	1.9 (−6.1, 10.0)	0.64
Pulse oximetry	−26.9 (−50.4, −3.4)	0.03
Auscultatory wheeze	204.8 (59.5, 350.1)	0.01
Any infiltrates in chest X-ray	106.8 (−37.7, 251.3)	0.15

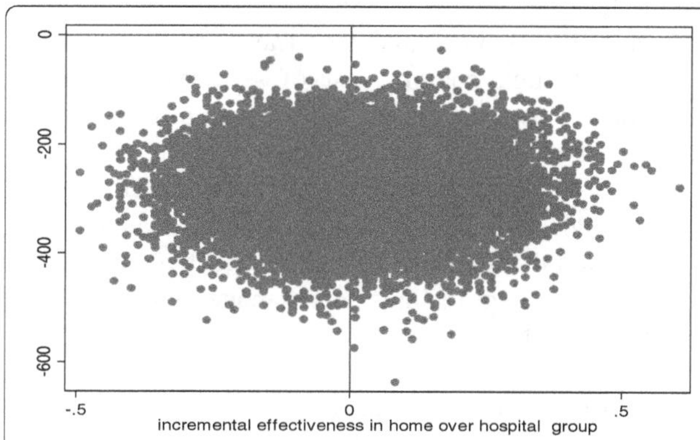

Fig. 3 20000 Bootstrap re-samples –cost-effectiveness plane

A recent systematic review has reported results of 4 trials, (2 multi-centric hospital based studies and 2 community based cluster trials) [19]. They reported non inferiority of Oral amoxicillin administered either in hospital or community for treatment of severe pneumonia as compared to standard treatment by injectable penicillin. The two community based cluster trials compared oral amoxicillin administered at home by community health workers to administration of cotrimoxazole in the community followed by standard of care of receiving parenteral therapy at hospital. The hospital based studies compared the use of oral amoxicillin for management of WHO defined severe pneumonia to either injectable penicillin or ampicillin for 48 h. None of these studies compared the use of oral amoxicillin administered for the first 48 h under hospital supervision to ambulatory management at home with oral amoxicillin. This is the only study that not only reports the overall response of severe pneumonia to oral amoxicillin whether administered at home or hospital but also provides the cost effectiveness of the treatment.

Is oral Amoxicillin cost effective?

The total cost of treating severe pneumonia in hospital for the first 48 h was significantly more than being treated at home. There were no significant differences between the two groups in costs of outpatient visits, but significantly higher costs were observed in the hospital group for the costs of hospitalization and for non-medical costs, which includes expenditure of the caregiver on travel or meal costs when taking care of the child. This was despite the fact that cost of hospitalization was perhaps an underestimate of the true costs as only variable costs were measured, and, because the costs of treatment and hospitalization are subsidized at Indian government hospitals. These results thus suggest that it will be cost efficient to manage children with WHO defined severe pneumonia at home with oral amoxicillin.

This is an important finding because WHO has recommended that children with severe pneumonia must be hospitalised which increases the cost of treatment due to daily bed charge, cost of services of medical personnel, cost of medications, monitoring, lost wages, cost of food for caretakers etc. If the treatment at home for a subgroup of severe pneumonia patients without high risk features, is as effective as treating in the hospital then it will be cost effective to recommend treatment guidelines for management of severe pneumonia at home.

Can these results be generalized?

Exclusion of children with additional risk factors such as measles, severe malnutrition, and those with radiological consolidation could apparently limit the external validity of the results. However, these were uncommon reasons for exclusion as most seriously ill children with presence of danger signs would be immediately admitted to hospital and would not undergo the screening process. Of the 6634 patients of severe pneumonia that presented to the 6 tertiary care hospitals, only 16.9 % were eligible to participate to receive oral amoxicillin. The most common reason for exclusion in this study at screening was refusal of consent to participate if the child were to be randomized to hospital group. This trend was also observed after the randomization to hospital group when a large number of children left against medical advice and were declared treatment failure by definition despite no clinical deterioration. The other reasons for exclusion were wheeze or lower chest indrawing responding to nebulization (11 %) or having received an antibiotic for longer than 48 h (4.7 %). Thus, since children with co-morbid conditions were not included in the trial these results are largely generalizable to patients with severe pneumonia who don't have co-morbidities or danger signs.

Limitations and strengths

Excluding patients with consolidation could also exclude those with bacterial pneumonia, while those children with fever, wheeze and infiltrates are more likely to be of nonbacterial causes or viral pneumonias.

Children with allergic bronchitis, asthma, bronchiolitis and viral pneumonia can also manifest with clinical signs of WHO defined severe pneumonia of cough with LCI. Excluding children whose LCI disappeared after nebulization with bronchodilators or those with a past history of wheeze or bronchodilators administration ensured that we minimize inclusion of children with allergic bronchitis or asthma. In developing countries, mixed viral and bacterial infections are not uncommon, and hence need to be treated with antibiotics. However, admitting these children as severe pneumonia will be an additional cost for the Government and for the patient's family.

The limitation in recording the cost data was that it was based partially on recall and partially on documents. It was also difficult to collect the cost data from patients who left against medical advice and those who had treatment failure. The sample size calculation was based on the clinical outcomes and not for the economic analysis. This may have influenced the validity of the cost effectiveness analysis.

Lastly, multiplicity of end points or a composite of end points of treatment failure that includes many conditions such as clinical deterioration, hospitalization, development of co-morbid conditions, changing antibiotics etc. do provide statistical efficiency but at the risk of difficulties with interpretation. Similarly, including treatment failures due to leaving against medical advice, lost to follow up or voluntary withdrawal can overestimate treatment failures and may not indicate true clinical deterioration, again causing difficulties with interpretation. Therefore, we analyzed treatment failure on intention to treat as well as per protocol basis.

Finally, this is the only trial that has evaluated the cost effectiveness and efficacy of oral amoxicillin administered at the hospital for first 48 h as compared to home administered oral amoxicillin to complete a course of 7 day treatment of WHO defined severe pneumonia in children at tertiary care hospitals as it not only reports the overall response of severe pneumonia to oral amoxicillin whether administered at home or hospital but also provides the costs of treatment and the differences in cost in the hospitalized and home group. This is an important strength of the study and will help greatly to guide policy for the case management of severe pneumonia in the developing countries.

Conclusions

The study results suggest that in selected children aged 3–59 months with chest indrawing pneumonia and without any of the study exclusion criteria, home based treatment of with oral amoxicillin is equivalent to 48 h of hospital administered oral amoxicillin followed by home based treatment. However, the results of this study should be generalized with due consideration of the fact that the selected participants had a limited spectrum of presentation which may not be true in the real life scenario.

This study also concludes that cost of treatment of severe pneumonia with oral amoxicillin in the hospital for initial 48 h followed by continuing it at home for 5 days is significantly more than the cost of treatment with oral amoxicillin at home for 7 days.

Hence, consistent with the recent WHO simplified guidelines, it will be cost effective to manage select stable children with only fast breathing and chest-indrawing or WHO defined chest indrawing pneumonia at home with oral amoxicillin.

Abbreviations

ANOVA: Analysis of variances; ITT: Intention to treat; LAMA: Left against medical advice; LCI: Lower chest indrawing; OLS: Ordinary Least Squares Regression; Rs: Rupees; WHO: World Health Organization.

Competing interests

The authors declare that they have no competing interests.

Authors' contributions

AP conceived the study and prepared the protocol; AP, AB, MS, LD, LRC, AM, SK, and all ISPOT study group members collected the data; LD developed the Manual of Operations and coordinated the staff training; AP did the statistical analysis and prepared the report; AP and AB wrote the manuscript; all the authors- AP, AB, MS, LD, LRC, AM, SK and ISPOT study group members read and approved the final version of the manuscript.

Acknowledgements

We thank the Data Safety and Monitoring Board members Dr William Macleod (chairperson), Dr Piyush Gupta, Dr Abhaya Indrayan, and Dr Varinder Singh for their oversight and guidance; the Protocol Development Committee members (see details in the Additional file 2) for reviewing the protocol and critically appraising it; Neetu Badhonia, Jitesh Borkar, and Amber Prakash for their help in the statistical analysis; and Dr Ashok K Patwari, Mr John M Pile, and Dr Avinash Ansingkar for reviewing the final report.
This study was funded with grants from MCH STAR, IndiaCLEN, and INCLEN. Amoxicillin was donated by Cipla Pharmaceuticals.
The funding source had no role in any study activities. The publication costs for this paper were funded by the Lata Medical Research Foundation, Nagpur, India.
The ISPOT Study Group Members: Archana Patel, Leena Dhande, Gopal Agrawal, Girish Charde (Indira Gandhi Government Medical College, Nagpur); Meenu Singh, Sadbhawna Pandit, Pallab Ray, Amit Agarwal (Post Graduate Institute of Medical Sciences, Chandigarh); Luke Ravi Chelliah, C. Ravichandran, Md. Meeran, Saradha Suresh (Institute of Child Health, Chennai); Akash Bang, Manish Jain, Krushna Vilhekar, Deepak Mendiratta, Vijayshree Khairkar (Mahatma Gandhi Institute of Medical Sciences, Sewagram); Ashraf Malik, Uzma Firdaus, Meher Rizvi (Jawaharlal Nehru Medical College, Aligarh); Sandhya Khadse, Chhaya Valvi (B.J. Medical College, Pune).
An additional file describes details of contributorship [See Additional file 2].

Author details

[1]Lata Medical Research Foundation and Indira Gandhi Government Medical College, Nagpur, India. [2]Mahatma Gandhi Institute of Medical Sciences, Sewagram, Maharashtra, India. [3]Post Graduate Institute of Medical Sciences, Chandigarh, India. [4]Institute of Child Health, Chennai, India. [5]Jawaharlal Nehru Medical College, Aligarh Muslim University, Aligarh, India. [6]B.J. Medical College, Pune, India.

References

1. Walker CL, Rudan I, Liu L, Nair H, Theodoratou E, Bhutta ZA, et al. Global burden of childhood pneumonia and diarrhea. Lancet. 2013;381:1405–16.
2. Rudan I, Boschi-Pinto C, Biloglav Z, Mulholland K, Campbell H. Epidemiology and etiology of childhood pneumonia. Bulletin of the World Health Organization. 2008;86:408–16.
3. International Institute for Population Sciences (IIPS) and ORC Macro. National Family Health Survey (NFHS-3), 2005–06, vol. 1. Mumbai: IIPS; 2007. p. 234–6.
4. World Health Organization: Technical bases for the WHO recommendations on the management of pneumonia in children at first-level health facilities. Geneva: World Health Organization; 1991. Available at: http://www.who.int/maternal_child_adolescent/documents/ari_91_20/en/. Accessed 17 November 2015.
5. World Health Organization: Home treatment of pneumonia safe and effective, finds study. Available at: http://www.who.int/mediacentre/news/releases/2008/pr01/en/. Accessed 17 November 2015.
6. Addo-Yobo E, Chisaka N, Hassan M, Hibberd P, Lozano JM, Jeena P, et al. Oral amoxicillin versus injectable penicillin for severe pneumonia in children aged 3 to 59 months: a randomised multicentre equivalency study. Lancet. 2004;364:1141–8.
7. Hazir T, Fox LM, Nisar YB, Fox MP, Ashraf YP, MacLeod WB, et al. Ambulatory short-course high-dose oral amoxicillin for treatment of severe pneumonia in children: a randomised equivalency trial. Lancet. 2008;371:49–56.
8. Addo-Yobo E, Anh DD, El-Sayed HF, Fox LM, Fox MP, MacLeod W, et al. Outpatient treatment of children with severe pneumonia with oral

amoxicillin in four countries: the MASS study. Trop Med Int Health. 2011;16: 995–1006.
9. Bhutta ZA, Das JK, Walker N, Rizvi A, Campbell H, Rudan I, et al. Interventions to address deaths from childhood pneumonia and diarrhoea equitably: what works and at what cost? Lancet. 2013;381:1417–29.
10. Cherian T, Mulholland EK, Carlin JB, Ostensen H, Amin R, de Campo M, et al. Standardized interpretation of paediatric chest radiographs for the diagnosis of pneumonia in epidemiological studies. Bulletin of the World Health Organization. 2005;83:353–9.
11. Luce BR, Manning WG, Seigel JE, Lipscomb L. Estimating costs in cost-effectiveness analysis. In: Gold MR, Siegel JE, Russel LB, Weinstein MC, editors. Cost-Effectiveness in Health and Medicine. New York: Oxford University Press; 1996.
12. Zhang Q, Guo Z, Bai Z, MacDonald NE. A 4 year prospective study to determine risk factors for severe community acquired pneumonia in children in southern China. Pediatr Pulmonol. 2013;48:390–7.
13. Basnet S, Adhikari RK, Gurung CK. Hypoxemia in children with pneumonia and its clinical predictors. Indian J Pediatr. 2006;73:777–81.
14. Jackson S, Mathews KH, Pulanic D, Falconer R, Rudan I, Campbell H, et al. Risk factors for severe acute lower respiratory infections in children: a systematic review and meta-analysis. Croat Med J. 2013;54:110–21.
15. Ramesh Bhat Y, Manjunath N, Sanjay D, Dhanya Y. Association of indoor air pollution with acute lower respiratory tract infections in children under 5 years of age. Paediatr Int Child Health. 2012;32:132–5.
16. Smith KR, McCracken JP, Weber MW, Hubbard A, Jenny A, Thompson LM, et al. Effect of reduction in household air pollution on childhood pneumonia in Guatemala (RESPIRE): a randomised controlled trial. Lancet. 2011;378:1717–26.
17. Mahalanabis D, Gupta S, Paul D, Gupta A, Lahiri M, Khaled MA. Risk factors for pneumonia in infants and young children and the role of solid fuel for cooking: a case–control study. Epidemiol Infect. 2002;129:65–71.
18. Hakim AK, Kharboush IF, Naguib KK, Mortada MM, Noweir KH, El Araby II. Indoor air pollution and acute lower respiratory infections in the first two years of life. J Egypt Public Health Assoc. 1995;70:661–78.
19. Das RR, Singh M. Treatment of severe community-acquired pneumonia with oral amoxicillin in under-five children in developing country: a systematic review. PLoS ONE. 2013;8, e66232.

6

Childhood asthma and physical activity: a systematic review with meta-analysis and Graphic Appraisal Tool for Epidemiology assessment

Lene Lochte[1*], Kim G. Nielsen[2], Poul Erik Petersen[1] and Thomas A. E. Platts-Mills[3]

Abstract

Background: Childhood asthma is a global problem affecting the respiratory health of children. Physical activity (PA) plays a role in the relationship between asthma and respiratory health. We hypothesized that a low level of PA would be associated with asthma in children and adolescents. The objectives of our study were to (1) summarize the evidence available on associations between PA and asthma prevalence in children and adolescents and (2) assess the role of PA in new-onset or incident asthma among children and adolescents.

Methods: We searched Medline, the Cochrane Library, and Embase and extracted data from original articles that met the inclusion criteria. Summary odds ratios (ORs) and confidence intervals (CIs) were used to express the results of the meta-analysis (forest plot). We explored heterogeneity using funnel plots and the Graphic Appraisal Tool for Epidemiology (GATE).

Results: We retrieved 1,571 titles and selected 11 articles describing three cohort and eight cross-sectional studies for inclusion. A meta-analysis of the cohort studies revealed a risk of new-onset asthma in children with low PA (OR [95 % CI] 1.32 [0.95; 1.84] [random effects] and 1.35 [1.13; 1.62] [fixed effects]). Three cross-sectional studies identified significant positive associations between childhood asthma or asthma symptoms and low PA.

Conclusions: Children and adolescents with low PA levels had an increased risk of new-onset asthma, and some had a higher risk of current asthma/or wheezing; however, there was some heterogeneity among the studies. This review reveals a critical need for future longitudinal assessments of low PA, its mechanisms, and its implications for incident asthma in children. The systematic review was prospectively registered at PROSPERO (registration number: CRD42014013761; available at: http://www.crd.york.ac.uk/PROSPERO [accessed: 24 March 2016]).

Keywords: Systematic review, Pediatric, Asthmatic disease, Exercise

Background

Asthma is one of the most common chronic pediatric diseases [1]. The prevalence of asthma in children has increased over the last thirty years in most developed countries [2, 3], although the prevalence has started to decrease in adolescents in Western countries [4, 5]. The etiology of childhood asthma is still not understood [6, 7], and the increase in prevalence has not been fully explained [8]. Physical activity (PA) is known to be associated with asthma symptoms in asthmatic children [9, 10], but its role in asthma prevention is unclear.

In Europe, PA levels have declined in children and adolescents [11]. Physical conditioning programs may reduce childhood asthma symptoms [12–14]; moreover, studies of asthmatic children have indicated that PA may induce anti-inflammatory effects [15, 16] such that brief intervals of PA alter the immune response [15]. However, whether such effects [17, 18] translate into a reduced risk of developing asthma also remains unclear.

* Correspondence: rkb664@alumni.ku.dk
[1]Department of Odontology, University of Copenhagen, Copenhagen 1014, Denmark
Full list of author information is available at the end of the article

The decline in PA may be linked to the increased prevalence and severity of childhood asthma [7, 9, 19, 20] or even to undiagnosed asthma [21]. Cross-sectional studies have shown inconsistent associations between PA and childhood asthma. In some studies, low levels of PA were related to a high asthma risk [22–24]; however, other studies did not find an association [25]. The few longitudinal studies on PA and childhood asthma have produced diverse results; in fact, one study showed that high levels of PA were related to an increase in diagnosed asthma [26].

Few authors [27] have collated the results of observational studies in this field. Therefore, our objectives were to (1) summarize the available evidence on associations between PA and asthma prevalence in children and adolescents and (2) assess the role of PA in new-onset or incident asthma in children and adolescents. We report the hypothesized associations between low PA and asthma in children and adolescents.

Methods

Design

This study was a systematic literature review that included a quantitative analysis (meta-analysis) and assessments using the Graphic Appraisal Tool for Epidemiology (GATE) [28]. We identified published studies examining the associations between PA and asthma in children and adolescents.

The protocol followed the Centre for Reviews and Dissemination (CRD) guidelines [29] for conducting systematic reviews: we (1) identified the available research and selected studies for inclusion, (2) extracted data, (3) assessed and described study quality, and (4) synthesized our findings. The reporting of our findings adhered to the Preferred Reporting Items for Systematic reviews and Meta-Analyses (PRISMA) statement [30] and, initially, to the consensus statement of the Meta-analysis Of Observational Studies in Epidemiology (MOOSE) Group [31]. Additional file 1 presents the PRISMA [32] checklist items that we examined. Additional file 2 presents the details obtained from using the Reporting Checklist of the MOOSE Group [31]. We used the GATE approach [28] to illustrate and assess the quality of the studies that did not qualify for the meta-analysis. When possible, we summarized the individual quality of these studies, assessing errors, effect sizes, and study applicability. For the meta-analysis, we used data on exposure to PA provided for asthma and control children; the outcomes were new-onset childhood asthma/or wheezing.

Ethical aspects

Since this is a systematic review based on published literature, the ethical requirements have been met previously for each individual study. Accordingly, the relevant approvals are stated in each original publication (article) included in our review. Written informed consent was obtained from the patient's guardian/parent/next of kin for the publication of each original article included in this report and any accompanying images.

Inclusion criteria for studies on PA and asthma diagnoses

We included longitudinal and cross-sectional studies that investigated asthma and PA in children and adolescents aged 0–18 years. PA was documented by either interviews or self-administered questionnaires. Childhood asthma was defined using parental reports of either physician diagnosis of asthma, "current" (within last 12 months) asthma, "ever" (lifetime) asthma, wheezing, exercise-induced asthma (EIA), or medical treatment of asthma symptoms. We defined new-onset asthma (incident asthma) as a physician diagnosis of asthma/or wheezing. Hence, for incident asthma, there was no sampling based on disease status [33]. We used asthma/or wheezing (a representative asthma symptom) [34] to capture the heterogeneous symptomatology of asthma in children [35].

We defined PA as a behavioral concept that varied according to "leisure time" or "sports and exercise" [36]. We recognized that PA can be further characterized by its dimensions as follows: (1) frequency, (2) intensity, (3) duration, and (4) type [37]. Intensity has been identified as the key dimension for possible dose-response relationships with either reduced or increased health risks for exercise-induced medical conditions [38]. This review did not distinguish between PA and exercise. The concept "PA" referred to general leisure-time PA, exercise, or sports during or outside of school hours [39]. High amounts of TV viewing (duration in hours) represented sedentary behavior [40, 41] and were used as a proxy for low PA. This approach was based on the previous use of TV viewing [24, 42] which validated that TV viewing could be used to represent PA in population surveys. It was beyond the scope of this review to discuss the scientific distinctions between sedentary activity and physical inactivity in children and adolescents.

Inclusion criteria for the meta-analysis

We adhered to appropriate standards [29] in defining our criteria for the meta-analysis, which were as follows: (1) broadly similar research questions, (2) comparable participant populations (children and adolescents), and (3) broadly similar research mechanisms.

Exclusion criteria

We excluded studies involving adults >18 years of age and non-English-language studies [43]. We also excluded single outcomes of intermediate phenotypes for childhood asthma (i.e., bronchial hyperresponsiveness [BHR], allergic rhinoconjunctivitis, atopic dermatitis, airway inflammation, eczema) and cumulative incidence along with studies that had fitness or body composition as their only outcomes. Studies that reported on only PA or asthma were excluded, as were clinical investigations (e.g., randomized controlled trial [RCT] designs) of training and/or medical treatment in children with asthma. If pediatric asthma or PA was explored using noncomparable (rare) methodologies or the studies excluded relevant participants, the studies were excluded. We excluded other reviews, methodology reports, validation studies, and studies that collected data for other purposes or had other non-applicable outcomes. The two stages of exclusion are illustrated in Fig. 1, and the articles excluded at each stage are grouped by exclusion rationale in Additional file 3A and B.

Search strategy

Identifying studies and study selection

We searched the following databases: Medline, National Library of Medicine (1946 to the last search date: 7 Jan 2014), the Cochrane Library (all Cochrane products to the last search date: 13 Jan 2014), and Embase/Excerpta Medica (2013 to the last search date: 17 Jan 2014). We used medical subject headings (MeSH) for asthma/or wheezing and PA. In Medline, "physical activity" was not available as a MeSH heading, and therefore we included the MeSH headings "physical fitness", "exercise", and "physical exertion"; we also restricted the search to English language, humans, and age 0–18 years. Table 1 illustrates the full electronic search strategy used in Medline. Initially, to expand the search, we conducted exploratory text, title, and adjacent word searches. Because we obtained large numbers of unrelated titles, these searches were subsequently omitted. One medical subject librarian (CFB) reviewed our search strategies for the Cochrane and Medline databases to ensure that the variation in search terms across the databases was taken into account. We read review articles and identified additional studies from the reference lists of retrieved full-text articles.

Table 1 Full Electronic Search Strategy for Medline

Action	Term
1	[a]asthma
2	[a]bronchial hyperreactivity
3	[a]bronchoconstriction
4	[a]respiratory hypersensitivity
5	[a]respiratory sounds
6	[a]dyspnea
7	[a]asthma, exercise-induced
8	[a]respiratory function tests
9	[a]exercise test
10	1 or 2 or 3 or 4 or 5 or 6 or 7 or 8 or 9
11	[a]physical fitness
12	[a]exercise
13	[a]physical exertion
14	11 or 12 or 13
15	10 and 14
16	Limit 15 to English language
17	Limit 16 to humans
18	Limit 17 to "all child (0 to 18 years)"

[a]Indicates a focused search using medical subject heading (MeSH) terms. "Or" was used to combine related search terms. "And" was used to combine two sets of terms for asthma and physical activity

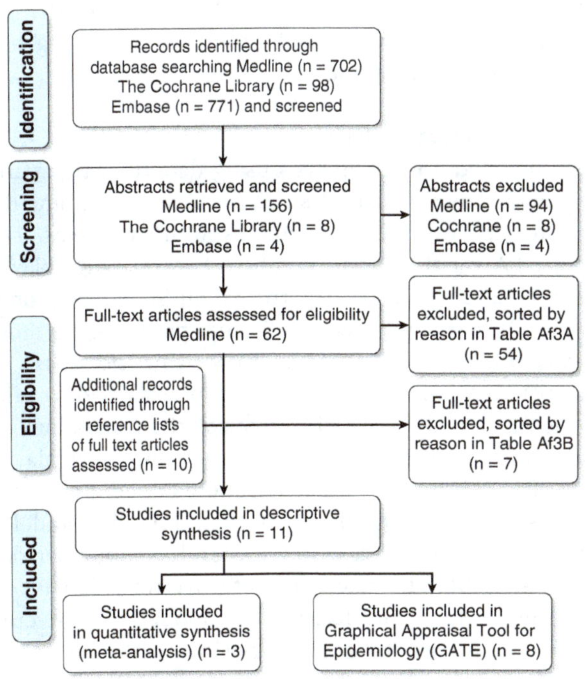

Fig. 1 Inclusion and Exclusion Criteria for Systematic Reviews. Numbers of search results from Medline, the Cochrane Library, and Embase

LL searched and screened studies by title and abstract for eligibility. Two medical students declined to be independent reviewers, and LL identified the articles for inclusion. When necessary, assessment was performed by the lead investigator (PEP). Figure 1 presents a flow diagram illustrating the studies identified by the database searches.

Data extraction and study quality

LL extracted information from the included studies. Table 2 shows the information points that were extracted from each study for the descriptive data synthesis. The extracted items represented adopted standards for methods, participants, outcomes, and results as defined in the checklist of The Cochrane Handbook for Systematic Review [44]. For the quantitative data synthesis (the meta-analysis), we extracted individual summary data [29] from each study that

Table 2 Data Extracted from Individual Studies in the Systematic Review

Data
Name of first author
Year of publication
Study design
Age (years) of study population: Mean (±2 SD) or range
Definition of physical activity
Definition of asthma
Number of children with asthma and total study population size
Main effect size and confidence interval
Adjustment covariates
Key conclusions of the study authors

met the criteria for meta-analysis. We excluded BHR as an asthma phenotype and consequently were only able to obtain asthma severity data from a few of the reviewed studies [22, 24, 45].

Using GATE [28] entailed documenting the study population, representativeness, measurement(s), and timing. All data that were extracted to electronic GATE forms [46] are illustrated in Additional file 4.

Statistical methods

The studies we examined followed different protocols, and therefore, we explored the clinical and methodological sources of their heterogeneity by reviewing the descriptive study characteristics that we extracted (Table 2). For the meta-analysis, we reported both random- and fixed-effects models (using inverse variance [29]) to illustrate the respective inter- and intra-study variability [47]. Technically, we produced 2 × 2 tables; i.e., we entered the numbers of children who developed asthma in the exposed (low PA) and unexposed (high PA) groups [48]. This approach produced summary statistics for each individual study and an overall estimate, both of which were expressed as odds ratios (ORs) and 95 % confidence intervals (CIs). Forest plots were used to illustrate these summary statistics and the variation (heterogeneity) across the studies. We expressed the percentages of variability in the effect estimates that were attributable to between-study variation (heterogeneity) rather than chance using I-squared (I^2), and the statistical assessment was performed using the chi-squared (χ^2) test [29, 47]. We assessed the risk of publication bias or selective outcome reporting [30] across studies by estimating the standard errors (SEs) of the logarithmic (log) scale ORs (logORs), and we depicted these graphically on the horizontal (logORs) and vertical (SEs) axes of a funnel plot. In addition, we assessed the funnel plot for asymmetry [49]. We used STATA™ version 12 (StataCorp, College Station, TX, US) [50] for the calculations and *P* set at 5 %.

Results

Identified studies

The searches yielded a total of 1,571 titles, and 11 studies that examined PA and childhood asthma met the inclusion criteria. Initially, we removed duplicates and contacted the authors of two articles to clarify details regarding the original data. Both authors responded, and we obtained the full texts of 62 studies. Of the 11 studies that met the inclusion criteria, three were cohort studies [45, 51, 52], and eight were cross-sectional studies [9, 22–25, 53–55]. We excluded 54 studies followed by seven additional studies at two different stages (Fig. 1). Tables 3 and 4 present the data extracted from each study sorted by study design. Below follow reports on the cohort studies (including meta-analysis) and the cross-sectional studies given in separate sections.

Cohort studies

Measurements of new-onset (incident) asthma/or wheezing

Two studies [45, 51] described cases of new-onset asthma using a physician's diagnosis of asthma (Table 3), and one study described new-onset wheezing [52]. We synthesized three cohort studies [45, 51, 52] that met the criteria for inclusion in our meta-analysis. The follow-up times (in years) were 6–7 [52], 10 [51], and 11.5 [45] (Table 3). In these studies [45, 51, 52], a total of 549 children had new-onset asthma/or wheezing, and the total number of cohort children studied was 6,037 (Table 3). The reported asthma prevalence was 6.0 % [45], the new-onset wheezing prevalence was 11.3 % [52], and the asthma incidence rate was 16.6 % per 1,000 person-years [51]. Overall, 57.7 % (317) of the cohort children with new-onset asthma/or wheezing had low PA [45, 51, 52] (Table 5).

Results from meta-analysis

We conducted a meta-analysis using data on asthma and PA provided by three articles [45, 51, 52]. To combine the study results, we reclassified the exposure variables. The original PA variables were number of team sports played (none, 1–2, >2) [51], sports participation frequency (≤once per month, ≤once per week, 2–3 times per week, >3 times per week) [52], and duration of TV viewing (not at all, <1 hour per day, 1–2 hours per day, >2 hours per day) [45]; for the meta-analysis, we dichotomized the results into no team sports played (low PA) and ≥1 team sport played (high PA) [51], sports participation ≤ once per week (low PA) and ≥2 times per week (high PA) [52], and TV viewing ≥1 hour per day (low PA) and <1 hour per day (high PA) [45]. The reference category was high PA in both the random- and fixed-effects models. The overall meta-analysis results showed positive risks for new-onset asthma (OR [95 % CI] 1.32 [0.95; 1.84] [random effects] and 1.35 [1.13; 1.62] [fixed effects]) in children with low PA compared with high PA (reference). These

Table 3 Cohort or Longitudinal Studies Included in the Systematic Review by Selected Study Information

Author	Year	Study design	Age[a] (years)	Definition		Number		Main effect size Adj OR/HR/GMR/mean	Adj covariates	Key conclusions reported by the study authors
				Physical activity	*Asthma*	*Asthma*	*Total*			
Vogelberg	2007	Cohort follow-up 6–7 years	16–18	Sports freq (questionnaire)	Physician diagnosed (wz)	329[wz,b]	2,858[b]	Risk (OR [95 % CI]) of incident wz by sports >3 times per wk vs ≤ once per month (rfgr): 0.8 (0.5–1.3)	Active and passive smoking, BMI, SES, gender	Inverse associations between wz and sport or PC
Sherriff	2009	Cohort follow-up 11.5 years	11.5	TV viewing (questionnaire)	Physician diagnosed	78[b]	1,599[b]	Associations (OR [95 % CI]) of asthma at age 11.5 years with TV viewing at age 3.5 years (>2 hrs/day) vs 1–2 hrs/day (rfgr): 1.8 (1.2–2.6) (P trend = 0.0003)	BMI, maternal asthma/ allergies and smoking, social variables	Longer duration of TV viewing associated with development of asthma in later childhood
Islam	2009	Cohort follow-up 10 years	7–11+	Team sports (questionnaire)	Physician diagnosed	142[b]	1,580[b]	Associations (HR [95 % CI]) of GSTP1[c] genotypes with new-onset asthma by > two team sports vs none (rfgr): 2.66 (1.2–5.9) (P < 0.05) [c]Subclass of GST	Ethnicity, community of residence, genetic information (GSTM1[c] and SNP1/SNP3) [c]Subclass of GST	Children with Val[105] variant allele may be protected against increased risk of asthma by exercise

Adj Adjusted or adjustment, *BMI* Body mass index, *CI* Confidence interval, *Freq* Frequency, *GST* Glutathione S-transferase, *Hr/hrs* Hour/hours, *HR* Hazard ratio, *OR* Odds ratio, *Rfgr* Reference group, *SD* Standard deviation, *SES* Socio-economic status, *SNP* Single nucleotide polymorphism, *Vs* Versus, *Wk* Week, *Wz* Wheezing
[a]Age: Mean (±2 SD) or range
[b]Those who contributed data on asthma/wheezing and physical activity to the meta-analysis
[c]Subclass of GST

results are illustrated in Fig. 2 (random effects) and Fig. 3 (fixed effects). I^2 was 60.6 % ($\chi^2 = 5.08$, $P = 0.079$) for both random and fixed effects.

Consistency of meta-analysis results: risk of bias across studies

In Fig. 4, the studies that included larger numbers of asthmatic participants [51, 52] were positioned toward the top, i.e., the upper two-thirds of the funnel, representing large sample sizes and small standard errors. Figure 4 also shows that the studies in the meta-analysis [45, 51, 52] were within the 95 % confidence limits (diagonal, dashed lines) around the summary estimate.

Validity and quality: risk of bias within studies

Our review showed that these three studies [45, 51, 52] explored the role of the temporal sequence following quantified PA exposure and its effect on new-onset asthma/or wheezing in children and adolescents.

Cross-sectional studies

Measurements of current or ever (prevalent) asthma/or wheezing

As shown in Table 4, two studies [22, 53] defined current asthma using questionnaires and a medical provider or physician diagnosis of asthma, whereas a majority [9, 23–25, 54, 55] used the International Study of Asthma and Allergies in Childhood (ISAAC) definitions.

Validity and quality: risk of bias within studies

We applied the GATE approach developed for the critical appraisal of quantitative studies (electronic forms) [28, 46]. When data were available, we first extracted study numbers regarding exposure, comparison, and outcomes for the association between PA and childhood asthma (Additional file 4). We first used the GATE calculator (one-page Microsoft Excel format) and then transferred the calculated results to the GATE-lite form (one-page Microsoft Word format) [46]. We used GATE to illustrate individual study designs and study details as recommended for gauging bias risks [56].

We illustrated the study design using the acronym PECOT, i.e., extracted data on **p**articipants, **e**xposure, **c**omparisons, **o**utcomes, and **t**ime. To assess study validity, we used the acronym RAMBOMAN, i.e., extracted data on **r**ecruitment, **a**llocation, **m**aintenance, **b**lind or **o**bjective **m**easurements, and **an**alyses.

We applied the GATE approach to a total of eight non-meta-analyzed cross-sectional studies [9, 22–25, 53–55] that investigated asthma prevalence or asthma symptoms. The studies included a total of 4,155 children with current asthma/or wheezing, and the total number of participants was 41,770 children (Table 4 and Additional file 4). Unfortunately, in one study [23], the absolute number of participants was not given. The prevalence of asthma/or wheezing in six of these studies

Table 4 Cross-Sectional Studies Included in the Systematic Review by Selected Study Information

Author	Year	Study design	Age* (years)	Definition		Number		Main effect size Adj OR	Adj covariates	Key conclusions reported by the study authors
				Physical activity	*Asthma*	*Asthma*	*Total*			
Nystad	1997	Cross-sectional	7–16 Area I–III	HBSC (WHO), two questions (hrs/wk and freq/wk)	ISAAC questionnaire and question on current asthma from reference	222 Area I: 123 II: 69 III: 30	4,021 Area I: 2,188 II: 1,045 III: 788	Association (OR [95%CI]) between current asthma and PA 1–3 hrs/wk vs ≤0.5 hr/wk (rfgr): 1.0 (0.6–1.5)	Age, gender, study area	Asthmatic children as physically active as peers
Nystad	2001	Cross-sectional	7–16	HBSC (WHO), two questions (hrs/wk and freq/wk); only hrs reported in article	ISAAC questionnaire plus question about current asthma (from ATS-MRC)	116[wz]	2,112	Associations (OR [95%CI]) wz or whistling (all children) and PA≤1 hr/wk: 1.9 (0.9–3.8)2–3 hrs/wk: 2.6 (1.3–5.2)≥4 hrs/wk: 2.5 (1.2–4.9)vs none (rfgr) "No clear dose-response relationship, but the effect was mainly among active vs inactive children"	Age, atopy (eczema and/or hay fever), current asthma, gender	Positive associations between PA and wz
Lang	2004	Cross-sectional	6–12	Questionnaire 1) total mins active in one (1) day; 2) number of days active in typical wk	Questionnaire. Medical provider ever-diagnosed asthma and some asthma symptoms in last 12 months	137	243	Association (OR [95%CI]) between mod/severe persistent asthma and PA <30 mins/day (inactivity) vs all other PA-groups (rfgr): 3.00 (1.19–7.52) (*P*<0.05)	Gender, health beliefs (e.g., child can do as much PA as children similar age without asthma or child upset with strenuous activity)	Disease severity and parental health beliefs contributed to lower activity levels of children with asthma
Jones	2006	Cross-sectional	9–12th grade	PA-levels (questionnaire)	Questionnaire. Physician-diagnosed asthma denoted lifetime asthma with/without current asthma last 12 months	1,943	13,553	Association (OR [95%CI]) between asthma status and sufficient mod PA: 1.1 (0.9–1.3)	Grade, race/ethnicity, gender	No differences in participation in vig or mod PA among students with and without current asthma
Priftis	2007	Cross-sectional	10–12	PA questionnaire (PANACEA)	ISAAC questionnaire. Asthma symptoms, e.g., ever asthma or ever wz	166[Symptoms]	700	Associations (OR [95%CI]) for asthma symptoms in boys; girls not participating in any PA vs no participation last wk (rfgr): 2.17 (1.34–3.54) (*P*<0.05); 1.63 (0.86–3.11)	Body weight (per 5 kg), time of watching TV or playing video games per day (per 1 hr)	PA associated with reduced odds of reporting asthma symptoms
Corbo	2008	Cross-sectional	6–7	PA levels in regular sports (i.e., formal games or other aerobic exercise) (questionnaire)	ISAAC questionnaire. Defined current asthma	1,343	20,016	Association (OR [95%CI]) between current asthma and low freq of regular sports (1–2 times per wk) vs none (rfgr): 1.13 (0.93–1.38) (*P* trend = 0.069)	Age, BMI, dietary variables, family asthma or rhinitis, mold, parental education and smoking, person filling questionnaire, regular sports, season, gender, study center, TV viewing	Wz or asthma not associated with regular sports activity
Kosti	2012	Cross-sectional	10–12	PA questionnaire (PANACEA)	ISAAC questionnaire. Asthma symptoms, e.g., ever asthma or ever wz	228	1,125	Association (OR [95%CI]) between leisure-time PA and asthma symptoms: 0.90 (0.79–1.03) (Ns)	Age, BMI, KIDMORE score, gender, urban/rural	Inverse relationship between asthma symptoms and leisure PA (rural)

Table 4 Cross-Sectional Studies Included in the Systematic Review by Selected Study Information *(Continued)*

Mitchell	2013	Cross-sectional	6–7 and 13–14	Weekly vig PA (freq) (questionnaire)	ISAAC questionnaire, i.e., ever asthma	Data not given	76,164(6–7 years)201,370 (13–14 years)	Associations (OR [95%CI]) between reported asthma ever and PA once or twice per wk vs vig PA never or occasionally each wk (rfgr): 0.96 (0.89–1.04) (6–7 years) 1.14 (1.08–1.20) (13–14 years)	BMI, income, language, region, gender, TV viewing	Vig PA positively associated with symptoms of asthma in adolescents but not in children

Adj Adjusted or adjustment, *Age: Range, *ATS-MRC* American Thoracic Society and Medical Research Council, *BMI* Body mass index, *CI* Confidence interval, *Freq* Frequency, *Hr/hrs* Hour/hours, *HBSC* Health Behaviour in School-aged Children, *ISAAC* International Study of Asthma and Allergies in Childhood (ever asthma and wz last 12 months) [2], *KIDMORE index* Mediterranean Diet Quality Index for children and adolescents (total scores and categories described in article), *Min/s* Minute/s, *Mod* Moderate, *Ns* Non-significant, *OR* Odds ratio, *PA* Physical activity, *PANACEA* The Physical Activity, Nutrition and Allergies in Children Examined in Athens Study, *Rfgr* Reference group, *Vig* Vigorous, *Vs* Versus, *Wk* Week, *Wz* Wheezing

Table 5 Distribution (N, %) of Children with New-Onset Asthma/or Wheezing and All Children According to PA

First author, publication year	PA-exposure levels	New-onset asthma outcome	New-onset asthma, N (%)	All children N (%)
Vogelberg et al., 2007 [52]	*Low PA if sport freq ≤ once/wk* High PA (rfgr) if sport freq ≥ two times/wk	Wheezing	*Low PA: 199 (60.5)* High PA: 130 (39.5)	*Low PA: 1,470 (51.4)* High PA: 1,388 (48.6)
Sherriff et al., 2009 [45]	*Low PA if TV viewing ≥1 hr/day* High PA (rfgr) if TV viewing = none or <1 hr/day	Asthma	*Low PA: 61 (78.2)* High PA: 17 (21.8)	*Low PA: 1,100 (68.8)* High PA: 499 (31.2)
Islam et al., 2009 [51]	*Low PA if number of team sports = none* High PA (rfgr) if number of team sports ≥1	Asthma	*Low PA: 57 (40.1)* High PA: 85 (59.9)	*Low PA: 648 (41.0)* High PA: 932 (59.0)

Details regarding data from the meta-analyzed studies
Freq Frequency, *Hr/hrs* Hour/hours, *N* Number, *PA* Physical activity, *Rfgr* Reference group, *Wk* Week

[9, 24, 25, 53–55] ranged from 3.8 % [55] to 23.7 % [24] (Table 4). Five cross-sectional studies originated from Europe [9, 24, 25, 54, 55], and two were from North America [22, 53]. One study was cross-national [23] and included data for 6–7-year-olds from 17 countries and data for 13–14-year-olds from 35 countries (Additional file 4). A majority of the eligible populations were derived from respective national surveys [9, 24, 25, 53–55] of children and adolescents (Additional file 4).

The GATE assessment showed that all eight studies [9, 22–25, 53–55] included measures of exposure and outcome and included a comparison group, and all authors reported the results of adjusted analyses; however, for six studies [22–25, 53, 54], we were unable to obtain data on either the exposure or the comparison groups (Additional file 4). The response rates were >50 % in seven [9, 23–25, 53–55] of the eight studies, although Mitchell et al. [23] observed a response rate <50 % for younger children (6–7 years of age) (Additional file 4). Two cross-sectional studies [22, 53] analyzed PA as an outcome.

The definitions of PA varied. Nystad [55] and Nystad et al. [9] measured PA outside of school hours (sports or exercise) that caused a child to become sweaty or out of breath. Lang et al. [22] registered the total minutes spent engaging in PA in one day, Jones at al. [53] assessed sufficient moderate PA (e.g., fast walking, slow bicycling), and Priftis et al. [24] examined sports-related PA (e.g., brisk walking, running, swimming). Corbo et al. [25] registered PA as regular sports, i.e., formal games or forms of aerobic exercise. Kosti et al. [54] observed leisure-time PA, i.e., unstructured outdoor PA involving play, walking, or cycling. Mitchell et al. [23] described PA as weekly vigorous activity that was sufficient to cause heavy breathing in the child.

Additionally, the definition of low PA varied, with some studies defining low PA as ≤1 hour per week [9], <30 min per day [22], once or twice per week [23], no participation in any PA [24], sports 1–2 times per week [25], sufficient moderate PA [53], leisure-time PA [54], and 1–3 h per week [55]. In four [9, 24, 25, 55], one [23], and one [54] of the eight [9, 22–25, 53–55] cross-sectional studies, the reference groups in the adjusted analyses were "low to no PA", "no vigorous PA", or "no leisure time", respectively (Additional file 4).

In four of the eight studies [9, 22, 53, 55], we were able to extract data for the GATE calculator to estimate occurrences in exposure groups and/or exposure effects. In the studies that investigated distinct low PA (≤1 h per week [9], 1–3 h per week [55], <30 min per day [22]), the occurrences per 100 persons in the exposure groups (EGO) were 6.2 [9], 4.1 [55], and 14.6 [22]. Two [9, 55] of these studies provided sufficient data to estimate exposure

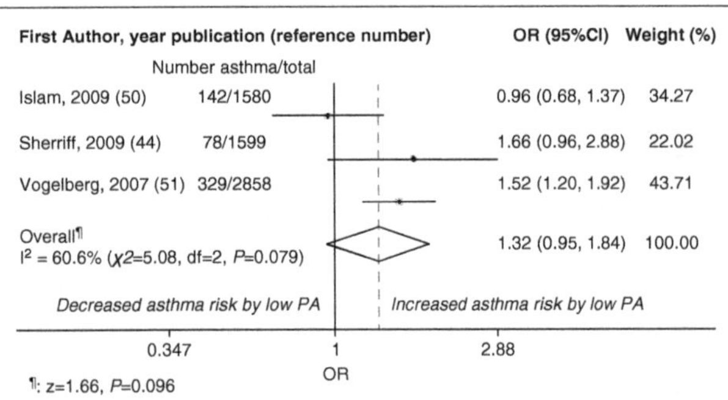

Fig. 2 Random-Effects Model: Study-Specific and Overall Odds Ratios (ORs) with 95 % Confidence Intervals (CIs). Data are derived from the meta-analysis of low physical activity (PA) and new-onset asthma during childhood. High PA: Reference category

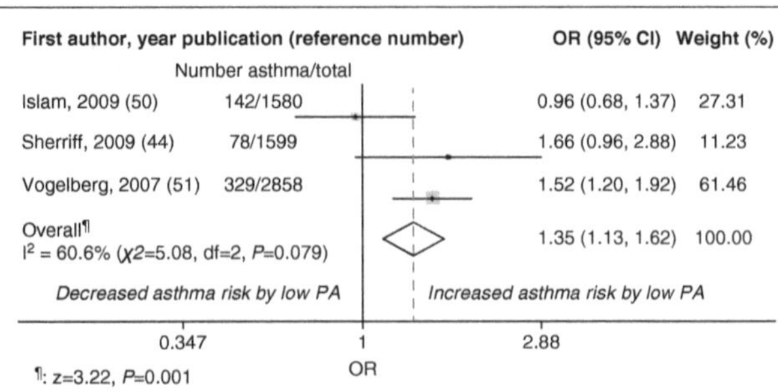

Fig. 3 Fixed-Effects Model: Study-Specific and Overall Odds Ratios (ORs) with 95 % Confidence Intervals (CIs). Data are from the meta-analysis of low physical activity (PA) and new-onset asthma during childhood. High PA: Reference category

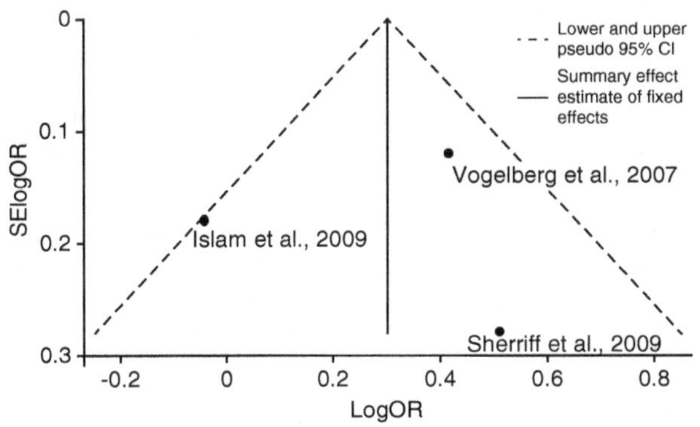

Fig. 4 Funnel Plot with 95 % Pseudo Confidence Intervals (CIs). Data are from the meta-analysis depicting the log-scale odds ratios (logORs) (horizontal axis) for new-onset childhood asthma by low physical activity (PA) using individual study effect size data plotted against the standard errors (SEs) (vertical axis) of the logORs

effects in terms of relative risk (RR) (Additional file 4). In the remaining four studies [23–25, 54], we could not derive appropriate data for the calculations.

Although we found each of the eight cross-sectional studies [9, 22–25, 53–55] applicable to practice (Additional file 4), the GATE analysis illustrated variations across the studies. We concluded that the quality of these studies was high for cross-sectional designs, but the variation among the studies confirmed that individual study analysis (e.g., GATE assessment) as opposed to common estimation across studies (e.g., meta-analysis) was a sound approach that agreed with recommendations [29, 49, 57].

All studies - measurements PA

In all but one study, PA was assessed using a questionnaire that asked about sports participation (Tables 3 and 4). One cohort study [45] reported TV viewing (Table 3).

Main effect size and adjustment covariates

Tables 3 and 4 show that six studies reported positive associations between asthma/or wheezing and low PA [9, 22, 24, 25, 45, 53], and one study showed that asthma/or wheezing was positively associated with high PA [51]. Of the eight cross-sectional studies [9, 22–25, 53–55], three [22–24] indicated significant positive associations between childhood asthma or asthma symptoms and low PA (of which one [23] reported this association for 13- to 14-year-olds only and one [24] reported this association for boys only).

The adjustment covariates applied in the multivariate analyses varied across the reviewed studies. All authors adjusted for age, gender, weight, and/or smoking measures (Tables 3 and 4), three studies included adjustments for asthma history [9, 25, 45], and eight studies adjusted for socioeconomic measures [23, 25, 45, 51–55].

Summarizing meta-analysis and GATE review

In each section, we first reported the descriptive data syntheses and then the analytical data syntheses based on quantitative (meta-analysis) and qualitative (GATE) approach. Meta-analysis was applied to three cohort studies while the GATE assessment was used to assess eight cross-sectional study designs.

Children and adolescents with low PA had increased risk of new-onset asthma, and some showed a higher risk of current asthma/or wheezing, but we found variations among the studies.

Discussion

The cohort studies showed that the overall risks of new-onset asthma/or wheezing increased up to 35 % in children with low PA, and three cross-sectional studies showed significant positive associations with low PA. Of the 11 studies we reviewed, more than 50 % suggested positive associations between childhood asthma and low PA. The critical problem was variation across the reviewed studies. We therefore applied appropriate epidemiological methods when performing meta-analysis of similar studies and when graphically assessing those that were dissimilar.

This systematic review followed established guidelines [29]. The review included >500 cases of new-onset (incident) asthma/or wheezing and approximately 4,000 current (prevalent) asthma cases. Although the number of studies was moderate, the inclusion of a variety of study designs may be advantageous. Previous investigations have produced contradictory results for the association under study, and the cross-sectional study design has limitations with respect to ruling out the directions of associations; therefore, we sought to identify studies with a longitudinal design. The longitudinal design of cohort studies overcomes the limitations of the cross-sectional design because measures of cause and effect are separated in time. Reverse causation (i.e., the notion that asthma causes low PA) was accounted for by the cohort studies [45, 51, 52]. For example, one study [45] included only asymptomatic children. Hence, we were able to derive some assessment of the directions of the associations. Other authors [58, 59] have proposed hypotheses fairly similar to ours; this review could confirm significant positive associations described by three [22–24] cross-sectional and two longitudinal [45, 52] studies.

The intensity of leisure-time activity studied by Vogelberg et al. [52] was similar to that of organized team sports studied by Islam et al. [51]. Although leisure-time activity differs from organized sports [37], they both fall along a spectrum of aerobic activities. The leisure activities included, e.g., running, bicycling, and swimming [52, 60], and the team sports encompassed a range of intensity from low to high [51, 61]. Thus, we could not identify systematic deviations in the PA definitions of these two studies [51, 52].

Generally, the quality of the reviewed studies was high. Although GATE does not provide one single quantitative assessment score [62], the observational studies appeared to reflect good standards for internal validity. We excluded ecological studies in an effort to retrieve studies with a rigorous design [63]. Although the clinical application of reviews is often overlooked [47], our results appear to align with those of others who have acknowledged the clinical importance of observational studies [64].

Recent systematic reviews have investigated the prevalence of wheezing in children [65] or PA in adolescents [66], but few have reviewed both. The asthma diagnosis was critical for our results. Asthma is a heterogeneous clinical syndrome [67], and because the diagnosis of asthma in children lacks a gold standard, it is ideally verified by uniform guidelines [68]. The asthma definitions in the current review were relatively uniform. Seven of the eleven studies used physician-confirmed asthma diagnoses, and our review populations were homogeneous (Europe and North America). Earlier reviews [65] that had to rely on less rigorous asthma symptom reports lack these characteristics.

All reviewed studies performed PA quantification. The cross-national survey, for example, used the ISAAC questionnaire [23] and showed a significant association between asthma and low PA in adolescents but not in children. Data on activity in young children are often difficult for parents to report, and in fact, some of the cross-sectional studies included 6-year-olds. The younger children in these studies received parental assistance with the questionnaire, and thus we cannot rule out information bias. Recent evidence has certainly suggested that parents and peers influence PA in both healthy [69–71] and asthmatic [72] children. Although we recognize that accelerometry still requires technical improvements for optimal use in the youngest children [71, 73, 74], the reported findings appear to align with earlier objective measurements that employed accelerometry [59].

The strength of the effect sizes varied, and the smaller studies [22, 24] yielded larger effect sizes, as expected. Moreover, low PA varied; for example, Lang et al. [22] analyzed daily PA durations as low as 30 min. Analogously, Nystad et al. [9] quantified "very low" PA (<1 h/week). Lang et al. [22] measured PA during the school day, whereas Nystad et al. [9] studied PA outside of school hours. This diurnal variation in PA could be of importance to the results because energy expended during seated school-day activities varies from that expended during leisure PA [75]. The reporting of PA also varied and included duration and frequency. Although protective associations between PA and current asthma were non-significant, Nystad [55] suggested that these associations could be a factor when PA frequency is analyzed. Therefore, although PA frequency and duration show correlations in children [76], it may be relevant to report both.

Our review may have certain limitations. Formal meta-analysis of the cross-sectional studies was not reasonable given that the overestimation of effects is well documented [57]. Although GATE is only one of a number of existing quality appraisal tools [62], we acknowledge that it provided some systematization to our assessments.

Limitations of the calculations were also made evident when individual patient data were not provided in the articles. We lacked some data on the exposed and non-exposed groups described in the cross-sectional studies. Although statistical methodology exists for imputing data [47], no such technique was used in the current analyses. Our meta-analysis was a two-stage process [48]. The first results produced were the summary statistics of each individual study that was included. These results agreed with the conclusions of each study. Because the meta-analysis inclusion criteria were met, we then combined the statistics. We have discussed the variation in the exposures (PA) and outcomes (asthma/or wheezing) of the meta-analyzed studies [45, 51, 52], but the basic cohort methodologies also appeared to be rather similar.

The meta-analysis revealed increased risks of new-onset asthma among children who reported low PA. The funnel plot showed that these three studies lay within the confidence intervals; this illustration may favor limited heterogeneity. Although we must expect some inter-study variability, the random-effects model could have assigned disproportionate influence to the studies with the smallest sample sizes. We cannot draw firm conclusions from the limited number of cohort studies available, but the parallel results for the fixed and random estimations may indicate only modest heterogeneity. We generated I-squared values of approximately 60 % (with non-significant chi-squared tests), and based on current guidelines [77], these findings may support our assumptions regarding heterogeneity. In the random- and fixed-effects models, this result implied that 60 % of the between-study heterogeneity could be explained by true study variation [47, 78].

Body composition was not reviewed in this study. Although obesity is related to childhood asthma [79, 80], the effects of asthma and weight on lung function are highly variable [81].

Future studies should involve the participation of clinical professionals. Clinicians (e.g., pediatricians or epidemiologists) may find our results useful when inquiring about the PA of their young patients who present with respiratory symptoms or asthma.

Conclusions

Of the 1,571 titles reviewed, we analyzed 11 original articles. Overall, we observed indications that children who were physically inactive may have a higher risk of asthma/or wheezing compared with active children. This review also revealed a critical need for future longitudinal assessments of low PA, its mechanisms, and its implications for incident asthma in children.

Additional files

Additional file 1: PRISMA Items Used in Reporting in the Current Systematic Literature Review. Additional file 1 presents the PRISMA checklist items that were examined, with the draft article page numbers.

Additional file 2: Reporting Items of the Meta-analysis Of Observational Studies in Epidemiology (MOOSE) Group.

Additional file 3: A. Articles Excluded ($n = 54$) from the Systematic Review Grouped by Exclusion Rationale. B. Articles Excluded ($n = 7$) from the Systematic Review after Review of the Reference Lists.

Additional file 4: Data from Eight Non-Meta-Analyzed Studies Extracted to the GATE Calculator and the GATE-Lite Appraisal Forms.

Abbreviations

BHR: bronchial hyperresponsiveness/or bronchial hyperresponsibility; BMI: body mass index; CI: confidence interval; EIA: exercise-induced asthma; GATE: Graphic Appraisal Tool for Epidemiology; HR: hazard ratio; ISAAC: International Study of Asthma and Allergies in Childhood; MeSH: medical subject heading; MET: metabolic equivalent; OR: odds ratio; PA: physical activity; RCT: randomised controlled trial; SE: standard error; SES: socio-economic status.

Competing interests

The authors declare that they have no competing interests.

Authors' contributions

LL developed the protocol, performed the literature searches, extracted the data for quantitative and qualitative syntheses, and conducted the data analyses. PEP was available for adjudication. KGN, PEP, and LL developed the strategy for GATE application and interpreted the results with assistance from RTJ. All authors (PEP, TAEPM, KGN, and LL) participated in the PROSPERO registration (University of York, UK) and are joint guarantors of this review. All authors also contributed to assessing the comprehensive results. LL drafted the initial manuscript, KGN and PEP revised the drafts critically, and all authors read and accepted the final manuscript.

Acknowledgements

The review commenced during LL's initial research program at the University of Bristol (UoB), Bristol, United Kingdom. Therefore, the authors wish to express thanks to Medical Subject Librarian CF Borwick (CFB), UoB, for assistance in refining the database search strategies. We also thank Prof RT Jackson (RTJ) of the University of Auckland (Auckland, New Zealand) for reviewing our data, providing helpful guidance (which included providing savable files for GATE), and offering suggestions regarding our application of the GATE tool.

Funding

LL received funding from one PhD Fellowship and two research awards (respective award dates: 13 May 2009, 9 Dec 2010, and 14 June 2011) from The Jubilee Foundation* and from four research grants of The Research Fund* dated 14 May 2008, 13 May 2009, 14 June 2011, and 10 Dec 2013. The funders had no role in the study design, data collection and analysis, decision to publish, or preparation of the manuscript.
*Danish Physiotherapy Organization

Author details

[1]Department of Odontology, University of Copenhagen, Copenhagen 1014, Denmark. [2]Department of Pediatrics and Adolescent Medicine, Copenhagen University Hospital, Rigshospitalet, Copenhagen 2100, Denmark. [3]Department of Medicine, Division of Allergy and Clinical Immunology, University of Virginia, Charlottesville 22908, VA, USA.

References

1. Papadopoulos NG, Arakawa H, Carlsen KH, Custovic A, Gern J, Lemanske R, et al. International consensus on (ICON) pediatric asthma. Allergy. 2012;67: 976–97.
2. Asher M, Keil U, Anderson H, Beasley R, Crane J, Martinez F, et al. International Study of Asthma and Allergies in Childhood (ISAAC): rationale and methods. Eur Respir J. 1995;8:483–91.
3. Burney PGJ, Chinn S, Rona RJ. Has the prevalence of asthma increased in children? Evidence from the National Study of Health and Growth 1973-86. BMJ. 1990;300:1306–10.
4. Ross Anderson H, Gupta R, Strachan DP, Limb ES. 50 years of asthma: UK trends from 1955 to 2004. Thorax. 2007;62:85–90.
5. Hill VL, Wood PR. Asthma epidemiology, pathophysiology, and initial evaluation. Pediatr Rev. 2009;30:331–6.
6. Asher M, Montefort S, Bjorksten B, Lai C, Strachan D, Weiland S, et al. Worldwide time trends in the prevalence of symptoms of asthma, allergic rhinoconjunctivitis, and eczema in childhood: ISAAC Phases One and Three repeat multicountry cross-sectional surveys. Lancet. 2006;368:733–43.
7. Platts-Mills TAE. Asthma severity and prevalence: an ongoing interaction between exposure, hygiene, and lifestyle. PLoS Med. 2005;2:e34.
8. Subbarao P, Mandhane PJ, Sears MR. Asthma: epidemiology, etiology and risk factors. CMAJ. 2009;181:E181–90.
9. Nystad W, Nafstad P, Harris J. Physical activity affects the prevalence of reported wheeze. Eur J Epidemiol. 2001;17:209–12.
10. Shaaban R, Leynaert B, Soussan D, Antó JM, Chinn S, de Marco R, et al. Physical activity and bronchial hyperresponsiveness: European Community Respiratory Health Survey II. Thorax. 2007;62:403–10.
11. World Health Organization. Children's environmental health: Children, mobility and environmental health. World Health Organization. http://www.who.int/ceh/risks/en/. Accessed 30 Mar 2016.
12. Cypcar D, Lemanske Jr RF. Asthma and exercise. Clin Chest Med. 1994;15: 351–68.
13. Matsumoto I, Araki H, Tsuda K, Odajima H, Nishima S, Higaki Y, et al. Effects of swimming training on aerobic capacity and exercise induced bronchoconstriction in children with bronchial asthma. Thorax. 1999;54:196–201.
14. Welsh L, Kemp JG, Roberts RGD. Effects of physical conditioning on children and adolescents with asthma. Sports Med. 2005;35:127–41.
15. Schwindt CD, Zaldivar F, Wilson L, Leu S-Y, Wang-Rodriguez J, Mills PJ, et al. Do circulating leucocytes and lymphocyte subtypes increase in response to brief exercise in children with and without asthma? Br J Sports Med. 2007;41:34–40.
16. Rosa J. Exercise leukocyte profiles in healthy, type 1 diabetic, overweight, and asthmatic children. Pediatr Exerc Sci. 2009;21:19–33.
17. Lucas SR, Platts-Mills TAE. Physical activity and exercise in asthma: relevance to etiology and treatment. J Allergy Clin Immunol. 2005;115: 928–34.
18. Cooper DM, Radom-Aizik S, Schwindt C, Zaldivar Jr F. Dangerous exercise: lessons learned from dysregulated inflammatory responses to physical activity. J Appl Physiol. 2007;103:700–9.
19. Platts-Mills TAE, Woodfolk JA, Chapman MD, Heymann PW. Changing concepts of allergic disease: The attempt to keep up with real changes in lifestyles. J Allergy Clin Immunol. 1996;98:S297–306.
20. Eijkemans M, Mommers M, de Vries SI, van Buuren S, Stafleu A, Bakker I, et al. Asthmatic symptoms, physical activity, and overweight in young children: a cohort study. Pediatrics. 2008;121:e666–72.
21. Siersted HC, Boldsen J, Hansen HS, Mostgaard G, Hyldebrandt N, Rees PJ, et al. Population based study of risk factors for underdiagnosis of asthma in adolescence: Odense schoolchild study. BMJ. 1998;316:651–7.

22. Lang DM, Butz AM, Duggan AK, Serwint JR. Physical activity in urban school-aged children with asthma. Pediatrics. 2004;113:e341–6.
23. Mitchell E, Beasley R, Björkstén B, Crane J, García-Marcos L, Keil U. The association between BMI, vigorous physical activity and television viewing and the risk of symptoms of asthma, rhinoconjunctivitis and eczema in children and adolescents: ISAAC Phase Three. Clin Exp Allergy. 2013;43:73–84.
24. Priftis K, Panagiotakos D, Antonogeorgos G, Papadopoulos M, Charisi M, Lagona E, et al. Factors associated with asthma symptoms in schoolchildren from Greece: The Physical Activity, Nutrition and Allergies in Children Examined in Athens (PANACEA) study. J Asthma. 2007;44:521–7.
25. Corbo G, Forastiere F, De Sario M, Brunetti L, Bonci E, Bugiani M, et al. Wheeze and asthma in children: associations with body mass index, sports, television viewing, and diet. Epidemiology. 2008;19:747–55.
26. Ownby D, Peterson E, Nelson D, Joseph C, Williams L, Johnson C. The relationship of physical activity and percentage of body fat to the risk of asthma in 8- to 10-year-old children. J Asthma. 2007;44:885–9.
27. Eijkemans M, Mommers M, Draaisma JM, Thijs C, Prins MH. Physical activity and asthma: a systematic review and meta-analysis. PLOS ONE. 2012;7:e50775.
28. Jackson R, Ameratunga S, Broad J, Connor J, Lethaby A, Robb G, et al. The GATE frame: critical appraisal with pictures. Evid Based Med. 2006;11:35–8.
29. Centre for Reviews and Dissemination. Systematic reviews: CRD's guidance for undertaking reviews in health care. York: University of York; 2009.
30. Moher D, Liberati A, Tetzlaff J, Altman DG, The Prisma Group. Preferred reporting items for systematic reviews and meta-analyses: the PRISMA statement. PLOS Med. 2009;6:e1000097.
31. Stroup DF, Berlin JA, Morton SC, Olkin I, Williamson GD, Rennie D, et al. Meta-analysis of observational studies in epidemiology: a proposal for reporting. JAMA. 2000;283:2008–12.
32. Liberati A, Altman DG, Tetzlaff J, Mulrow C, Gøtzsche PC, Ioannidis JPA, et al. The PRISMA statement for reporting systematic reviews and meta-analyses of studies that evaluate health care interventions: explanation and elaboration. J Clin Epidemiol. 2009;62:e1–e34.
33. Pearce N. Classification of epidemiological study designs. Int J Epidemiol. 2012;41:393–7.
34. Duijts L. Fetal and infant origins of asthma. Eur J Epidemiol. 2012;27:5–14.
35. Lee DA, Winslow NR, Speight AN, Hey EN. Prevalence and spectrum of asthma in childhood. BMJ. 1983;286:1256–8.
36. Sallis JF, Saelens BE. Assessment of physical activity by self-report: status, limitations, and future directions. Res Q Exercise Sport. 2000;71:S1–S14.
37. Howley E. Type of activity: resistance, aerobic and leisure versus occupational physical activity. Med Sci Sports Exerc. 2001;33:S364–S9.
38. Haskell WL. What to look for in assessing responsiveness to exercise in a health context. Med Sci Sports Exerc. 2001;33:S454–S8.
39. Hickmann M, Roberts C, de Matos M. Exercise and leisure-time activities. In: Currie C, Hurrelmann K, Settertobulte W, Smith R, Todd J, editors. Health and health behaviour among young people. Health behaviour in school-aged children: a WHO Cross-National Study (HBSC) International Report. Copenhagen: World Health Organization; 2000. p. 73–82.
40. Owen N, Healy GN, Matthews CE, Dunstan DW. Too much sitting: the population health science of sedentary behavior. Exerc Sports Sci Rev. 2010;38:105–13.
41. Pettee Gabriel KK, Morrow Jr JR, Woolsey AL. Framework for physical activity as a complex and multidimensional behavior. J Phys Act Health. 2012;9 Suppl 1:S11–S8.
42. Romieu I, Mannino DM, Redd SC, McGeehin MA. Dietary intake, physical activity, body mass index, and childhood asthma in the third national health and nutrition survey (NHANES III). Pediatr Pulmonol. 2004;38:31–42.
43. Moher D, Pham B, Klassen TP, Schulz KF, Berlin JA, Jadad AR, et al. What contributions do languages other than English make on the results of meta-analyses? J Clin Epidemiol. 2000;53:964–72.
44. Higgins JPT, Deeks JJ. Table 7.3.a. Checklist for items to consider in data collection or data extraction. In: Higgins J, Green S, editors. Cochrane handbook for systematic reviews of interventions, Version 5.1.0 [updated March 2011]. Baltimore: The Cochrane Collaboration; 2011. http://handbook.cochrane.org/. Accessed 30 Mar 2016.
45. Sherriff A, Maitra A, Ness AR, Mattocks C, Riddoch C, Reilly JJ, et al. Association of duration of television viewing in early childhood with the subsequent development of asthma. Thorax. 2009;64:321–5.
46. University of Auckland. Evidence-based practice and critical appraisal. Auckland, NZ: University of Auckland. https://www.fmhs.auckland.ac.nz/en/soph/about/our-departments/epidemiology-and-biostatistics/research/epiq/2015-evidence-based-practice-and-cats.html. Accessed 30 Mar 2016.
47. Riley RD, Higgins JPT, Deeks JJ. Interpretation of random effects meta-analyses. BMJ. 2011;342:d549.
48. Deeks JJ, Altman DG, Bradburn MJ. Statistical methods for examining heterogeneity and combining results from several studies in meta-analysis. In: Egger M, Davey Smith G, Altman DG, editors. Systematic reviews in health care: meta-analysis in context. 2nd ed. London: BMJ; 2008. p. 285–312.
49. Liberati A, Altman DG, Tetzlaff J, Mulrow C, Gotzsche PC, Ioannidis JP, et al. The PRISMA statement for reporting systematic reviews and meta-analyses of studies that evaluate health care interventions: explanation and elaboration. PLOS Med. 2009;6:e1000100.
50. StataCorp. http://www.stata.com/. Accessed 30 Mar 2016.
51. Islam T, Berhane K, McConnell R, Gauderman WJ, Avol E, Peters JM, et al. Glutathione-S-transferase (GST) P1, GSTM1, exercise, ozone and asthma incidence in school children. Thorax. 2009;64:197–202.
52. Vogelberg C, Hirsch T, Radon K, Dressel H, Windstetter D, Weinmayr G, et al. Leisure time activity and new onset of wheezing during adolescence. Eur Respir J. 2007;30:672–6.
53. Jones S, Merkle S, Fulton J, Wheeler L, Mannino D. Relationship between asthma, overweight, and physical activity among U.S. high school students. J Commun Health. 2006;31:469–78.
54. Kosti R, Priftis K, Anthracopoulos M, Papadimitriou A, Grigoropoulou D, Lentzas Y, et al. The association between leisure-time physical activities and asthma symptoms among 10- to 12-year-old children: the effect of living environment in the PANACEA study. J Asthma. 2012;49:342–8.
55. Nystad W. The physical activity level in children with asthma based on a survey among 7–16-year-old school children. Scand J Med Sci Sports. 1997;7:331–5.
56. Wood L, Egger M, Gluud LL, Schulz KF, Jüni P, Altman DG, et al. Empirical evidence of bias in treatment effect estimates in controlled trials with different interventions and outcomes: meta-epidemiological study. BMJ. 2008;336:601–5.
57. Egger M, Davey Smith G, Altman DG. Systematic reviews in health care: meta-analysis in context. London: BMJ Books; 2001.
58. Firrincieli V, Keller A, Ehrensberger R, Platts-Mills J, Shufflebarger C, Geldmaker B, et al. Decreased physical activity among headstart children with a history of wheezing: use of an accelerometer to measure activity. Pediatr Pulm. 2005;40:57–63.
59. Rundle A, Goldstein IF, Mellins RB, Ashby-Thompson M, Hoepner L, Jacobson JS. Physical activity and asthma symptoms among New York City head start children. J Asthma. 2009;46:803–9.
60. Radon K, Dressel H, Hümmer S, Riu E, Nowak D, Weinmayr G, et al. Berufliche allergierisiken-die SOLAR-kohortenstudie. University of Munich. BAuA - Forschungsberichte 2005/Forschungsberichte/Schriftenreihe der BAuA/Publikationen/Bundesanstalt für Arbeitsschutz und Arbeitsmedizin - Berufliche Allergierisiken. Accessed 21 Aug 2015.
61. McConnell R, Berhane K, Gilliland F, London SJ, Islam T, Gauderman WJ, et al. Asthma in exercising children exposed to ozone: a cohort study. Lancet. 2002;359:386–91.
62. Voss PH, Rehfuess EA. Quality appraisal in systematic reviews of public health interventions: an empirical study on the impact of choice of tool on meta-analysis. J Epidemiol Commun H. 2013;67:98–104.
63. Pearce N. Epidemiology in a changing world: variation, causation and ubiquitous risk factors. Int J Epidemiol. 2011;40:503–12.
64. Black N. Why we need observational studies to evaluate the effectiveness of health care. BMJ. 1996;312:1215–8.
65. Patel S, Jarvelin M-R, Little M. Systematic review of worldwide variations of the prevalence of wheezing symptoms in children. Environ Health. 2008;7:57.
66. Dumith SC, Gigante DP, Domingues MR, Kohl 3rd HW. Physical activity change during adolescence: a systematic review and a pooled analysis. Int J Epidemiol. 2011;40:685–98.
67. Eder W, Ege MJ, von Mutius E. The asthma epidemic. New Engl J Med. 2006;355:2226–35.
68. The British Thoracic Society and Scottish Intercollegiate Guidelines Network. British guideline on the management of asthma. Quick reference guide, guideline no. 141. London: British Thoracic Society, Scottish Intercollegiate Guidelines Network; 2014. http://www.sign.ac.uk/guidelines/fulltext/141/index.html. Accessed 30 Mar 2016.
69. Alderman BL, Benham-Deal TB, Jenkins JM. Change in parental influence on children's physical activity over time. J Phys Act Health. 2010;7:60–7.
70. Jago R, Page AS, Cooper AR. Friends and physical activity during the transition from primary to secondary school. Med Sci Sports Exerc. 2012;44:111–7.

71. Warren JM, Ekelund U, Besson H, Mezzani A, Geladas N, Vanhees L. Assessment of physical activity – a review of methodologies with reference to epidemiological research: a report of the exercise physiology section of the European Association of Cardiovascular Prevention and Rehabilitation. Eur J Cardiov Prev R. 2010;17:127–39.
72. Dantas F, Correia M, Silva A, Peixoto D, Sarinho E, Rizzo J. Mothers impose physical activity restrictions on their asthmatic children and adolescents: an analytical cross-sectional study. BMC Public Health. 2014;14:287.
73. Cliff DP, Reilly JJ, Okely AD. Methodological considerations in using accelerometers to assess habitual physical activity in children aged 0–5 years. J Sci Med Sport. 2009;12:557–67.
74. Bornstein DB, Beets MW, Byun W, McIver K. Accelerometer-derived physical activity levels of preschoolers: A meta-analysis. J Sci Med Sport. 2011;14:504–11.
75. Ainsworth BE, Haskell WL, Whitt MC, Irwin ML, Swartz AM, Strath SJ, et al. Compendium of physical activities: an update of activity codes and MET intensities. Med Sci Sports Exerc. 2000;32:S498–S516.
76. Booth ML, Okely AD, Chey T, Bauman A. The reliability and validity of the physical activity questions in the WHO health behaviour in schoolchildren (HBSC) survey: a population study. Br J Sports Med. 2001;35:263–7.
77. Higgins JPT, Deeks JJ. 9.5.4 Incorporating heterogeneity into random-effects models. In: Higgins J, Green S, editors. Cochrane handbook for systematic reviews of interventions, Version 5.1.0 [updated March 2011]. Baltimore: The Cochrane Collaboration; 2011. http://handbook.cochrane.org/. Accessed 30 Mar 2016.
78. Higgins JPT, Thompson SG, Deeks JJ, Altman DG. Measuring inconsistency in meta-analyses. BMJ. 2003;327:557–60.
79. Quinto KB, Zuraw BL, Poon KY, Chen W, Schatz M, Christiansen SC. The association of obesity and asthma severity and control in children. J Allergy Clin Immunol. 2011;128:964–9.
80. Saint-Pierre P, Bourdin A, Chanez P, Daures JP, Godard P. Are overweight asthmatics more difficult to control? Allergy. 2006;61:79–84.
81. Nicolacakis K, Skowronski ME, Coreno AJ, West E, Nader NZ, Smith RL, et al. Observations on the physiological interactions between obesity and asthma. J Appl Physiol. 2008;105:1533–41.

7

Comparison of the frequency of bacterial and viral infections among children with community-acquired pneumonia hospitalized across distinct severity categories

Amanda C. Nascimento-Carvalho[1], Olli Ruuskanen[2] and Cristiana M. Nascimento-Carvalho[3*]

Abstract

Background: The comparison of the frequencies of bacterial and viral infections among children with community-acquired pneumonia (CAP) admitted in distinct severity categories, in an original study, is lacking in literature to-date. We aimed to achieve this goal.

Methods: Children aged 2-59-months-old hospitalized with CAP were included in this prospective study in Salvador, Brazil. Clinical data and biological samples were collected to investigate 11 viruses and 8 bacteria. Severity was assessed by using the World Health Organization criteria.

Results: One hundred eighty-one patients were classified as "non-severe" ($n = 53$; 29.3 %), "severe" ($n = 111$; 61.3 %), or "very severe" ($n = 17$; 9.4 %) CAP. Overall, aetiology was detected among 156 (86.2 %) cases; viral ($n = 84$; 46.4 %), bacterial ($n = 26$; 14.4 %) and viral-bacterial ($n = 46$; 25.4 %) infections were identified. Viral infection frequency was similar in severe/very severe and non-severe cases (46.1 % *vs.* 47.2 %; $p = 0.9$). Pneumococcal infection increased across "non-severe" (13.2 %), "severe" (23.4 %), and "very severe" (35.3 %) cases (qui-squared test for trend $p = 0.04$). Among patients with detected aetiology, after excluding cases with co-infection, the frequency of sole bacterial infection was different ($p = 0.04$) among the categories; non-severe (12.5 %), severe (29.3 %) or very severe (55.6 %). Among these patients, sole bacterial infection was independently associated with severity (OR = 4.4 [95 % CI:1.1–17.6]; $p = 0.04$) in a model controlled for age (OR = 0.7 [95 % CI:0.5–1.1]; $p = 0.1$).

Conclusions: A substantial proportion of cases in distinct severity subgroups had respiratory viral infections, which did not differ between severity categories. Bacterial infection, particularly pneumococcal infection, was more likely among severe/very severe cases.

Keywords: Acute respiratory infection, Lower respiratory tract infection, Lung disease, Respiratory viruses, Severity assessment

* Correspondence: nascimentocarvalho@hotmail.com
[3]Department of Paediatrics, Federal University of Bahia School of Medicine, Salvador, Bahia, Brazil
Full list of author information is available at the end of the article

Background

Community-acquired pneumonia (CAP) continues to be a major cause of death among children aged under-5 years worldwide and almost all of these deaths occur in developing countries [1]. In the 1980s, it was established that most children dying from CAP in these regions had bacterial infection. Such assumption was based on the results of bacterial culture of lung aspirates from cases in these developing countries, as well as of lung aspiration studies and post-mortem studies from cases in developed countries in the pre-antimicrobial era [2, 3]. During the last decade, a wide range of studies have been conducted across different continents with the purpose of investigating the aetiology of childhood CAP [4]. Of note, while in the former set of studies only conventional bacteriological methods were employed, new molecular tests have been used in recent investigations, which consequently increased the yield of microbiological results [5, 6]. In this latter group, children with different categories of severity have been included, either with non-severe, severe, or very severe disease [4]. However, the comparison of the frequencies of different aetiologies among children with CAP in distinct severity categories in an original study is lacking in literature to-date.

In this context, we assessed whether there was difference in the frequency of bacterial and viral infections among children with CAP in distinct severity subgroups.

Methods

This was a prospective cross-sectional study conducted at the Federal University of Bahia Hospital, in Salvador, North-eastern Brazil, where community-dwelling children from the low income population were first seen at the hospital's Emergency Room. This is a public service. Data were prospectively collected from September 2003 to May 2005. CAP diagnosis was based on the report of respiratory complaints and fever or difficulty breathing plus the detection of pulmonary infiltrate or pleural effusion on the chest radiograph taken at the initial evaluation and read by the paediatrician on duty. For the purpose of this analysis, only children with tachypnoea or chest indrawing were included. Every child under-5-years-old hospitalized due to CAP diagnosis at the Emergency Room, based on the aforementioned criteria, was enrolled. Those with chronic lung disease except asthma, underlying comorbidities (cancer, organ dysfunction like cardiac, hepatic, respiratory or renal insufficiency), any other concurrent infections (for example, measles, chickenpox, tuberculosis, whooping cough, otitis, gastroenteritis, pyodermitis, meningitis), suspected or diagnosed immunodeficiency (including children born to an HIV-infected mother), or transferred from other health-care units were excluded. The applied exclusion criteria assured that only previously healthy children were enrolled and the clinical characteristics were exclusively attributable to the current CAP episode.

Upon hospital admission, demographic and clinical data and biological samples were collected by the research team, after receiving written informed consent by parents or legal guardians. Detailed interviews regarding the current illness, general medical history and thorough physical examinations were performed to complete a standardized questionnaire and assure eligibility. Data on clinical evolution and outcome were not collected because treatment may influence them. Therefore, the focus of this investigation was the severity presented by patients upon admission to hospital. Nasopharyngeal aspirates (NPA) collected through the nostrils were stored (−70 °C) until virologic tests were performed. Blood was collected for blood culture (BACTEC automatic system), buffy-coat (-70 °C) and serum (−20 °C) storage. Follow-up visits occurred between 2 and 4 weeks after enrolment when blood was also collected for serum storage (−20 °C). This procedure allowed the comparison of specific IgG titres as an investigational tool to detect several aetiologies. Everyone in the study had to have both NPA and paired serum samples collected to assure the same opportunity for investigation of all pathogens included in the panel.

Nineteen aetiological agents were investigated: 11 viruses and 8 bacteria. *Streptococcus pneumoniae*, *Haemophilus influenzae*, and *Moraxella catarrhalis* infections were investigated by blood culture and by searching for specific IgG increase tested by an in-house enzyme immune assay (ELISA) in paired serum samples. For pneumococcal infections, IgG antibodies to pneumococcal pneumolysin and pneumococcal C-polysaccharide were used; a ≥2-fold or ≥3-fold increase, respectively, in antibody titres, between paired serum samples, was considered diagnostic [7].

For *H. influenzae* and *M. catarrhalis* infections, Ig (polyvalent) antibodies against whole bacterial cell antigens were measured and a ≥3-fold antibody increase between paired serum samples was considered diagnostic [7]. Pneumococcal infection was also sought by pneumolysin-polymerase chain reaction (PCR) performed in acute buffy-coat for the detection of pneumococcal DNA [8]. *Staphylococcus aureus* infection was investigated by blood culture. *Mycoplasma pneumoniae* infection was investigated by testing for specific IgM by using a commercial ELISA kit (Platelia, Bio-Rad, Marnes La Coquette, France) [9]. *Chlamydia trachomatis* IgG antibodies were measured by a commercial, solid-phase ELISA (Ani Labsystems Ltd., Vantaa, Finland). The laboratory diagnosis was based on signal to cut-off (S/CO) values, which were ≥1.4 S/CO [10]. An in-house micro-immunofluorescence (MIF) test was used to measure

IgG, IgA and IgM antibodies to *Chlamydophila pneumoniae* and *Simkania negevensis*, using purified, formalized elementary bodies of strains Kajaani 6 in *C. pneumoniae* and ATCC strain Z (ATCC, Catalog no. VR-1471) in *S. negevensis* tests. The diagnosis was based on a ≥4-fold increase in IgG or IgA antibodies between the paired serum samples or on the presence of IgM antibodies (a titre of ≥10) [11]. Rhinovirus, enterovirus, and human metapneumovirus were investigated by reverse transcriptase PCR in NPA. Parainfluenza virus 1, 2, 3, respiratory syncytial virus (RSV), influenza virus A and B, and adenovirus were investigated by viral antigen identification in the NPA by time-resolved fluoroimmunoassay with monoclonal antibodies; additionally, virus-specific serum antibody titres were determined in paired serum samples using an ELISA with an antigen-coated solid phase and horseradish peroxidase conjugated rabbit anti-human IgG; a ≥3-fold antibody titres increase was considered diagnostic [12]. Human bocavirus was investigated by quantitative PCR of NPA and serum, IgG increase determination in paired serum samples and searching for IgM and IgG avidity by ELISA [13]. Frequencies of these aetiological agents analysed by age distribution have been published [14–17].

The patients were grouped into three distinct severity subgroups according to the World Health Organization (WHO) severity criteria for children aged 2 months and above available in the 2000 decade; patients with "non-severe" CAP had tachypnoea neither with chest indrawing nor with any danger signs, patients with "severe" CAP had chest indrawing or supraclavicular recession without any danger signs, and patients with "very severe" CAP presented any danger signs, which were inability to drink, convulsions, lethargy, stridor in a calm child, or central cyanosis [18]. Tachypnoea was defined as respiratory rate ≥50 breaths/min in children aged 2–11 months and respiratory rate ≥40 breaths/min in children aged 12–59 months [18]. Therefore, children aged under-

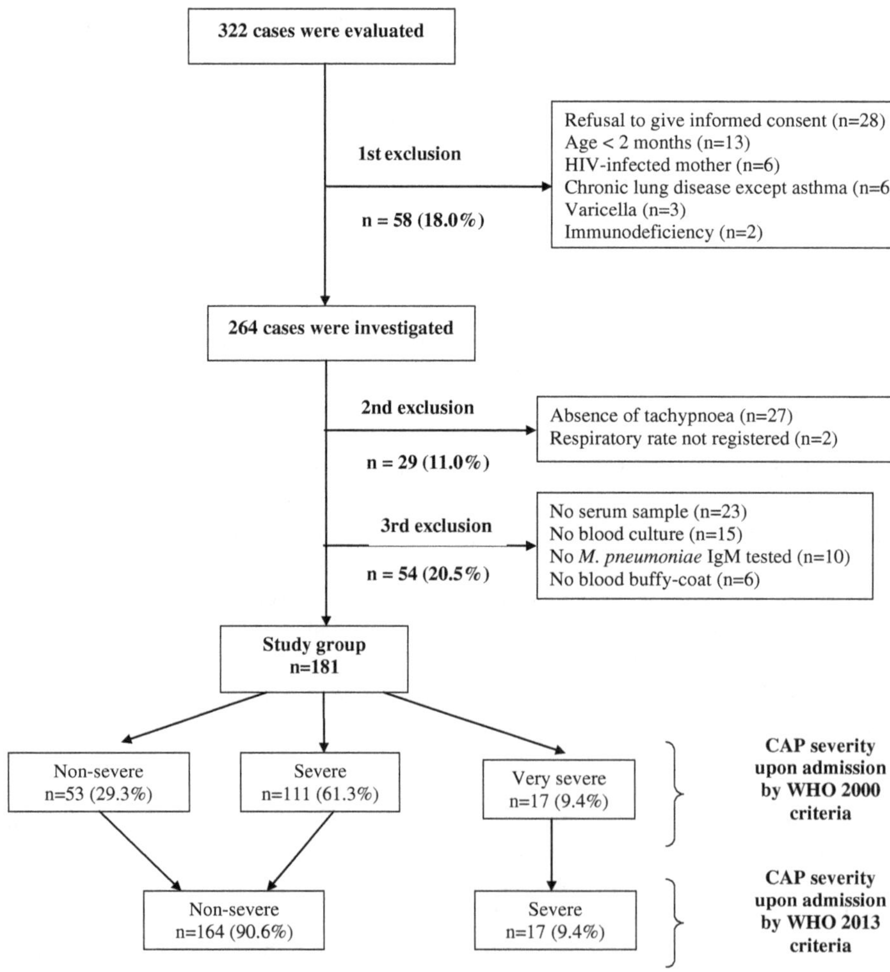

Fig. 1 Flow-chart of recruitment of children hospitalized with community-acquired pneumonia referred for aetiology investigation and grouped according to severity upon admission

2 months, or without tachypnoea, or with missing respiratory rate, or missing danger signs were excluded. Severity classification was performed by a researcher blinded to the aetiological tests' results, who had previously received training regarding the WHO severity criteria. Additionally, the patients were further grouped into two distinct severity subgroups according to the current WHO severity criteria published in 2013 [19]. According to these latter criteria, children with "non-severe" pneumonia have tachypnoea or chest wall indrawing, and children with "severe" pneumonia have central cyanosis, stridor in a calm child, inability to drink, lethargy, or convulsions, besides having tachypnoea or chest wall indrawing. That is, the subgroups "non-severe" and "severe" in the former criteria were grouped into the subgroup "non-severe" in the latter criteria; the subgroup labelled "very severe" in the former criteria was re-named "severe" in the latter criteria. Invasive disease was defined as positive blood culture (bacteraemia) or positive blood pneumococcal PCR.

For the purpose of analysis, the cases were classified as viral infection when only viral infection was detected, bacterial infection when bacterial infection was diagnosed irrespective of also viral infection having been detected; this last subgroup was split into two others: typical bacterial infection if infection by *S. pneumoniae*, *H. influenzae*, *M. catarrhalis* or *S. aureus* was found irrespective of other agents; atypical bacterial infection if infection by *M. pneumoniae*, *C. trachomatis*, *C. pneumoniae* or *S. negevensis* was detected irrespective of viral infection.

Continuous variables showed non-parametric distribution and were presented as median [interquartile range (IQR)]. Categorical variables were compared using chi-square or Fisher's exact test, as appropriate. A trend analysis for bacterial, typical bacterial, and pneumococcal

Table 1 Demographic and clinical characteristics of children with non-severe, severe or very severe community-acquired pneumonia

Characteristics	Severity by the World Health Organization 2000 criteria		
	Non-severe ($n = 53$)	Severe ($n = 111$)	Very severe ($n = 17$)
Age (months)[a, b]	23 (13–35)	16 (9–26)	18 (13–26)
Length of disease (days)[a, c]	7 (5–13)	7 (4–11)	8 (4–11)
Tachypnoea[d]	53 (100.0)	97 (87.4)	15 (88.2)
Chest indrawing[d]	0	109 (98.2)	7 (41.2)
Supraclavicular recession[d]	0	4 (3.6)	0
Inability to drink[d]	0	0	17 (100.0)

[a]Median (interquartile range)
[b]Children with non-severe community-acquired pneumonia *versus* those with severe ($p = 0.03$) or *versus* those with severe and very severe CAP ($p = 0.04$)
[c]No significant difference was found
[d]Results in n (%)

Table 2 Overall frequency of aetiological agents detected among 181 children hospitalized with community-acquired pneumonia

Aetiological agents	Frequency
S. pneumoniae	39 (21.5)
positive blood culture	8 (4.4)
positive blood PCR	7 (3.9)
invasive infection[a]	13 (7.2)
increased paired IgG titres only	26 (14.4)
H. influenzae	13 (7.2)
M. pneumoniae	11 (6.1)
C. trachomatis	9 (5.0)
M. catarrhalis	4 (2.2)
S. negevensis[b]	3 (1.7)
Rhinovirus	39 (21.5)
RSV	36 (19.9)
antigen in NPA and increased paired IgG titres	17 (9.4)
antigen in NPA	11 (6.1)
increased paired IgG titres	8 (4.4)
Parainfluenza 1, 2, 3	35 (19.3)
antigen in NPA and increased paired IgG titres	11 (6.0)
antigen in NPA	2 (1.1)
increased paired IgG titres	22 (12.2)
Influenza A, B	15 (8.3)
antigen in NPA and increased paired IgG titres	3 (1.65)
antigen in NPA	3 (1.65)
increased paired IgG titres	9 (5.0)
Human bocavirus	17 (9.4)
low IgG avidity (<15)	17 (9.4)
positive IgM	16 (8.8)
qPCR in NPA >10E + 4/ml	15 (8.3)
positive qPCR in serum	4 (2.2)
IgG seroconversion	3 (1.65)
increased paired IgG titres	2 (1.1)
Adenovirus	10 (5.5)
antigen in NPA and increased paired IgG titres	3 (1.65)
antigen in NPA	1 (0.55)
increased paired IgG titres	6 (3.3)
Enterovirus	10 (5.5)
Human metapneumovirus	8 (4.4)

Results in n (%)
RSV respiratory syncytial virus
NPA nasopharyngeal aspirate
qPCR quantitative polymerase chain reaction
[a]Invasive disease was defined as positive blood culture (bacteraemia) and/or positive blood PCR for pneumococcus
[b]All three cases had IgM against *S. negevensis* detected

infection across 3 different severity categories was performed using qui-squared test for trend. Continuous variables were assessed using Mann–Whitney U. Analysis was stratified by age. Multivariable logistic regression analysis by enter method assessed the potential impact of bacterial infection (predictor variable) on clinical severity upon admission (outcome variable) in an age adjusted model. Statistical tests were two-tailed, at significance level of 0.05. SPSS software (version 9.0, IBM, Armonk, New York) was used for analysis. Sample size was estimated considering a smaller frequency of bacterial infection in non-severe cases of 30 % and an expected frequency of bacterial infection in severe/very severe cases of 45 %. Thus, the sample size was estimated as 162 cases, considering a significance level of 0.05 (95 % Confidence Interval [95 % CI]) and power of 80 %. Exclusion criteria were chosen to address potential confounders. Blinding at severity classification was performed to address potential bias. Cases with any missing biological sample or data were excluded.

Different data from the same research project have already been published. The novelty in this paper is the presentation of clinical characteristics which were used to group the cases in distinct severity categories, along with the analysis of the aetiological data across these distinct severity categories.

Results

Overall, 322 patients were evaluated, out of which 141 (43.8 %) were excluded due to different reasons (Fig. 1). Therefore, the study group comprised 181 patients (Fig. 1). There were no additional diagnoses as reasons for hospitalization. The overall median (IQR) age was 17 (10–27) months and there were 113 (62.4 %) boys. No patient had previously received either pneumococcal or influenza vaccines. On the contrary, 85.0 % had received

Table 3 Comparison between frequencies of different aetiologies among children with non-severe or severe and/or very severe community-acquired pneumonia according to the World Health Organization 2000 criteria

Aetiology	Overall frequency (*n* = 181)	Severity by the World Health Organization 2000 criteria						
		Non-severe (*n* = 53)	Severe or very severe (*n* = 128)	*p*	Severe (*n* = 111)	*p*	Very severe (*n* = 17)	*p*
Subgroups								
Detected	156 (86)	41 (77.4)	115 (89.8)	0.03	101 (91.0)	0.017	14 (82.4)	1
Viral infection	84 (46.4)	25 (47.2)	59 (46.1)	0.9	54 (48.6)	0.9	5 (29.4)	0.2
Bacterial infection	72 (39.8)	16 (30.2)	56 (43.8)	0.09	47 (42.3)	0.1	9 (52.9)	0.09
Typical bacterial infection	54 (29.8)	11 (20.8)	43 (33.6)	0.09	36 (32.4)	0.1	7 (41.2)	0.1
Atypical bacterial infection	18 (9.9)	5 (9.4)	13 (10.2)	0.9	11 (9.9)	0.9	2 (11.8)	1
Pathogens								
S. pneumoniae	39 (21.5)	7 (13.2)	32 (25.0)	0.08	26 (23.4)	0.1	6 (35.3)	0.07
Positive blood culture	8 (4.4)	3 (5.7)	5 (3.9)	0.7	3 (2.7)	0.4	2 (11.8)	0.6
Positive blood PCR	7 (3.9)	1 (1.9)	6 (4.7)	0.7	5 (4.5)	0.7	1 (5.9)	0.4
Invasive infection[a]	13 (7.2)	3 (5.7)	10 (7.8)	0.8	8 (7.2)	1	2 (11.8)	0.6
H. influenzae	13 (7.2)	4 (7.5)	9 (7.0)	1	8 (7.2)	1	1 (5.9)	1
M. pneumoniae	11 (6.1)	6 (11.3)	5 (3.9)	0.08	4 (3.6)	0.08	1 (5.9)	1
C. trachomatis	9 (5.0)	0	9 (7.0)	0.06	9 (8.1)	0.03	0	-
M. catarrhalis	4 (2.2)	0	4 (3.1)	0.3	4 (3.6)	0.3	0	-
S. negevensis	3 (1.7)	0	3 (2.3)	0.6	2 (1.8)	1	1 (5.9)	0.2
Rhinovirus	39 (21.5)	13 (24.5)	26 (20.3)	0.5	26 (23.4)	0.9	0	0.03
RSV	36 (19.9)	13 (24.5)	23 (18.0)	0.3	20 (18.0)	0.3	3 (17.6)	0.7
Parainfuenza 1, 2, 3	35 (19.3)	11 (20.8)	24 (18.8)	0.8	21 (18.9)	0.8	3 (17.6)	1
Influenza A, B	15 (8.3)	2 (3.8)	13 (10.2)	0.2	12 (10.8)	0.2	1 (5.9)	1
Human bocavirus	17 (9.4)	3 (5.7)	14 (10.9)	0.4	14 (12.6)	0.2	0	1
Adenovirus	10 (5.5)	2 (3.8)	8 (6.3)	0.7	7 (6.3)	0.7	1 (5.9)	1
Enterovirus	10 (5.5)	1 (1.9)	9 (7.0)	0.3	8 (7.2)	0.3	1 (5.9)	0.4
Human metapneumovirus	8 (4.4)	0	8 (6.3)	0.1	7 (6.3)	0.1	1 (5.9)	0.2

Results in n (%)

RSV respiratory syncytial virus

[a]Invasive disease was defined as positive blood culture (bacteraemia) and/or positive blood PCR for pneumococcus

H. influenzae type b vaccine according to information retrieved from their vaccination cards. Cough (98.9 %), fever (96.7 %), and difficulty breathing (86.1 %) were the most frequent complaints. Antibiotic use in the previous 72 h (21.3 %) and asthma (23.9 %) were reported.

The patients were classified as non-severe ($n = 53$; 29.3 %), severe ($n = 111$; 61.3 %), or very severe ($n = 17$; 9.4 %) CAP (Fig. 1) in accordance with the WHO severity criteria available in the 2000 decade. Table 1 shows demographic and clinical characteristics of patients in each severity subgroup. Children with non-severe CAP were older than those with severe or severe plus very severe CAP. No significant differences were found among distinct severity subgroups in regard to duration of illness prior to hospitalization. Likewise, no difference was found when the frequency of asthma was compared between children with non-severe or severe plus very severe CAP (23.1 % *vs.* 24.2 %, $p = 0.9$), as well as when the frequency of antibiotic use in the previous 72 h was compared (13.7 % *vs.* 24.4 %, $p = 0.1$).

Overall, 156 (86.2 %) patients had detected aetiology. Viral infection ($n = 84$; 46.4 %), bacterial infection ($n = 26$; 14.4 %) and mixed viral-bacterial infection ($n = 46$; 25.4 %) were identified. Table 2 depicts the overall frequency of the found aetiological agents along with the frequency of the positive laboratory tests. No significant difference was found in the frequency of detected aetiology when children who did or did not receive antibiotic in the 72 h prior to hospital admission were compared (86.8 % *vs.* 86.4 %, $p = 0.9$). Table 3 presents the comparison of different aetiologies among patients across distinct severity subgroups according to the WHO severity criteria in the 2000 decade. Aetiology was more likely to be determined in severe or very severe cases (89.8 %) compared to non-severe cases (77.4 %; $p = 0.03$). *C. trachomatis* infection was more frequent among severe (8.1 %) than non-severe (0 %) cases ($p = 0.03$). Rhinovirus was significantly uncommon ($p = 0.03$) among very severe cases (0 %) whereas 24.5 % of non-severe cases had rhinovirus found. Human metapneumovirus was detected only among severe (6.3 %) and very severe (5.9 %) patients. Pneumococcal infection increased across "non-severe" (13.2 %), "severe" (23.4 %), and "very severe" (35.3 %) cases (qui-squared test for trend $p = 0.04$). The frequency of bacterial and typical bacterial infection showed the same trend, being the statistical result borderline ($p = 0.06$). Infection by *C. pneumoniae* or *S. aureus* was not detected. Table 4 compares the frequency of the different aetiologies among patients across dinstict severity subgroups according to the WHO severity criteria published in the year 2013. In such analysis, rhinovirus was also significantly uncommon among severe cases in comparison with non-severe ones (0 % *vs.* 23.8 %; $p = 0.03$)

Table 4 Comparison between frequencies of different aetiologies among children with non-severe or severe and/or very severe community-acquired pneumonia according to the World Health Organization 2013 criteria

Aetiology	Severity by the World Health Organization 2013 criteria		
	Non-severe ($n = 164$)	Severe ($n = 17$)	p
Subgroups			
Detected	142 (86.6)	14 (82.4)	0.7
Viral infection	79 (48.2)	5 (29.4)	0.1
Bacterial infection	63 (38.4)	9 (52.9)	0.2
Typical bacterial infection	47 (28.7)	7 (41.2)	0.3
Atypical bacterial infection	16 (9.8)	2 (11.8)	0.7
Pathogens			
S. pneumoniae	33 (20.1)	6 (35.3)	0.2
Positive blood culture	6 (3.7)	2 (11.8)	0.2
Positive blood PCR	6 (3.7)	1 (5.9)	0.5
Invasive infection[a]	11 (6.7)	2 (11.8)	0.4
H. influenzae	12 (7.3)	1 (5.9)	1.0
M. pneumoniae	10 (6.1)	1 (5.9)	1.0
C. trachomatis	9 (5.5)	-	1.0
M. catarrhalis	4 (2.4)	-	1.0
S. negevensis	2 (1.2)	1 (5.9)	0.3
Rhinovirus	39 (23.8)	-	0.03
RSV	33 (20.1)	3 (17.6)	1.0
Parainfuenza 1, 2, 3	32 (19.5)	3 (17.6)	1.0
Influenza A, B	14 (8.5)	1 (5.9)	1.0
Human bocavirus	17 (10.4)	-	0.4
Adenovirus	9 (5.5)	1 (5.9)	1.0
Enterovirus	9 (5.5)	1 (5.9)	1.0
Human metapneumovirus	7 (4.3)	1 (5.9)	0.6

Results in n (%)
RSV respiratory syncytial virus
[a]Invasive disease was defined as positive blood culture (bacteraemia) and/or positive blood PCR for pneumococcus

Because of the difference in age distribution in regard to different severity subgroups, we analysed age in regard to detected aetiology, pneumococcal, *C. trachomatis*, rhinovirus, or human metapneumovirus infection (Table 5). Age distribution was only different when children infected with human metapneumovirus were analysed: they were younger than those without it ($p = 0.046$).

Among children with detected aetiology, by grouping cases with sole bacterial infection together with cases with mixed viral-bacterial infection in a subgroup labeled bacterial infection, in multivariable analysis controlled for age, bacterial infection did not affect severity upon admission, using the WHO severity criteria availabe either in the 2000 decade or in 2013 (Table 6).

Table 5 Comparison of age among children with or without specific aetiology

Characteristics	Compared subgroups		p
Detected aetiology	Yes ($n = 156$)	No ($n = 25$)	
Age (months)[a]	17 (10–27)	19 (11–30)	0.5
Pneumococcal infection	Yes ($n = 39$)	No ($n = 142$)	
Age (months)[a]	21 (11–31)	17 (10–27)	0.8
C. trachomatis	Yes ($n = 9$)	No ($n = 172$)	
Age (months)[a]	15 (4–23)	21 (10–28)	0.2
Rhinovirus infection	Yes ($n = 39$)	No ($n = 142$)	
Age (months)[a]	17 (9–34)	18 (11–27)	0.7
Human metapneumovirus infection	Yes ($n = 8$)	No ($n = 173$)	
Age (months)[a]	10 (5–18)	18 (11–28)	0.046

[a]Median (interquartile range)

Out of 156 patients with established aetiology, 91 (58.3 %) had infection caused by one pathogen and 65 (41.7 %) had infection caused by two or more pathogens. In the former group, 25 (27.5 %) cases had bacterial infection and 66 (72.5 %) had viral infection. Conversely, in the latter group, 46 (70.8 %) had viral-bacterial infection, 18 (27.7 %) had viral-viral infection, and 1 (1.5 %) had bacterial-bacterial infection. Severe or very severe CAP was detected among 67 (73.6 %) patients with single infection, and among 48 (73.8 %) patients with co-infections ($p = 1$). Among patients with detected aetiology, after excluding cases with co-infection, the frequency of sole bacterial infection was different among children with non-severe (12.5 %), severe (29.3 %) or very severe (55.6 %) CAP cases ($p = 0.04$) (Table 7). Furthermore, by considering only the 91 cases with aetiology detected and without co-infection, sole bacterial infection was directly and independently associated with severity when the patients were grouped according to the WHO severity criteria available in the 2000 decade (Table 8). In this latter analysis, children with sole bacterial infection were compared with children with sole viral infection. The identified aetiological agents in the 25 cases with sole bacterial infection were *S. pneumoniae* ($n = 12$), *H. influenzae* ($n = 4$), *M. pneumoniae* ($n = 4$), *M. catarrhalis* ($n = 2$), *C. trachomatis* ($n = 2$), and *S. negevensis* ($n = 1$).

Cases with incomplete specimen collection (Fig. 1) were at random. In order to address systematic bias, the whole analysis was repeated with the inclusion of these cases and the results were the same (Additional file 1).

Discussion

This study showed that respiratory viral infections were detected in a reasonable proportion of cases in each severity subgroup. The frequencies of these infections did not differ across the distinct severity categories. Notably, one third to half of the cases classified as severe CAP had respiratory viral infections (Tables 3 and 4). Human metapneumovirus was the only viral pathogen exclusively found in the severe or very severe categories (Table 3). However, the difference was not significant. Pneumococcal infection increased across "non-severe", "severe", and "very severe" cases (Table 3). Only after excluding co-infections, sole bacterial infection was significantly more frequent among children with severe or very severe CAP (Table 8). No difference was found in the frequency of invasive typical bacterial infection (Tables 3 and 4).

Viral CAP has been recognized as a frequent entity among children, with an estimated occurrence of 100 million cases annually of which one third presents viral-bacterial co-infection [20]. Molecular diagnostics have played a fundamental role in obtaining these findings [21]. Indeed, viruses currently account for the largest proportion of CAP in preschool children in both developed and developing countries [22]. However, the pathogenesis and clinical impact of viral lung infection is not well understood [23]. Interestingly, herein, human metapneumovirus infection was only identified among severe or very severe cases. Human metapneumovirus has been identified as a single pathogen in childhood

Table 6 Multivariable logistic regression analysis of bacterial infection and age (predictors) and severity (outcome) upon admission of hospitalized children with community-acquired pneumonia

Predictors	Severity by the World Health Organization 2000 criteria		unadjOR (95 % CI)	p	adjustOR (95 % CI)	p
	Non-severe ($n = 53$)	Severe or very severe ($n = 128$)				
Bacterial infection[a]	16 (30.2)	56 (43.8)	1.5 (0.7–3.1)	0.3	1.7 (0.8–3.5)	0.2
Age (months)[b]	23 (13–35)	16 (9–26)	0.8 (0.6–0.99)	0.04	0.7 (0.5–1.0)	0.07
	Severity by the World Health Organization 2013 criteria					
	Non-severe ($n = 164$)	Severe ($n = 17$)				
Bacterial infection[a]	63 (38.4)	9 (52.9)	2.3 (0.7–7.1)	0.2	2.3 (0.7–7.3)	0.2
Age (months)[b]	17 (10–27)	18 (13–24)	1.0 (0.6–1.6)	1.0	0.9 (0.6–1.6)	0.8

[a]Results in n (%)
[b]Median (interquartile range)

Table 7 Comparison between frequencies of sole bacterial and sole viral infection among 91 children hospitalized with community-acquired pneumonia and detected aetiology, after excluding cases with co-infection

Aetiology	Severity by the World Health Organization 2000 criteria		
	Non-severe ($n = 24$)	Severe ($n = 58$)	Very severe ($n = 9$)
Sole bacterial infection	3 (12.5)	17 (29.3)	5 (55.6)
Sole viral infection	21 (87.5)	41 (70.7)	4 (44.4)

Results in n (%)
$p = 0.04$ for the frequency of sole bacterial infection across three distinct severity categories among patients with sole aetiological agent infection

CAP [24] and it was found more frequently among children with alveolar CAP than in controls [25]. Disease caused by human metapneumovirus may be severe enough to require hospitalization or even admission to a paediatric intensive care unit [26]. Our results support the importance of viral respiratory pathogens contributing to CAP severity.

Noteworthily, pneumococcal infection frequency increased across "non-severe", "severe", and "very severe" cases. Additionally, after excluding the cases with co-infection, sole bacterial infection was independently associated with severity (Table 8), that is, sole bacterial infection is associated with severe CAP when compared with sole viral infection. This finding suggests that bacteria may be more aggressive than viruses when there is one sole pathogen related to the CAP illness. These results are in accordance with the classical association between clinical severity and bacterial infection [4]. A recent systematic and meta-analysis reported an estimated increase in the rate of bacterial infection among severe cases in relation to patients with non-severe CAP. This rate was found to be even more important in the subgroup of the children who eventually die of the disease [27]. Nonetheless, no differences were found in the frequency of invasive bacterial disease (Tables 3 and 4). Figures from studies conducted among adults have shown that pneumococcal bacteraemia increases the risk of mortality and extra-pulmonary involvement in patients with pneumococcal CAP which was attributable to their older age and higher frequency of underlying medical conditions [28]. Host factors related to severity of disease have been recognized as confounders of the association between pneumococcal bacteraemia (invasive disease) and poor outcomes [29]. Herein, we excluded children with possible confounders for opportunistic infections and with co-morbidities.

Aetiology was more likely to be determined in severe or very severe cases (Table 3). Despite using an expanded range of diagnostic tests to search for each pathogen by different tools, aetiology was not detected in all cases. This finding may be attributable to unrecognized aetiological agents, or limitation of the employed methods, or both. Patients diagnosed as either severe or very severe cases were younger than those non-severe patients (Table 1). During the first three years of life whilst the immune system is maturing, particularly the production of IgG, the host is more vulnerable to infections [30]. Moreover, the first two years are often regarded as the most vulnerable period, especially for infections due to capsulated bacteria as pneumococcus and capsulated *H. influenzae.*

Our results must be viewed with caution. A higher number of cases would provide more precise results for comparing each pathogen's frequencies. That is, low statistical power due to relatively small sample size is the main limitation of this study. Although a wide range of tests to investigate a big number of aetiological agents was performed, it was difficult to assign causality even if aetiology was known, especially when there were co-detections. Aetiology was established as probable because lung tissue was not studied, for ethical reasons. However, different techniques were used, sometimes searching for the same pathogen to strengthen each result. Besides searching for the pathogen (by blood culture or PCR or antigen detection) we also searched for the host's

Table 8 Multivariable logistic regression analysis of bacterial infection and age (predictors) and severity (outcome) upon admission of hospitalized children with community-acquired pneumonia with documented infection by only one pathogen

Predictors	Severity by the World Health Organization 2000 criteria		unadjOR (95 % CI)	p	adjustOR (95 % CI)	p
	Non-severe ($n = 24$)	Severe or very severe ($n = 67$)				
Bacterial infection[a]	3 (12.5)	22 (32.8)	3.4 (0.9–12.7)	0.07	4.4 (1.1–17.6)	0.04
Age (months)[b]	19 (12–35)	17 (7–26)	0.8 (0.6–1.2)	0.3	0.7 (0.5–1.1)	0.1
	Severity by the World Health Organization 2013 criteria					
	Non-severe ($n = 82$)	Severe ($n = 9$)				
Bacterial infection[a]	20 (24.4)	5 (55.6)	3.9 (0.9–15.8)	0.06	3.8 (0.9–16.0)	0.07
Age (months)[b]	18 (10–26)	19 (14–31)	1.2 (0.7–2.1)	0.5	1.1 (0.6–1.9)	0.9

[a]Results in n (%)
[b]Median (interquartile range)

response to the presence of the pathogen. Pneumococcal aetiology was assessed by blood culture, paired pneumococcal antibodies titres and buffy-coat PCR. This approach is better than culturing or performing PCR of respiratory samples as *S. pneumoniae* commonly colonizes children's nasopharynx [31]. Antibody increase in paired serum samples due to acquisition of a new pneumococcal colonizing strain has been described to occur in <1 % to 3 % of the healthy children [32]. However, the final roles of pneumococcal serology and buffy-coat PCR are still open for discussion. The roles of non-capsulated *H. influenzae, M. catarrhalis,* and *S. negevensis* are less clear in the aetiology of childhood CAP. Likewise, serological diagnoses of Mycoplasma and Chlamydia infections are difficult. This approach may be acceptable, as no better approaches are currently available, particularly because Mycoplasma strains found in the upper respiratory samples can be detected by PCR without any relation to the current illness [33]. Additionally, the lack of pneumococcal and influenza vaccines resulted in difficulty to extend our findings to regions with high vaccine coverage. As such, in these regions, it is expected that the role of respiratory viruses is even more remarkable among children hospitalized with CAP, whilst pneumococcal infection is supposedly less frequent. In a recent study on CAP among 2,222 U.S. hospitalized children, viral (66 %), bacterial (8 %), or viral-bacterial (7 %) infections were reported [34]. However, the relative positivity rates between non-pneumococcal and non-influenza pathogens reported herein are still of interest. Additionally, it is important to note that severity was assessed on the basis of clinical findings present upon admission and not inferred from the evolution of the patients, as well as, severity was measured by using standardized protocols by a blinded investigator.

The WHO changed the severity CAP criteria in 2013 in order to make feasible the treatment at home of cases previously labeled as severe [19]. Several differences in the aetiologies frequencies were found when we used the WHO severity criteria available in the 2000 decade [18], but not all these differences were found when we used the WHO severity criteria published in 2013 [19] (Tables 3, 4 and 8). This finding raises the question about possible true differences among the subgroups formed by using the 2000 WHO severity criteria, as WHO changed these criteria to facilitate treatment logistic.

Conclusions

Respiratory viral infections were detected in a reasonable proportion of cases in each severity subgroup. A high proportion of patients with viral detections supports the need for more antiviral medicines and vaccines. Bacterial infection, particularly pneumococcal infection, was more likely among severe/very severe cases. This finding supports the use of empiric antibiotics to treat these patients, as it has been done in clinical practice.

Abbreviations

95 % CI, 95 % confidence interval; CAP, community-acquired pneumonia; ELISA, enzyme immune assay; IQR, interquartile range; MIF, microimmunofluorescence; NPA, nasopharyngeal aspirate; PCR, polymerase chain reaction; RSV, respiratory syncytial virus; WHO, World Health Organization.

Acknowledgements

Not applicable.

Funding

This study was supported by the Bahia State Agency for Research Funding (FAPESB) [grant number 52/2004] and the Brazilian Council for Scientific and Technological Development (CNPq) [grant number 303551/2011-9]. CMN-C is an investigator at CNPq. The funding agencies had no role in the design of the study and collection, analysis and interpretation of data and in writing the manuscript.

Authors' contributions

CMN-C designed the study and conducted the collection of data. OR contributed to the study design, data analysis and interpretation. ACN-C analysed the data and drafted the manuscript. CMN-C and OR proofread the manuscript. All authors read and approved the final manuscript.

Authors' information

Not applicable.

Competing interests

The authors declare that they have no competing interests.

Author details

[1]Bahiana School of Medicine, Bahiana Foundation for Science Development, Salvador, Bahia, Brazil. [2]Department of Paediatrics, Turku University and University Hospital, Turku, Finland. [3]Department of Paediatrics, Federal University of Bahia School of Medicine, Salvador, Bahia, Brazil.

References

1. Walker CL, Rudan I, Liu L, Nair H, Theodoratou E, Bhutta ZA, et al. Global burden of childhood pneumonia and diarrhoea. Lancet. 2013;381:1405–16.
2. Shann F. Etiology of severe pneumonia in children in developing countries. Pediatr Infect Dis. 1986;5:247–52.

3. Vuori-Holopainen E, Peltola H. Reappraisal of lung tap: review of an old method for better etiologic diagnosis of childhood pneumonia. Clin Infect Dis. 2001;32:715–26.
4. Gilani Z, Kwong YD, Levine OS, Deloria-Knoll M, Scott JA, O'Brien KL, et al. A literature review and survey of childhood pneumonia etiology studies: 2000-2010. Clin Infect Dis. 2012;54 Suppl 2:102–8.
5. Johansson N, Kalin M, Tiveljung-Lindell A, Giske CG, Hedlund J. Etiology of community-acquired pneumonia: increased microbiological yield with new diagnostic methods. Clin Infect Dis. 2010;50:202–9.
6. Howie SR, Morris GA, Tokarz R, Ebruke BE, Machuka EM, Ideh RC, et al. Etiology of severe childhood pneumonia in The Gambia West Africa determined by conventional and molecular microbiological analyses of lung and pleural aspirate samples. Clin Infect Dis. 2014;59:682–5.
7. Nohynek H, Eskola J, Kleemola M, Jalonen E, Saikku P, Leinonen M. Bacterial antibody assays in the diagnosis of acute lower respiratory tract infection in children. Pediatr Infect Dis J. 1995;14:478–84.
8. Saukkoriipi A, Palmu A, Kilpi T, Leinonen M. Real-time quantitative PCR for the detection of *Streptococcus pneumoniae* in the middle ear fluid of children with acute otitis media. Mol Cell Probes. 2002;16:385–90.
9. Atkinson TP, Waites KB. Mycoplasma pneumoniae infections in childhood. Pediatr Infect Dis J. 2014;33:92–4.
10. Morré SA, Munk C, Persson K, Krüger-Kjaer S, van Dijk R, Meijer CJ, et al. Comparison of three commercially available peptide-based immunoglobulin G (IgG) and IgA assays to microimmunofluorescence assay for detection of Chlamydia trachomatis antibodies. J Clin Microbiol. 2002;40:584–7.
11. Yamaguchi T, Yamazaki T, Inoue M, Mashida C, Kawagoe K, Ogawa M, et al. Prevalence of antibodies against Simkania negevensis in a healthy Japanese population determined by the microimmunofluorescence test. FEMS Immunol Med Microbiol. 2005;43:21–7.
12. Mäkelä MJ, Puhakka T, Ruuskanen O, Leinonen M, Saikku P, Kimpimäki M, et al. Viruses and bacteria in the etiology of the common cold. J Clin Microbiol. 1998;36:539–42.
13. Korppi M, Jartti T, Hedman K, Söderlund-Venermo M. Serologic diagnosis of human bocavirus infection in children. Pediatr Infect Dis J. 2010;29:387.
14. Nascimento-Carvalho CM, Ribeiro CT, Cardoso MR, Barral A, Araújo-Neto CA, Oliveira JR, et al. The role of respiratory viral infections among children hospitalized for community-acquired pneumonia in a developing country. Pediatr Infect Dis J. 2008;27:939–41.
15. Nascimento-Carvalho CM, Cardoso MR, Paldanius M, Barral A, Araújo-Neto CA, Saukkoriipi A, et al. Simkania negevensis infection among Brazilian children hospitalized with community-acquired pneumonia. J Infect. 2009;58:250–3.
16. Nascimento-Carvalho CM, Cardoso MR, Ruuskanen O, Lappalainen M. Sole infection by human metapneumovirus among children with radiographically diagnosed community-acquired pneumonia in a tropical region. Influenza Other Respir Viruses. 2011;5:285–7.
17. Nascimento-Carvalho CM, Cardoso MR, Meriluoto M, Kemppainen K, Kantola K, Ruuskanen O, et al. Human bocavirus infection diagnosed serologically among children admitted to hospital with community-acquired pneumonia in a tropical region. J Med Virol. 2012;84:253–8.
18. World Health Organization. Management of the child with a serious infection or severe malnutrition: guidelines for care at the first-referral level in developing countries. 2000. http://apps.who.int/iris/bitstream/10665/42335/1/WHO_FCH_CAH_00.1.pdf. Page 20. Accessed 2 May 2003.
19. World Health Organization. Pocket book of hospital care for children. Guidelines for the management of common childhood illnesses. 2nd ed. 2013. http://www.who.int/maternal_child_adolescent/documents/child_hospital_care/en/index.html. Page 81. Accessed 7 June 2013.
20. Ruuskanen O, Lahti E, Jennings LC, Murdoch DR. Viral pneumonia. Lancet. 2011;377:1264–75.
21. Nolte FS. Molecular diagnostics for detection of bacterial and viral pathogens in community-acquired pneumonia. Clin Infect Dis. 2008;47 Suppl 3:123–6.
22. Mameli C, Zuccotti GV. The impact of viral infections in children with community-acquired pneumonia. Curr Infect Dis Rep. 2013;15:197–202.
23. Ruuskanen O, Jarvinen A. What is the real role of respiratory viruses in severe community-acquired pneumonia? Clin Infec Dis. 2014;59:71–3.
24. Woods CR, Bryant KA. Viral infections in children with community-acquired pneumonia. Curr Infect Dis Rep. 2013;15:177–83.
25. Wolf DG, Greenberg D, Shemer-Avni Y, Givon-Lavi N, Bar-Ziv J, Dagan R. Association of human metapneumovirus with radiologically diagnosed community-acquired alveolar pneumonia in young children. J Pediatr. 2010;156:115–20.
26. Principi N, Esposito S. Paediatric human metapneumovirus infection: epidemiology, prevention and therapy. J Clin Virol. 2014;59:141–7.
27. Rudan I, O'Brien KL, Nair H, Liu L, Theodoratou E, Qazi S, et al. Epidemiology and etiology of childhood pneumonia in 2010: estimates of incidence, severe morbidity, mortality, underlying risk factors and causative pathogens for 192 countries. J Glob Health. 2013;3:010401.
28. Lin SH, Lai CC, Tan CK, Liao WH, Hsueh PR. Outcomes of hospitalized patients with bacteraemic and non-bacteraemic community-acquired pneumonia caused by Streptococcus pneumoniae. Epidemiol Infect. 2011;139:1307–16.
29. Bordón J, Peyrani P, Brock GN, Blasi F, Rello J, File T, et al. The presence of pneumococcal bacteremia does not influence clinical outcomes in patients with community-acquired pneumonia: results from the Community-Acquired-Pneumonia Organization (CAPO) International Cohort study. Chest. 2008;133:618–24.
30. Ishimine P. Fever without source in children 0 to 36 months of age. Pediatr Clin North Am. 2006;53:167–94.
31. Bogaert D, Sluijter M, Toom NL, Mitchell TJ, Goessens WH, Clarke SC, et al. Dynamics of pneumococcal colonization in healthy Dutch children. Microbiology. 2006;152:377–85.
32. Korppi M, Leinonen M, Ruuskanen O. Pneumococcal serology in children's respiratory infections. Eur J Clin Microbiol Infect Dis. 2008;27:167–75.
33. Spuesens EB, Fraaij PL, Visser EG, Hoogenboezem T, Hop WC, van Adrichem LN, et al. Carriage of Mycoplasma pneumoniae in the upper respiratory tract of symptomatic and asymptomatic children: an observational study. PLoS Med. 2013;10:e1001444.
34. Jain S, Williams DJ, Arnold SR, Ampofo K, Bramley AM, Reed C, et al. Community-acquired pneumonia requiring hospitalization among U.S. children. N Engl J Med. 2015;372:835–45.

8

Appraisal of clinical practice guidelines on community-acquired pneumonia in children with AGREE II instrument

Zhenwei Xie[1,2†], Xiaoling Wang[1†], Lin Sun[3], Jun Liu[4], Yan Guo[4], Baoping Xu[4], Libo Zhao[1*] and Adong Shen[3*]

Abstract

Background: Community-acquired pneumonia (CAP) remains a major cause of morbidity and mortality worldwide among children. The growing number of guidelines have been accompanied with a growing concern about variance and conflicts among guideline recommendations. There is a need to critically appraise clinical practice guidelines (CPGs) in order to ensure safe and effective practices.

Methods: A literature search was systematically conducted in English and Chinese major academic databases (from January 2000 to March 2015). CPGs related to CAP in children were evaluated by four independent assessors, according to AGREE II instruments. Standardized domain scores were calculated for each guideline. Inter-rater reliability was assessed by intraclass correlation coefficient. The software used for analysis was SPSS 17.0.

Results: A total of 10 guidelines met the inclusion criteria and were appraised. Scope and purpose (69.03 %) and clarity of presentation (83.33 %) achieved relative high scores, while the scores of the other four domains were low: stakeholder involvement (42.78 %), rigour of development (44.95 %), applicability (37.60 %), and editorial independence (23.74 %). 3 guidelines were strongly recommended as a result of the overall scores were greater than 60 %.

Conclusion: The qualities of CPGs for CAP in children were generally acceptable with several flaws. Stakeholder involvement, rigour of development, applicability and editorial independence should be considered and well described in the future development of CPGs.

Keywords: Clinical practice guidelines, Community-acquired pneumonia, Children, Quality assessment, AGREE II

Background

Community-acquired pneumonia (CAP) is defined as an acute infection of lower respiratory tract occurring outside hospital. It remains a major cause of morbidity and mortality among children in developing and developed countries. In developing countries, CAP has an incidence of 0.29 episodes per child-year and a mortality rate of 1.3–2.6 % [1, 2]. The incidence of CAP is lower in developed countries, with an incidence of about 0.05 episodes per child-year, however, it is still one of the leading causes of hospitalization [3, 4]. In certain conditions, it would occur repeatedly and cause harm to children without proper and complete treatments. Meantime, it will bring heavy burden for national public health care systems.

Guidelines for the management of CAP in children have been increasingly produced and disseminated in recent years. Generally, globalization and uniformity between centers worldwide in patient management has become a trend. However, acceptance of evidence-based medicine (EBM) varies around the world. The growing number of guidelines has been accompanied with a growing concern about variance and conflicts among guideline recommendations. Therefore, there can be huge differences between countries or regions in respect

* Correspondence: libozhao2011@163.com; shenad16@hotmail.com
†Equal contributors
[1]Department of Pharmacy, Beijing Children's Hospital, Capital Medical University, Beijing 100045, China
[3]Key Laboratory of Pediatric Respiratory Infection Diseases, Beijing Pediatric Research Institute, Beijing Children's Hospital, Capital Medical University, Beijing 100045, China
Full list of author information is available at the end of the article

to guideline qualities. Hence, it is urgent to identify existing high quality guidelines and make guideline developers follow methodological standards while developing guidelines.

The appraisal of guidelines for research and evaluation II (AGREE II), consisting of 6 domains covering 23 key items, is initially developed from AGREE and updated in 2010. The purpose of this instrument is to evaluate the strengths and limitations of guidelines; to provide methodology for development of guidelines; and to present guidance for reporting recommendations. It is a widely-used instrument and remains the current golden standard for guideline appraisal [5, 6].

The quality of CAP guidelines has not been systematically evaluated till now. Thus, the aim of this study was to access the available guidelines for the treatment of children with CAP and to determine the methodological quality and reliability of guidelines.

Methods

Literature search

A literature search was systematically conducted in English and Chinese major academic databases (from January 2000 to March 2015). English databases were MEDLINE, EMBASE, Guidelines International Network (GIN), National Guideline Clearinghouse (NGC), Chinese databases were Chinese Biomedical Literature Database (CBM), China National Knowledge Internet (CNKI), VIP Database and Wanfang Database. Key words were "community-acquired", "pneumonia", "children", "pediatric", "guideline", "guidance", "recommendation", "management", and "consensus".

Inclusion and exclusion criteria

Guidelines published in Chinese or English, which addressed diagnoses and treatments of CAP for children under 18 years of age were included. Guidelines that are systematic reviews, editorials, short summaries, and other literature explaining or evaluating guidelines were excluded. If guidelines have been fully updated, the latest version were evaluated and the old versions were excluded.

Data extraction

Two of the investigators (Z.W.X and L.B.Z) searched the database, selected guidelines independently and determined if they warranted inclusion in this study and then extracted general characteristics of the guideline. Disagreements were resolved by consulting a third expert opinion (A.D.S). The following information was extracted, such as title of guidelines, country or region, publication date, affiliation or organization, developed method, quality of evidence and filled in an established standard table on Microsoft Excel 2013.

Appraisal guidelines

The AGREE II instrument was used to assess the methodological quality of included guidelines. It contains 23 key items of 6 domains, such as scope and purpose, stakeholder involvement, rigour of development, clarity of presentation, applicability, editorial independence, and overall guideline assessment. Each item was scored on a scale of 1–7, with 1 being strongly disagree and 7 being strongly agree. Each domain was calculated by summing up all the scores of the individual items in a domain and then standardizing as follows: (obtained score - minimal possible score) / (maximal possible score - minimal possible score).

Quality assessment were performed independently by four trained reviewers (Z.W. X, L.S, J.L, and Y.G). They conducted an independent review of the quality of each eligible guideline. Disagreement between reviewers was resolved through consensus or by consulting an independent expert adjudicator (L.B.Z). Final average appraisal scores and standard deviations for each domain and scaled domain percentages were calculated.

Intraclass correlation coefficient (ICC) was used as a measure of agreement between reviewers. The ICC values was carried out by SPSS v.17.0 and applied to each guidelines.

Finally, the overall guideline assessment was evaluated. A guideline would be "recommended" if overall scores were greater than 60 %, "recommended with modifications" at scores between 30 % and 60 %, and "not recommended" at scores less than 30 %.

Statistical analysis

Standardized domain scores were calculated according to methods described in the AGREE II user manual. A descriptive statistical analysis was used to summarize the data. Subgroup comparison between evidence-based guidelines and non evidence-based guidelines were performed by t-test. All tests were two-sided, and P values < 0.05 were considered statistically significant. All statistics were calculated using SPSS v.17.0.

Results

A total of 827 records were identified through comprehensive database search and 22 additional records more were identified through Google search engine. 56 were exclude due to duplication, and the remaining 771 were screened by titles and abstracts. 88 were screened by full text articles for eligibility. 42 review articles, 6 guidelines before 2000, 13 interpretation of guidelines, 9 outcome on empirical treatments, 2 old version, 1 involving other disease guideline, 2 adult guidelines, 2 old version (Canadian 97, and Thorax 2009) and 3 other foreign languages (Brazilian, Spanish and Italian guidelines) were excluded. Finally, 10 guidelines were identified and involved in the analysis [7–17]. The details of review process was summarized in Fig. 1. The characteristics of each included guideline were presented in Table 1.

Scope and purpose

This domain addressed the overall objectives, health issues and target population. The score of this domain was relatively high (mean 69.03 %, range: 23.61–95.83 %), indicating most guidelines met the criteria of this domain.

Stakeholder involvement

This domain assess whether the relevant professional group is represented, the patients' views and preference has been sought, and the definition of target users of the guideline are clearly defined. The score of this domain was 42.78 % (range: 9.70–76.39 %). A few guidelines [7, 8, 10, 13, 16, 17] could describe the relevant professional group, however, few guidelines seek the preference of target populations.

Rigour of development

This domain is the core of guideline methodology and mainly focus on the method of evidence search, grading, summarizing and the formulation of the recommendation. The score of scope was 44.95 % (range: 17.19–79.69 %).

Clarify of presentation

This domain evaluates the presentation and the format. The score of this domain was 83.33 % (range: 69.44–94.44 %). Most guidelines recommendations were specific. Different options for management of the condition were clearly presented, and key recommendation was easily identifiable.

Applicability

This domain discusses the organization barriers, cost implications and monitoring criteria. The assessment result was 37.50 % (range: 17.71–61.46 %). Most guidelines failed to consider it during the guideline development.

Editorial independence

This domain focuses on the funding issues and competing interests of all contributing members. The score of this domain was 23.74 % (range: 0–87.50 %). Both evidence-based guidelines and non evidence-based guidelines achieved low scores in this domain.

Agreement among reviewers

ICC for each guideline is listed in Table 2. Eight of 10 ICC values were (>75 %) excellent. No ICC values were less than 45 %. The reliability of this reviewers were acceptable.

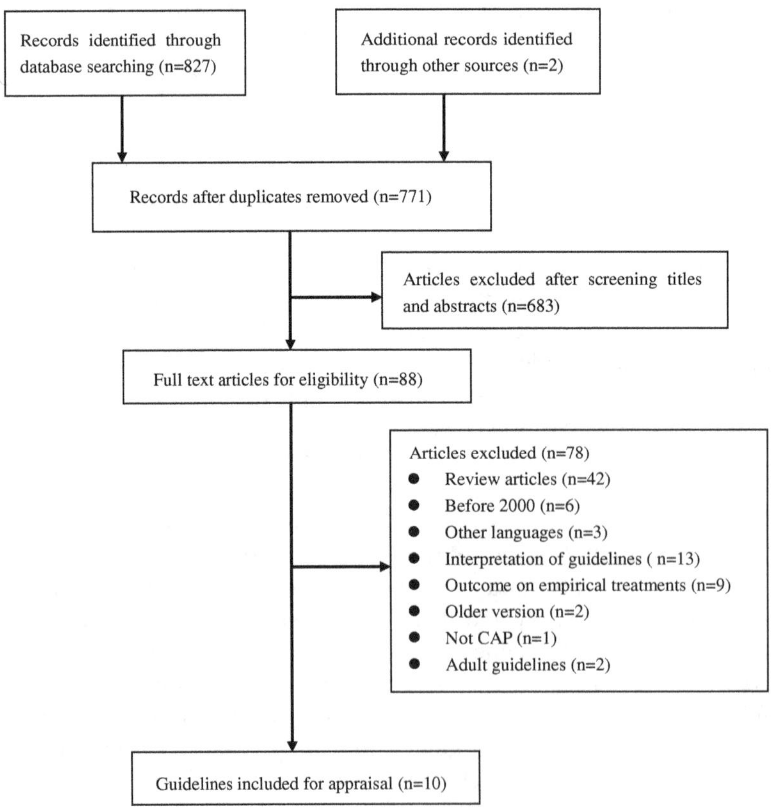

Fig. 1 Flow chart of searching and selecting guidelines

Table 1 Characteristics of 10 included guidelines

Clinical practice guideline	Country or region	Language of guidelines	Publication date	Affiliation or organization	Developed method	Quality of evidence
[7]	United States	English	2011	Pediatric Infectious Diseases Society and the Infectious Diseases Society of America	Evidenced-based	GRADE
[8]	United Kingdom	English	2011	British Thoracic Society Community Acquired Pneumonia in Children Guideline Group	Evidenced-based	Self designed grading system
[10]	South African	English	2005	Working Groups of the Paediatric Assembly of the South African Thoracic Society	Literature review	Not mentioned
[13, 14]	China	Chinese	2013	Subspecialty Group of Respiratory Diseases, The Society of Pediatrics, Chinese Medical Association	Literature review	Self designed grading system
[16]	Malaysia	English	2004	Ministry of Health Malaysia Academy of Medicine Maylaysia	Evidenced-based	SIGN
[12]	Taiwan	English	2007	Taiwan Pediatric Working Group for "Guideline on the management of CAP in children"	Literature review	Not mentioned
[9]	Japan	English	2007	Japanese Society of Pediatric Pulmonology and the Japanese Society for Pediatric Infectious Diseases	Literature review	Not mentioned
[15]	WHO	English	2013	Word Health Organization	Literature review	Not mentioned
[11]	Canada	English	2011	Canadian Paediatric Society, Infectious Diseases and Immunization Committee	Literature review	Not mentioned
[17]	United States	English	2006	Cincinnati children's hospital medical center	Evidenced-based	Self designed grading system

Overall quality assessment of guideline

3 CPGs [7, 8, 17] were strongly recommended as results of the overall scores greater than 60 %. 4 CPGs [10, 13, 15, 16] were "recommended with modifications", whose scores between 30 % and 60 %. 3 CPGs [9, 11, 12] were "not recommended" due to all items scores being less than 30 %. Finally, IDSA guideline [7] achieved a relative high score among the 10 guidelines. This provides a reference of methodology for developing other CAP guidelines. The details of the appraisal results are presented in Table 2. AGREE II domain scores are plotted for each guideline for comparison are showed in Fig. 2.

Table 2 Standardized scores of each domain by AGREE II of guidelines

Guideline	Scope and purpose (%)	Stakeholder involvement (%)	Rigor of development (%)	Clarity of presentation (%)	Applicability (%)	Editorial independence (%)	ICC	Overall assessment
[7]	95.83	73.61	79.17	94.44	54.17	87.50	0.82	Strongly recommended
[8]	93.06	37.50	79.69	93.06	61.46	58.33	0.73	Strongly recommended
[10]	81.95	34.72	32.29	76.39	35.41	33.33	0.88	Recommended with modifications
[13, 14]	80.56	45.83	30.21	80.56	33.33	0	0.88	Recommended with modifications
[16]	79.17	76.39	60.94	86.11	33.33	0	0.84	Recommended with modifications
[12]	23.61	11.11	19.27	86.11	17.71	0	0.91	Not recommended
[9]	61.11	9.70	23.44	83.33	25.00	0	0.91	Not recommended
[15]	52.78	48.61	32.81	73.61	35.42	29.1	0.69	Recommended with modifications
[11]	30.56	15.28	17.19	69.44	31.25	0	0.86	Not recommended
[17]	91.67	75.00	74.48	90.28	47.92	29.17	0.82	Strongly recommended
Mean (range)	69.03 (23.61–95.83)	42.78 (9.70–76.39)	44.95 (17.19–79.69)	83.33 (69.44–94.44)	37.50 (17.71–61.46)	23.74 (0–87.50)	/	/

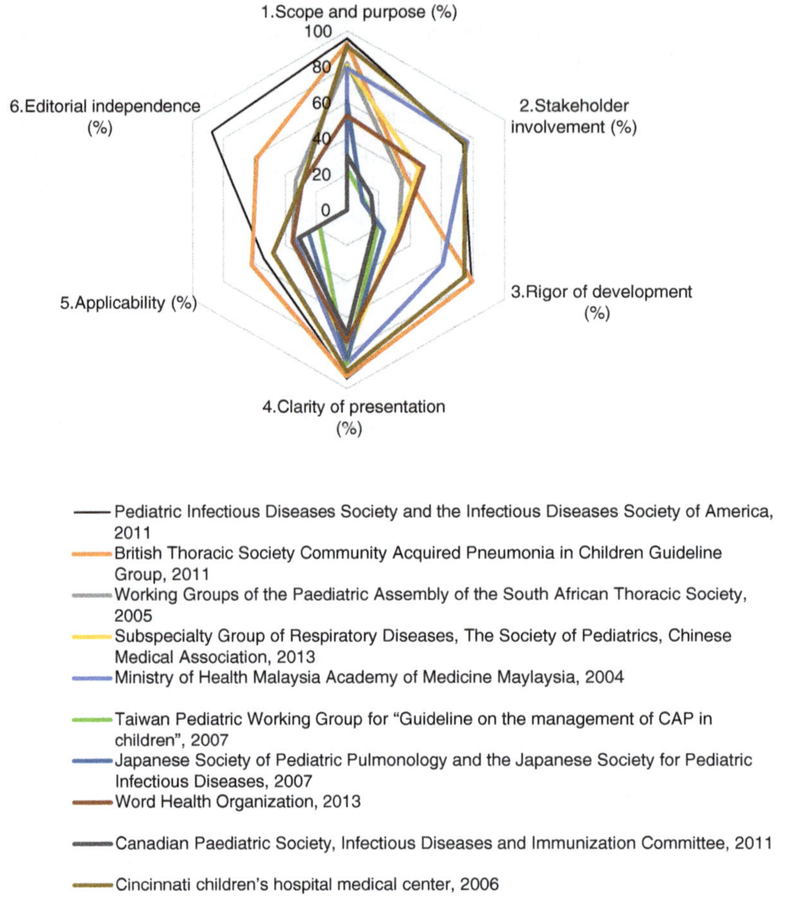

Fig. 2 AGREE II domain scores are plotted for each guideline for comparison

Of the guidelines involved, 4 were evidence-based guidelines which processed details of evidence scale, on the other hand, the remaining 6 were more consensuses than evidence-based guidelines. Compared with non evidence-based guidelines, evidence-based guidelines obtained significant higher scores in nearly all domains except "editorial independence". Table 3 shows a subgroup analysis of the involved guidelines.

Discussion

This study discussed a qualitative evaluation of the CPGs on CAP in children with the AGREE II guideline assessment. Eventually, 10 guidelines were included. In this study, we demonstrated that the scores of CAP guidelines were higher than an average international quality level [18], especially "Scope and purpose" and "Clarity of presentation". Compared to the guidelines published from 1980 to 2007, current guidelines could specifically describe the purpose of the guidelines and also clearly present the recommendation. However, in some domains the scores were much lower when compared with contemporary guidelines in respect to pediatric infectious diseases [19], such as "rigour of development" and "editorial independence". The average

Table 3 Comparison of mean quality scores among evidence-based guidelines and non evidence-based guidelines

Subgroup	Domain (Mean ± SD)					
	Scope and purpose (%)	Stakeholder involvement (%)	Rigor of development (%)	Clarity of presentation (%)	Applicability (%)	Editorial independence %
Evidence-based guideline	89.93 ± 7.38	65.63 ± 18.78	73.57 ± 8.74	90.97 ± 3.67	49.22 ± 11.95	43.75 ± 37.65
Non Evidence-based guideline	55.10 ± 24.51*	27.54 ± 17.71*	25.87 ± 6.83*	78.24 ± 6.25*	29.69 ± 7.02*	10.41 ± 16.17

Data are presented as mean ± standard deviation. *$P < 0.05$

score of the evidence-based guidelines on pediatric infectious diseases respectively was 76.04 % and 81.25 %. Hence, there is still potential improvement with respect to qualities of pediatric CAP guidelines.

It was concluded from our results that CPGs tackling CAP on children account for a small amount compared with adults. A great number of countries or associations ignored to develop guidelines which are targeted to this particular group. Pediatric patients are tend to be more vulnerable in nature, therefore, it is essential to ensure that guidelines are developed under strict criteria. On the other hand, a great number of organizations failed to translate the CAP guidelines into English and hindered the efficiency of health science communication. Efforts are needed to translate guideline into a universal language and to assist health professions in better mastering strictly developed guidelines and to rectify discrepancies and promote evidence-based practices to enhance patient outcomes.

In our study, it should be noted that "scope and purpose" and "clarity of presentation" achieved a relative high scores among the six domains, which indicated that most guidelines fully satisfied this criteria. Most guidelines could fully describe the overall objective and their specific clinical issues. For "stakeholder involvement", relevant professionals in the development process were involved in most guidelines and target population was declared. However, the guideline developers did not seek the preference of target populations resulting in a decrease in score of this domain.

"Rigour of development" was considered to be one of the most crucial domain for the assessment of guideline development. In our study, this domain varied in guidelines, for evidence based guideline, it obtained higher scores, while consensus not. A strong recommendation should not solely be based on expert opinion. Guideline developers should adhere to a standardized evidence-based evaluation system. In this study, only 4 [7, 8, 16, 17] guidelines clearly described the criteria for selecting the evidence, as well as strengths and limitations of the evidence. The quality may be improved by involving methodologists in the guideline development. It is also expected that CPGs should grade the quality of evidence on an existing well recognized grading system such as GRADE (Grading of Recommendations Assessment, Development and Evaluation). GRADE grading system was first introduced in 2004 for access the quality of evidence and strength of recommendation. Gradually, it was recognized by more than 30 organizations including WHO and Cochrane Collaboration. Although the 10 guidelines included in our study were published after 2005, only 1 CPG [7] use the GRADE system. 1 CPG [16] use SIGN (The Scottish Intercollegiate Guidelines Network) and 3 CPGs [8, 13, 17] guidelines used their own developing system. We suggest further guidelines should use a comparable uniform grading system to evaluate the quality of evidence and strength of recommendations. In this domain, a procedure of updating the guidelines was neglected in most guidelines. Only 2 CPGs [16, 17] referred the updating procedures. It is recommended that guidelines be updated at 3-year intervals, as new evidence may result in substantial changes to the recommendations [20].

Our study found that "applicability" scored low among the six domains. A great number of guidelines lack of describing facilitators and barriers to its application, advice and/or tools on how the recommendations can be put into practice. Guideline would rate high if the potential resource implications of applying the recommendations had been considered, such as a summary document, a quick reference guide, and educational tool. In order to ensure the feasibility of clinical practice, it is also suggested that a pilot test for the applicability of new guidelines should be performed before its publication. These items should be taken into consideration when the following guidelines are developing.

Editorial independence was also neglected in a great deal of guidelines. Only 3 [7, 10, 17] guidelines reported detailed information on potential conflicts of interest. Conflicts of interest are the most common source of bias in guideline development [21]. There should be an explicit statement that all group members have declared whether they have any competing interests. It may be suggested by making it mandatory for guideline developers to list the potential competing interests in the documents.

A strength of our study is that we used AGREE II instrument to assess the methodological quality of guidelines related to CAP in children, which has no related appraisal research on this particular group. Furthermore, our team consisted of pediatric clinical experts and pharmacist with extensive experience in clinical guidelines appraisal.

There are limitations within this study that should be noted. Firstly, the guidelines involved are confined to English and Chinese. Secondly, the literature search only identified published guidelines in pediatric pneumonia. It is possible that some guidelines may have been missed by the search, especially those that combined pediatric and adult recommendations. Thirdly, the AGREE II instrument is a tool that assesses the methodological rigour and transparency in which a guideline is developed [22, 23]. It informs what information and how information ought to be reported in guideline. However, there is no threshold for discrimination from high quality to low quality CPGs. Thus, the guidelines quality would be left to the appraisers to identify and the scores of an AGREE II evaluation have to be interpreted with caution and confined to a particular situation.

Conclusion

Overall, this study appraised quality scores of the CPGs on CAP in children. The appraisal results showed acceptable. The developers are suggested to pay more attention to rigour of development, applicability, and editorial independence during the development process. The AGREE II instrument should be adopted by guideline developers to improve the applicability of guidelines.

Abbreviations

AGREE II, the appraisal of guidelines for research and evaluation II; CAP, community-acquired pneumonia; CBM, Chinese databases were Chinese Biomedical Literature Database; CNKI, China National Knowledge Internet; CPGs, clinical practice guidelines; EBM, evidence-based medicine; GIN, Guidelines International Network; GRADE, Grading of Recommendations Assessment, Development and Evaluation; ICC, intraclass correlation coefficient; IDSA, Infectious Diseases Society of America; NGC, National Guideline Clearinghouse; SIGN, The Scottish Intercollegiate Guidelines Network

Acknowledgements

The authors gratefully acknowledge the support by WHO-China Biennial Collaborative Projects 2014–2015.

Funding

The Project was supported by WHO-China Biennial Collaborative Projects 2014–2015.

Authors' contributions

LBZ and XLW conceived and designed the study. ZWX and LBZ searched the database and consulting ADS when there was a disagreement. ZWX, LS, JL and YG appraised the guidelines. XLW, ADS and BPX participated in the phase of discussion on results and critically reviewed the work. ZWX wrote the initial draft and was responsible for data management. LBZ, ADS and XLW provided critical revision on subsequent drafts and approved of the manuscript in its final form. All authors read and approved the final manuscript.

Competing interests

The authors declare that they have no competing interests.

Author details

[1]Department of Pharmacy, Beijing Children's Hospital, Capital Medical University, Beijing 100045, China. [2]School of Pharmaceutical Science, Peking University, Beijing 100191, China. [3]Key Laboratory of Pediatric Respiratory Infection Diseases, Beijing Pediatric Research Institute, Beijing Children's Hospital, Capital Medical University, Beijing 100045, China. [4]Department of Respiratory, Beijing Children's Hospital, Capital Medical University, Beijing 100045, China.

References

1. Ranganathan SC, Sonnappa S. Pneumonia and other respiratory infections. Pediatr Clin North Am. 2009;56(1):135–56. xi.
2. Chisti MJ, Tebruegge M, La Vincente S, Graham SM, Duke T. Pneumonia in severely malnourished children in developing countries - mortality risk, aetiology and validity of WHO clinical signs: a systematic review. Tropical Med Int Health. 2009;14(10):1173–89.
3. Atkinson M, Yanney M, Stephenson T, Smyth A. Effective treatment strategies for paediatric community-acquired pneumonia. Expert Opin Pharmacother. 2007;8(8):1091–101.
4. Rudan I, Boschi-Pinto C, Biloglav Z, Mulholland K, Campbell H. Epidemiology and etiology of childhood pneumonia. Bull World Health Organ. 2008;86(5):408–16.
5. Brouwers MC, Kho ME, Browman GP, Burgers JS, Cluzeau F, Feder G, Fervers B, Graham ID, Grimshaw J, Hanna SE, et al. AGREE II: advancing guideline development, reporting, and evaluation in health care. Prev Med. 2010;51(5):421–4.
6. Vlayen J, Aertgeerts B, Hannes K, Sermeus W, Ramaekers D. A systematic review of appraisal tools for clinical practice guidelines: multiple similarities and one common deficit. Int J Qual Health Care. 2005;17(3):235–42.
7. Bradley JS, Byington CL, Shah SS, Alverson B, Carter ER, Harrison C, Kaplan SL, Mace SE, McCracken Jr GH, Moore MR, et al. The management of community-acquired pneumonia in infants and children older than 3 months of age: clinical practice guidelines by the Pediatric Infectious Diseases Society and the Infectious Diseases Society of America. Clin Infect Dis. 2011;53(7):e25–76.
8. Harris M, Clark J, Coote N, Fletcher P, Harnden A, McKean M, Thomson A, British Thoracic Society Standards of Care C. British Thoracic Society guidelines for the management of community acquired pneumonia in children: update 2011. Thorax. 2011;66 Suppl 2:ii1–23.
9. Uehara S, Sunakawa K, Eguchi H, Ouchi K, Okada K, Kurosaki T, Suzuki H, Tsutsumi H, Haruta T, Mitsuda T, et al. Japanese Guidelines for the Management of Respiratory Infectious Diseases in Children 2007 with focus on pneumonia. Pediatr Int. 2011;53(2):264–76.
10. Zar HJ, Jeena P, Argent A, Gie R, Madhi SA, Working Groups of the Paediatric Assembly of the South African Thoracic S. Diagnosis and management of community-acquired pneumonia in childhood–South African Thoracic Society Guidelines. S Afr Med J. 2005;95(12 Pt 2):977–81. 984–990.
11. Le Saux N, Robinson J. Pneumonia in healthy Canadian children and youth: Practice points for management. Paediatr Child Health. 2011;16(7):417–24.
12. Lee PI, Chiu CH, Chen PY, Lee CY, Lin TY, Taiwan Pediatric Working Group for Guideline on the Management of CAPiC. Guidelines for the management of community-acquired pneumonia in children. Acta Paediatr Taiwan. 2007;48(4):167–80.
13. Subspecialty Group of Respiratory Diseases TSoPCMA, Editorial Board CJoP. Guidelines for management of community acquired pneumonia in children (the revised edition of 2013) (I). Zhonghua Er Ke Za Zhi. 2013;51(10):745–52.
14. Subspecialty Group of Respiratory Diseases TSoP, Chinese Medical Association The Editorial Board CJoP. Guidelines for management of community acquired pneumonia in children (the revised edition of 2013) (II). Zhonghua Er Ke Za Zhi. 2013;51(11):856–62.
15. World Health Organization. Pocket book of hospital care for children. Guidelines for the management of common illnesses with limited resources. Geneva: WHO Press; 2005. p. 72–81.
16. Azizi H NM, Bilkis B: Clinical Practice Guidelines on pneumonia and respiratory tract infections in children. Academy of Medicine of Malaysia Clinical Practice Guidelines (CPGs). 2002, Available at: http://pdfsr.com/pdf/2004-cpg-rational-antibiotic-utilisation-in-selected-paediatric-conditions. (accessed Jan10,2013).
17. Community Acquired Pneumonia Guideline Team Cincinnati Children's Hospital Medical Center: Evidence-based care guideline for medical management of Community Acquired Pneumonia in children 60 days to 17 years of age. http://www.docin.com/p-375158193.html (Guideline 14):1–16.
18. Alonso-Coello P, Irfan A, Sola I, Gich I, Delgado-Noguera M, Rigau D, Tort S, Bonfill X, Burgers J, Schunemann H. The quality of clinical practice guidelines over the last two decades: a systematic review of guideline appraisal studies. Qual Saf Health Care. 2010;19(6):e58.
19. Wilby KJ, Black EK, MacLeod C, Wiens M, Lau TT, Paiva MA, Gorman S. Critical appraisal of clinical practice guidelines in pediatric infectious diseases. Int J Clin Pharm. 2015;37(5):1-9.
20. Shekelle PG, Ortiz E, Rhodes S, Morton SC, Eccles MP, Grimshaw JM, Woolf SH. Validity of the Agency for Healthcare Research and Quality clinical practice guidelines: how quickly do guidelines become outdated? JAMA. 2001;286(12):1461–7.

21. Detsky AS. Sources of bias for authors of clinical practice guidelines. CMAJ. 2006;175(9):1033–5.
22. Brouwers MC, Kho ME, Browman GP, Burgers JS, Cluzeau F, Feder G, Fervers B, Graham ID, Grimshaw J, Hanna SE, et al. AGREE II: advancing guideline development, reporting and evaluation in health care. CMAJ. 2010;182(18):E839–842.
23. MacDermid JC, Brooks D, Solway S, Switzer-McIntyre S, Brosseau L, Graham ID. Reliability and validity of the AGREE instrument used by physical therapists in assessment of clinical practice guidelines. BMC Health Serv Res. 2005;5(1):18.

9

Refractory wheezing in Chinese children under 3 years of age: bronchial inflammation and airway malformation

Wenjing Gu[1], Wujun Jiang[1], Xinxing Zhang[1], Zhengrong Chen[1], Yongdong Yan[1], Li Huang[1], Meijuan Wang[1], Xuejun Shao[2], Shuhui Wang[1] and Wei Ji[1*]

Abstract

Background: Wheezing is a common symptom in early childhood. However, refractory wheezing is difficult to treat, and it may thus account for extensive use of medical resources. It is therefore important to improve our understanding of the pathophysiology of refractory childhood wheezing.

Methods: In this descriptive study, we studied 156 children with refractory wheezing using fiberoptic bronchoscopy and bronchoalveolar lavage (BAL), and compared the results with a control group of 46 children with various pulmonary diseases but no wheezing. Etiology and cell classification were analyzed for each BAL sample.

Results: Overall, 21.8 % of children with refractory wheezing had airway malformations including tracheomalacia, airway stenosis, and tracheal bronchus. The incidence of airway malformations increased to 31 % in infants under 12 months of age. A significant increase in neutrophil ratio and decrease in macrophage ratio were observed in BAL from children with refractory wheezing compared with controls. Pathogen infection led to a higher ratio of neutrophils in the wheezing group compared with controls. However, there were no significant differences in neutrophil ratios among children with various pathogen infections. Furthermore, children with refractory wheezing had a high rate of *Mycoplasma pneumoniae* infection.

Conclusions: Airway malformations might play an important role in children under 3 years of age with refractory wheezing, especially in infants under 12 months of age. Neutrophil-mediated airway inflammation was characteristic of refractory wheezing in children under 3 years of age. In addition, infections such as *M. pneumoniae* may aggravate airway inflammation and affect refractory wheezing.

Keywords: Bronchoalveolar lavage, Neutrophil-mediated inflammation, Infant, Refractory wheezing, Airway malformation

Abbreviations: BAL, Bronchoalveolar lavage; ECP, Eosinophil cationic protein; FB, Fiberoptic bronchoscopy

Background

Wheezing in early childhood is a common but poorly characterized symptom, with a third of infants reported to experience multiple episodes of wheezing in their first 3 years [1]. Lower-airway inflammation, especially neutrophil-mediated inflammation, occurs in young children with recurrent wheezing [2, 3]. Compared with recurrent wheezing, refractory wheezing is more difficult to treat effectively and often accounts for extensive use of medical resources. It is therefore important to improve our understanding of the pathophysiology of refractory wheezing.

Congenital malformations of the lungs and airways are among several causes of irreversible airway obstruction in children who may develop various symptoms such as recurrent wheezing, cough, recurrent lower airway infection, severe dyspnea, and respiratory insufficiency [4–7].

* Correspondence: szdxjiwei@163.com
[1]Department of Respiration, Children's Hospital of Soochow University, Suzhou 215003, China
[2]Department of Clinical laboratory, Children's Hospital, Children's Hospital of Soochow University, Suzhou 215003, China

We speculate that airway morphology may play an important role in refractory wheezing.

Fiberoptic bronchoscopy (FB) and bronchoalveolar lavage (BAL) are indispensable techniques for investigating pediatric patients with airway abnormalities and pulmonary infiltrates, and both are carried out as routine procedures in many health centers [8]. The aim of this study was to determine the cellular profile of BAL from infants with refractory wheezing in the Suzhou area, China, and to investigate airway malformations and neutrophil ratios to determine if ongoing inflammation plays a role in the development of this condition.

Methods

Inclusion and exclusion criteria

This descriptive, retrospective study enrolled children under 3 years of age with refractory wheezing, defined as persistent wheezing requiring at least 4 weeks of oral corticosteroid treatment after poor responses to an initial inhaled combination of corticosteroids and bronchodilators. Additionally, the symptom-free time during which children had no wheezing symptoms was no longer than 3 days in the study population. Children were excluded from the study group if they met any of the following conditions: 1) wheezing symptoms lasted for <1 month; 2) had an apparent recovery period; 3) were severely sick and unable to tolerate FB; 4) had a family history of smoking; and 5) were premature or low birthweight babies. All the participants' parents or guardians gave their written informed consent for participation in the study. The study was approved by the ethics committee of Soochow University.

Children with wheezing

Based on the inclusion and exclusion criteria, 156 children with wheezing who were hospitalized in the Children's Hospital of Soochow University, China, from September 2011 to May 2014 were chosen for this study. All included patients received oral steroids. A wheezing infant was considered to be atopic if they had a strong family history of atopy (two or more direct relatives with atopy), atopic dermatitis, or a prior positive allergen test consisting of a prick test with an allergen on the skin or a radioallergosorbent test.

Control group

There are ethical problems associated with conducting BAL cell analysis in healthy children. The control group therefore consisted of children sampled during the same period with the following conditions, in which the BAL cell analysis was relatively normal: 1) recurrent bronchitis without wheezing ($n = 11$); 2) persistent pulmonary atelectasis for at least 1 month ($n = 3$); 3) suspicion of foreign-body aspiration ($n = 7$); 4) persistent cough and final diagnosis of psychogenic cough ($n = 12$); 5) persistent laryngeal stridor with suspected laryngomalacia ($n = 10$); or 6) hemoptysis with suspected lung disease and final diagnosis of epistaxis ($n = 3$). Children in the first three groups underwent FB during remission. Children were excluded from the control group if they met any of the following criteria: 1) history of wheezing; 2) endoscopic bronchial inflammation; 3) endoscopic airway malformation; and/or 4) personal or familial history of atopy.

Initial evaluation

Demographic, clinical, and laboratory data were collected after admission. White blood cell count, platelets, neutrophil ratio, and lymphocyte ratio were tested within 4 h after admission.

Fiberoptic bronchoscopy

Parents/guardians were informed about the surgical risks of FB and signed consent was obtained prior to the procedure. Children were fasted for both solids and liquids for at least 6 h prior to the procedure. Intramuscular atropine sulfate 0.01–0.02 mg/kg and midazolam 0.2–0.4 mg/kg were administered as premedication. Upper and lower airway anesthesia was achieved with 2 % lidocaine. A flexible bronchoscope (Olympus CV260, Tokyo, Japan or Fujinon EB-270P, Miyoshi, Japan) was wedged into each lobe. The airways were washed three times with 1 ml/kg of prewarmed sterile 0.9 % saline solution, which was then collected by a sterile sputum-collecting pipe (Falcon 50 ml, Becton-Dickinson, Rutherford, NJ, USA). The collected BAL was used for cell counts, viral analysis, and microbiological analysis (bacteria and *Mycoplasma pneumoniae*).

Cell counts

Differential cell counts were obtained using a modified version of Wright–Giemsa staining (Wright–Giemsa Stain, Baso Diagnostics Inc., Taiwan, China). At least 500 cells were examined for each specimen. The ratios of various cell types in total cell counts were reported.

Microbiological analysis

BAL samples from wheezing and control children were tested for 10 types of viruses and bacteria, as well as *M. pneumoniae*. Bacteria were tested by inoculating BAL onto blood plates and examining them after incubation for 18–20 h. Bacterial growth $>10^3$ colony-forming units/ml was considered significant. Viruses, including respiratory syncytial virus, adenovirus, influenza virus (A, B), and parainfluenza virus (1, 2, 3) were investigated by immunofluorescence tests using D^3 Ultra Respiratory Virus Screening and LD Kit (Diagnostic Hybrids, OH, USA). Positive results were defined as more than five inclusion bodies detected under a fluorescence microscope. *M. pneumoniae* and viruses including rhinovirus, human metapneumovirus, and bocavirus were examined by polymerase chain reaction using a Nucleic Acid Amplification Fluorescent Reagent Kit (Ann Gene Co., Guangdong, China) according to the manufacturer's instructions.

Statistical analysis

Cell counts were presented as the mean ± standard deviation (SD) and as medians (25 % to 75 %). The wheezing and control groups were compared using nonparametric Mann–Whitney two-sample U-tests, and Mann–Whitney U-tests were used for unpaired data. χ^2 tests were used for categorical variables. A P value < 0.05 was considered statistically significant.

Results

Demographic information

Overall, 5830 children under 3 years old were hospitalized because of wheezing between September 2011 and May 2014. Among these, 356 had refractory wheezing for at least 4 weeks (6.1 %), 54 had an apparent recovery period, 120 had a family history of smoking, and 32 were premature or low-birthweight babies. According to the exclusion criteria, 156 children with refractory wheezing were ultimately enrolled in the study (age range, 3–36 months; mean ± SD, 13.68 ± 7.08 months), of whom 121 (77.6 %) were male. The control group was aged 1–36 months (mean ± SD, 13.08 ± 10.56 months), including 35 male children (76.1 %). The age, sex ratio, and weight were similar in the wheezing and control groups ($P >$ 0.05). The white blood cell count was significantly higher in the wheezing group compared with the control group (11.44 ± 4.97 vs 10.39 ± 4.28, $P < 0.001$). The neutrophil ratio was significantly higher and the lymphocyte ratio significantly lower in the wheezing group compared with the controls (36.82 ± 14.97 vs 29.00 ± 13.47 and 53.38 ± 14.38 vs 60.31 ± 13.22, respectively, $P < 0.001$). The blood platelet count was significantly higher in the wheezing group compared with the controls (394.44 ± 120.19 vs 381.48 ± 131.09, respectively, $P < 0.001$) (Table 1).

Fiberoptic bronchoscopy findings

FB and BAL were well tolerated by both groups of children, and no major complications were observed. Thirty-four children (21.8 %) in the wheezing group had airway malformations including tracheomalacia ($n = 24$), airway stenosis ($n = 6$), and tracheal bronchus ($n = 7$). Among these 34 had airway malformations, 28 (82.4 %) were male and 27 (79.4 %) were under 12 months of age.

We further studied the characteristics of the airway inflammation in the wheezing group. A previous study reported that airway malformation alone could cause refractory childhood wheezing [4], and that these children might not have typical airway inflammation. We therefore analyzed the cellular contents of BAL from children with refractory wheezing without airway malformation and compared the results with the control group. We also performed a subject-to-subject comparison in the wheezing group.

Table 1 Demographic data for children with refractory wheezing and controls

	Wheezing group ($n = 156$)	Control group ($n = 46$)	P value
Age, months	13.68 ± 7.08	13.08 ± 10.56	0.262
Sex, M/F	121/35	35/11	0.843
Weight, kg	10.56 ± 2.13	9.74 ± 3.72	0.115
Breastfeeding, Y/N	98/58	35/11	0.095
Whole blood cell analysis			
White blood cell, $\times 10^9$	11.44 ± 4.97	10.39 ± 4.28	<0.001
Neutrophils, %	36.82 ± 14.97	29.00 ± 13.47	<0.001
Lymphocytes, %	53.38 ± 14.38	60.31 ± 13.22	<0.001
Blood platelet, $\times 10^9$	394.44 ± 120.19	381.48 ± 131.09	<0.001

The median recovery rate was 70 % (range, 45 %–80 %), with very little variation between the two compared groups. However, the recovered cell ratio showed a wide distribution in the wheezing group (Table 2).

Comparison between wheezing and control subjects

The neutrophil ratio was significantly higher (31.26 ± 28.10 % vs 6.38 ± 6.59 %, respectively, $P < 0.001$) and the macrophage ratio was significantly lower (60.80 ± 29.20 % vs 87.06 ± 8.22 %, respectively, $P < 0.001$) in the wheezing group compared with the control group. The eosinophil ratio was also higher in the wheezing group (0.75 ± 2.76 % vs 0.08 ± 0.27 %, respectively, $P = 0.040$). There was no significant difference in BAL lymphocyte ratio between the two groups.

Comparisons within the wheezing group

Eighty-one of 122 (66.4 %) wheezing children were atopic and had no airway malformations. There was no significant difference in the ratio of macrophages, lymphocytes, eosinophils, or neutrophils in the BAL between atopic and nonatopic children in the wheezing group (Table 3).

In terms of pathogen analysis, we performed viral analysis, and *M. pneumoniae* and microbiological cultures for the wheezing and control groups. No pathogens were detected in the control group. Virus detection was positive in 17 (13.9 %) of the wheezing children without airway malformations, and microbiological findings were positive in 78 (63.9 %). Among them, *M. pneumoniae* showed the highest detection rate ($n = 63$, 51.6 %). In

Table 2 BAL cellular contents in children with refractory wheezing and controls[a]

	Refractory wheezing children without airway malformation ($n = 122$)	Control group ($n = 46$)	P value
Alveolar macrophages, %	60.80 ± 29.20, 67 (35.0 ~ 88.25)	87.06 ± 8.22, 90 (82.5 ~ 93.0)	<0.001
Lymphocytes, %	7.20 ± 6.46, 5 (2.0–10.0)	6.48 ± 5.52, 5 (2.0 ~ 8.0)	0.314
Neutrophils, %	31.26 ± 28.10, 25 (6.0 ~ 49.25)	6.38 ± 6.59, 4 (2.0 ~ 9.0)	<0.001
Eosinophils, %	0.75 ± 2.76, 0.0 (0.0 ~ 0.0)	0.08 ± 0.27, 0.0 (0.0 ~ 0.0)	0.040

[a]Data presented as mean ± SD, median (25th to 75th percentiles)

addition, other bacteria were detected in 30 wheezing children (24.6 %), including *Haemophilus influenzae* ($n = 12$), *Streptococcus pneumoniae* ($n = 12$), *Escherichia coli* ($n = 2$), *Burkholderia cepacia* ($n = 1$), *Pseudomonas aeruginosa* ($n = 1$), *Serratia marcescens* ($n = 1$), and *Enterobacter aerogenes* ($n = 1$).

We further investigated how the BAL cellular content was affected by pathogens by categorizing wheezing children into three groups: 1) non-infection group (N, $n = 40$), no pathogens detected; 2) bacterial-infection group (B, $n = 78$), bacterial infection detected (including *M. pneumoniae*); and (3) virus-infection group (V, $n = 17$), virus infection detected. We then compared the BAL cellular content between each of these groups and the control group (C, $n = 46$) (Fig. 1). The lowest neutrophil ratio was found in the control group, followed by the non-infection group, with the highest neutrophil ratios in the infection groups. There was no significant difference among the various bacterial ratios. The highest alveolar macrophage ratio was found in the control group, and the lowest in the infection groups, while the eosinophil ratio was highest in the infection groups. Of note, there was no significant difference in lymphocyte ratios among the four groups.

Discussion

Wheezing is a common clinical symptom in infants. Its long disease course, slow recovery, and risk of relapse mean that refractory wheezing is difficult to treat, resulting in high medical-resource utilization. In our department, 6.1 % of children under 3 years of age had refractory wheezing for at least 4 weeks. Although various treatments have been used, including inhaled and systemic corticosteroids, and montelukast, they have little effect on preventing the recurrence of refractory wheezing [9]. These medications may influence eosinophilic airway inflammation but have limited impact on noneosinophilic airway inflammation. It has therefore been speculated that refractory wheezing may have a different pathophysiologic mechanism.

Airway malformation is one cause of irreversible airway obstruction in children and is accompanied by many clinical symptoms [10]. The incidence of congenital pulmonary airway malformation is one per 8300–35,000. It usually affects a single lobe and has no sex bias [11]. In this study, 21.8 % of children with refractory wheezing had airway malformations including tracheomalacia, airway stenosis, and tracheal bronchus, and 27 of 87 (31 %) wheezing children under 12 months of age had airway malformations, suggesting that airway malformations may play an important role in refractory wheezing.

A literature search [12, 13] revealed differing total BAL cell counts, though they generally fell within the range 0.5–57.1 × 10^4/ml. Of the total BAL cells, >85 % are alveolar macrophages, <12 % are lymphocytes, <2 % are neutrophils, and <1 % are eosinophils [8, 10]. The classification of BAL cells in pathological conditions varies, and BAL analysis can provide important reference information on the nature of lung diseases, the inflammation process, and disease activity. BAL fluid analysis has recently been used globally for diagnostic and prognostic purposes, and to observe the curative effect of respiratory disease treatments. However, although it is theoretically important to study the cellular profile of BAL in healthy children, this is ethically difficult. We therefore used BAL from relatively normal children as a control, as in previous studies [3]. BAL cell analysis in our control group was comparable to that reported for healthy children [3], suggesting that the results in the control group were representative of the endotracheal cell ratio in a normal child. In the current study, we compared the BAL inflammatory cell profiles between

Table 3 BAL cellular content in atopic and nonatopic children[a]

Variables	Atopic children ($n = 81$)	Nonatopic children ($n = 41$)	P value
Alveolar macrophages, %	56.86 ± 30.28, 61.0(33.5 ~ 85.5)	68.56 ± 25.60, 77.0 (53.5 ~ 90.0)	0.052
Lymphocytes, %	7.75 ± 7.28, 5.0 (2.0 ~ 12.0)	6.10 ± 4.30, 5.0 (2.0 ~ 10.0)	0.366
Neutrophils, %	34.89 ± 29.61, 30.0 (7.0 ~ 54.0)	24.10 ± 23.57, 15.0 (5.0 ~ 35.5)	0.062
Eosinophils, %	0.51 ± 1.28, 0.0 (0.0 ~ 0.0)	1.24 ± 4.40, 0.0 (0.0 ~ 0.0)	0.305

[a]Data presented as mean ± SD, median (25th to 75th percentiles)

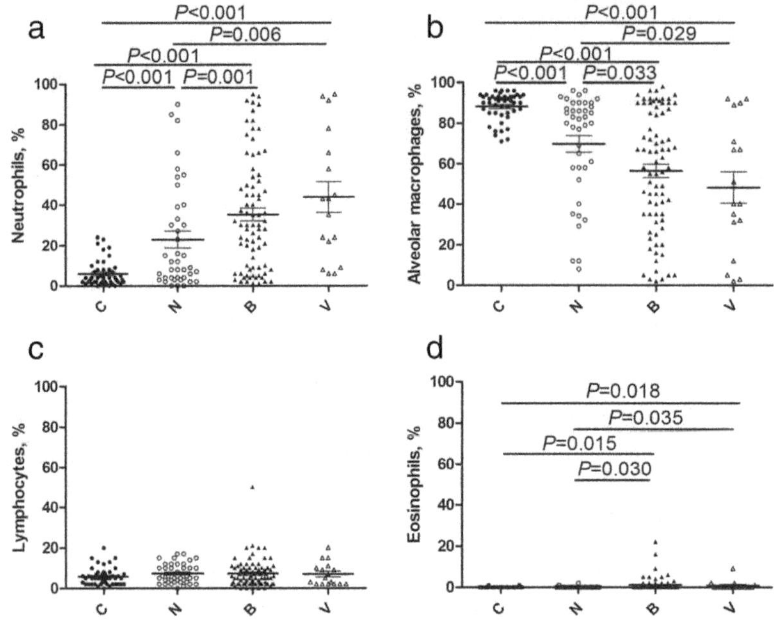

Fig. 1 BAL cellular content. The percentages of neutrophils (**a**), alveolar macrophages (**b**), lymphocytes (**c**) and eosinophils (**d**) in the BAL in the control (C, $n = 46$), non-pathogen (N, $n = 40$), bacterial-infection (including *M. pneumoniae*) (B, $n = 78$), and virus-infection groups (V, $n = 17$). Horizontal bars indicate the median for each group of patients

122 children with severe refractory wheezing and 46 control children. The BAL neutrophil ratio was significantly increased and the macrophage ratio was significantly decreased in the wheezing group compared with controls, suggesting that granulocytes contribute to airway inflammation. The mechanism of neutrophil influx and activation may be mediated by interleukin (IL)-8 secretion [14]. Studies on neutrophilic inflammation and persistent asthma by Gibson et al. revealed that sputum IL-8 levels were higher in patients with noneosinophilic asthma [15]. Neutrophils showed a close correlation with IL-8 levels [15]. Similarly, neutrophil levels were significantly higher in 83 wheezing infants compared with 10 control subjects [3]. Marguet et al. compared BAL cell profiles in children with asthma, infantile wheeze, chronic cough, and cystic fibrosis, and reported a significantly higher level of neutrophils in wheezing infants [2].

Previous studies indicated that airway virus infection and bacterial colonization can increase the risk of wheezing [16, 17]. In this study, virus detection was positive in 17 children with refractory wheezing and no airway malformation, but who had the highest bocavirus ratios. *M. pneumoniae* was positive in 63 wheezing children, and other culture findings were positive in 30 wheezing children. The *M. pneumoniae* infection rate was high in children with refractory wheezing in the current study, and previous studies also suggested that *M. pneumoniae* could cause childhood wheezing [18, 19]. However, the *M. pneumoniae* status in infants is often ignored in clinical practice. These results suggest that children with refractory wheezing should be prescribed macrolides to treat *M. pneumoniae* infection and help reduce clinical symptoms.

A high level of neutrophils in the BAL might correlate with infection. The relationships between various BAL cells counts and infection indicated a significantly higher neutrophil ratio and lower alveolar macrophage ratio in children with refractory wheezing compared with the control group, but this result was not affected by pathogen infection. However, children with a pathogenic infection had a higher neutrophil ratio and lower alveolar macrophage ratio than those without positive pathogen detection. We speculated that neutrophil-mediated chronic inflammation in the airways may also play an important role in refractory wheezing, regardless of pathogen infection, though infection may potentially aggravate the airway inflammation.

Irrespective of the pathogens, the neutrophil ratio was always higher in infected compared with uninfected children. Furthermore, there was no difference in neutrophil numbers between those infected with bacteria (including *M. pneumoniae*) or virus. Bacteria, viruses, and *M. pneumoniae* have been shown to increase the BAL neutrophil ratio. A previous study [20] found that BAL neutrophilia was associated with bacterial pulmonary infection. The neutrophil ratio has shown a tendency to increase with the occurrence of viral infection [21, 22]. This may be correlated with IL-8 and leukotriene B4, which favor the recruitment of neutrophils in airways [23–25]. *M. pneumoniae* has been studied intensively in recent years, and children with *M. pneumoniae* infection had an increased BAL cell count, which was attributed to an increase in neutrophils [26]. In contrast, other previous studies indicated that the BAL neutrophil ratio was not correlated with bacteriological results, implying that neutrophil-mediated inflammation was independent of bacterial infection [2, 3, 27] in wheezy infants.

Cellular BAL levels may be related to allergy. In our study, wheezing children were further categorized as atopic or nonatopic, and there were no significant differences in cell counts (macrophages, lymphocytes, eosinophils, and neutrophils) between the atopic and nonatopic groups. This was similar to the results of Le Bourgeois et al. [3], who observed normal BAL cell levels in atopic children. However, other studies revealed that children with atopy had higher eosinophil levels [2]. Marguet et al. [2] reported that eosinophils, which are characteristic of asthma, were rarely seen in wheezing infants. However, normal eosinophil levels do not exclude the possibility of their involvement in the physiopathology of atopic wheezing, and further studies are needed to examine the roles of activated and degranulated eosinophils. Eosinophil cationic protein (ECP) is released by activated eosinophils and is used as a marker of eosinophilic inflammation. High ECP levels have been reported in patients with active asthma and other allergic diseases [28]. The detection of ECP levels in BAL would thus be valuable [29].

Conclusions

It is important to identify the causes associated with the pathogenesis of refractory wheezing in children. In this descriptive study, some children with refractory wheezing had airway malformations, with children under 12 months of age having a particularly high proportion of airway anomalies. Neutrophil-mediated airway inflammation might also play an important role in the pathophysiology of refractory wheezing, while infections might aggravate airway inflammation. The bacterial-detection rate (especially *M. pneumoniae*) was high among wheezing children. Further research on infants with refractory wheezing is needed to develop specific inflammatory markers.

Acknowledgments

We gratefully acknowledge the valuable cooperation of Mrs. Xiuping Gu and the members of her team in helping us accomplish fiberoptic bronchoscopy and collecting bronchoalveolar lavage.

Funding

This work was supported by the National Natural Science Foundation of China (Grant to Wei Ji, No. 81570016).

Authors' contributions

WJ, ZC and WG conceived and designed the experiments. XS, LH, MW and YY performed the experiments. XZ and SW analyzed the data. WG, LH and WJ drafted the manuscript. All authors read and approved the final manuscript.

Competing interests

The authors declare that they have no competing interests.

References

1. Schwerk N, Brinkmann F, Soudah B, Kabesch M, Hansen G. Wheeze in preschool age is associated with pulmonary bacterial infection and resolves after antibiotic therapy. PLoS One. 2011;6, e27913.
2. Marguet C, Jouen-Boedes F, Dean TP, Warner JO. Bronchoalveolar cell profiles in children with asthma, infantile wheeze, chronic cough, or cystic fibrosis. Am J Respir Crit Care Med. 1999;159:1533–40.
3. Le Bourgeois M, Goncalves M, Le Clainche L, Benoist MR, Fournet JC, Scheinmann P, et al. Bronchoalveolar cells in children < 3 years old with severe recurrent wheezing. Chest. 2002;122:791–7.
4. Carden KA, Boiselle PM, Waltz DA, Ernst A. Tracheomalacia and tracheobronchomalacia in children and adults: an in-depth review. Chest. 2005;127:984–1005.
5. Wood RE. Localized tracheomalacia or bronchomalacia in children with intractable cough. J Pediatr. 1990;116:404–6.
6. Irwin RS, Madison JM. The persistently troublesome cough. Am J Respir Crit Care Med. 2002;165:1469–74.
7. McNamara VM, Crabbe DC. Tracheomalacia. Paediatr Respir Rev. 2004;5:147–54.
8. Efrati O, Sadeh-Gornik U, Modan-Moses D, Barak A, Szeinberg A, Vardi A, et al. Flexible bronchoscopy and bronchoalveolar lavage in pediatric patients with lung disease. Pediatr Crit Care Med. 2009;10:80–4.
9. Beigelman A, Isaacson-Schmid M, Sajol G, Baty J, Rodriguez OM, Leege E, et al. Randomized trial to evaluate azithromycin's effects on serum and upper airway IL-8 levels and recurrent wheezing in infants with respiratory syncytial virus bronchiolitis. J Allergy Clin Immunol. 2014.
10. Boogaard R, Huijsmans SH, Pijnenburg MW, Tiddens HA, de Jongste JC, Merkus PJ. Tracheomalacia and bronchomalacia in children: incidence and patient characteristics. Chest. 2005;128:3391–7.
11. Nadeem M, Elnazir B, Greally P. Congenital pulmonary malformation in children. Scientifica (Cairo). 2012;2012:209896.
12. de Blic J, Midulla F, Barbato A, Clement A, Dab I, Eber E, et al. Bronchoalveolar lavage in children. ERS Task Force on bronchoalveolar lavage in children. European Respiratory Society. Eur Respir J. 2000;15:217–31.
13. Ratjen F, Bredendiek M, Brendel M, Meltzer J, Costabel U. Differential cytology of bronchoalveolar lavage fluid in normal children. Eur Respir J. 1994;7:1865–70.
14. Ordonez CL, Shaughnessy TE, Matthay MA, Fahy JV. Increased neutrophil numbers and IL-8 levels in airway secretions in acute severe asthma: Clinical and biologic significance. Am J Respir Crit Care Med. 2000;161:1185–90.
15. Gibson PG, Simpson JL, Saltos N. Heterogeneity of airway inflammation in persistent asthma : evidence of neutrophilic inflammation and increased sputum interleukin-8. Chest. 2001;119:1329–36.
16. Jartti T, Lehtinen P, Vuorinen T, Ruuskanen O. Bronchiolitis: age and previous wheezing episodes are linked to viral etiology and atopic characteristics. Pediatr Infect Dis J. 2009;28:311–7.
17. Bisgaard H, Hermansen MN, Buchvald F, Loland L, Halkjaer LB, Bonnelykke K, et al. Childhood asthma after bacterial colonization of the airway in neonates. N Engl J Med. 2007;357:1487–95.
18. Chen GD, Chen AH. The wheezing associated with Mycoplasma pneumoniae infection in children. Zhonghua Er Ke Za Zhi. 2012;50:756–8. 9.
19. Chung HL, Kim SG, Shin IH. The relationship between serum endothelin (ET)-1 and wheezing status in the children with Mycoplasma pneumoniae pneumonia. Pediatr Allergy Immunol. 2006;17:285–90.
20. Stolz D, Stulz A, Muller B, Gratwohl A, Tamm M. BAL neutrophils, serum procalcitonin, and C-reactive protein to predict bacterial infection in the immunocompromised host. Chest. 2007;132:504–14.
21. Schellhase DE, Fawcett DD, Schutze GE, Lensing SY, Tryka AF. Clinical utility of flexible bronchoscopy and bronchoalveolar lavage in young children with recurrent wheezing. J Pediatr. 1998;132:312–8.
22. Everard ML, Swarbrick A, Wrightham M, McIntyre J, Dunkley C, James PD, et al. Analysis of cells obtained by bronchial lavage of infants with respiratory syncytial virus infection. Arch Dis Child. 1994;71:428–32.
23. Becker S, Koren HS, Henke DC. Interleukin-8 expression in normal nasal epithelium and its modulation by infection with respiratory syncytial virus and cytokines tumor necrosis factor, interleukin-1, and interleukin-6. Am J Respir Cell Mol Biol. 1993;8:20–7.

24. Becker S, Quay J, Soukup J. Cytokine (tumor necrosis factor, IL-6, and IL-8) production by respiratory syncytial virus-infected human alveolar macrophages. J Immunol. 1991;147:4307–12.
25. Jarjour NN, Gern JE, Kelly EA, Swenson CA, Dick CR, Busse WW. The effect of an experimental rhinovirus 16 infection on bronchial lavage neutrophils. J Allergy Clin Immunol. 2000;105:1169–77.
26. Huang H, Zhong LL, Peng L, Li J, Lin L. Levels of interleukin-4 and interferon-gamma in the bronchoalveolar lavage fluid of children with refractory Mycoplasma pneumoniae pneumonia. Zhongguo Dang Dai Er Ke Za Zhi. 2012;14:581–4.
27. Fayon M, Just J, Thien HV, Chiba T, Pascual L, Sandouk G, et al. Bacterial flora of the lower respiratory tract in children with bronchial asthma. Acta Paediatr. 1999;88:1216–22.
28. Munthe-Kaas MC, Gerritsen J, Carlsen KH, Undlien D, Egeland T, Skinningsrud B, et al. Eosinophil cationic protein (ECP) polymorphisms and association with asthma, s-ECP levels and related phenotypes. Allergy. 2007;62:429–36.
29. Bjornsson E, Janson C, Hakansson L, Enander I, Venge P, Boman G. Serum eosinophil cationic protein in relation to bronchial asthma in a young Swedish population. Allergy. 1994;49:730–6.

10

Non-invasive respiratory support for infants with bronchiolitis

H. Turnham[1], R. S. Agbeko[2,3], J. Furness[4], J. Pappachan[5], A. G. Sutcliffe[6*] and P. Ramnarayan[7]

Abstract

Background: Bronchiolitis is a common respiratory illness of early childhood. For most children it is a mild self-limiting disease but a small number of children develop respiratory failure. Nasal continuous positive airway pressure (nCPAP) has traditionally been used to provide non-invasive respiratory support in these children, but there is little clinical trial evidence to support its use. More recently, high-flow nasal cannula therapy (HFNC) has emerged as a novel respiratory support modality. Our study aims to describe current national practice and clinician preferences relating to use of non-invasive respiratory support (nCPAP and HFNC) in the management of infants (<12 months old) with acute bronchiolitis.

Methods: We performed a cross-sectional web-based survey of hospitals with inpatient paediatric facilities in England and Wales. Responses were elicited from one senior doctor and one senior nurse at each hospital. We analysed the proportion of hospitals using HFNC and nCPAP; clinical thresholds for their initiation; and clinician preferences regarding first-line support modality and future research.

Results: The survey was distributed to 117 of 171 eligible hospitals; 97 hospitals provided responses (response rate: 83%). The majority of hospitals were able to provide nCPAP (89/97, 91.7%) or HFNC (71/97, 73.2%); both were available at 65 hospitals (67%). nCPAP was more likely to be delivered in a ward setting in a general hospital, and in a high dependency setting in a tertiary centre. There were differences in the oxygenation and acidosis thresholds, and clinical triggers such as recurrent apnoeas or work of breathing that influenced clinical decisions, regarding when to start nCPAP or HFNC. More individual respondents with access to both modalities (74/106, 69.8%) would choose HFNC over nCPAP as their first-line treatment option in a deteriorating child with bronchiolitis.

Conclusions: Despite lack of randomised trial evidence, nCPAP and HFNC are commonly used in British hospitals to support infants with acute bronchiolitis. HFNC appears to be currently the preferred first-line modality for non-invasive respiratory support due to perceived ease of use.

Keywords: Bronchiolitis, Respiratory failure, Non-invasive respiratory support, Critical care

Background

Bronchiolitis is a common respiratory illness of young childhood caused by viruses such as Respiratory Syncytial Virus (RSV) [1]. Bronchiolitis is usually a mild, self-limiting disease, but 2–5% of children require hospitalisation [1–6], while 1–2.7% need critical care support [7, 8].

Nasal continuous positive airway pressure (nCPAP) has been used as a mode of non-invasive respiratory support for infants with bronchiolitis-induced respiratory failure for over two decades [9–13], and is increasingly being used in a ward setting [14]. Recently, high-flow nasal cannula therapy (HFNC) has become a popular alternative [15]. However, investment and training in new equipment is expensive, and concerns persist regarding the safety of HFNC (risk of pneumothorax or pneumomediastinum and nosocomial infection) and the potential for delay in initiating invasive ventilation for high-risk children [16–20].

* Correspondence: a.sutcliffe@ucl.ac.uk
[6]Institute of Child Health, University College London, GAP unit, Institute of Child Health, 30 Guilford Street, London WC1N 1EH, UK
Full list of author information is available at the end of the article

A previous survey of UK neonatal units demonstrated widespread adoption of HFNC despite the absence of robust clinical trial evidence [21]. We aimed to establish current national practice in the management of infants with acute bronchiolitis by conducting a cross-sectional survey of clinicians working in hospitals in England and Wales. We also aimed to determine clinician preferences regarding clinical triggers to initiate nCPAP and HFNC, and to ascertain if clinical equipoise existed to support a multicentre trial of non-invasive respiratory support in acute bronchiolitis.

Methods

Survey

We designed a cross-sectional survey of hospitals with inpatient paediatric facilities. An online questionnaire using Survey Monkey software (www.surveymonkey.com, Survey Monkey, Palo Alto, USA) was piloted by three senior doctors from different parts of England (authors JP, AS and JF). Feedback from the pilot was used to finalise the questionnaire used in the study. The final questionnaire covered three main themes: availability and use of nCPAP and HFNC at hospital level, clinical criteria for the initiation of nCPAP and HFNC, and clinician preferences towards future research. The final questionnaire is available as Additional file 1. Survey responses were elicited using two methods: a) a survey link emailed to the lead consultant and lead nurse in all 25 tertiary paediatric hospitals and b) a survey link sent to each of the 12 regional paediatric intensive care retrieval services, who were asked to forward the questionnaire to the designated consultant and senior nurse at each of the district general hospitals in their regional network. Completion of the survey was voluntary and consent was implied though completion and submission of the survey. The initial survey distribution was followed up by reminder emails 4 and 8 weeks later. Survey data were collected between June and October 2014.

Data collected by the Royal College of Paediatrics and Child Health for the Medical Workforce Census 2013 was used to provide data regarding the number and size of all hospitals admitting children as in-patients in the United Kingdom [22]. We used the definition of High Dependency Care (HDC) as that defined in England and Wales by the Royal College of Paediatrics and Child Health: 'care for a child who requires enhanced observation, monitoring or intervention than cannot be delivered on a standard paediatric ward' [23]. The Royal College of Nursing have published recommendations for minimum nurse staffing levels for general paediatric wards (1 nurse per 3 infants), high dependency units (1 nurse per 2 patients) and intensive care units (1 nurse per patient) [24].

Data analysis

We used the hospital as the unit of analysis for questions relating to hospital practice. If discrepancies were identified between respondents from the same hospital, we chose to use the senior doctor's response for this analysis. We used the respondent as the unit of analysis for questions relating to clinical thresholds and beliefs regarding clinical equipoise. Results are reported as proportions and/or means as appropriate. Significance testing for differences in proportions were performed using the chi-square test, and for differences in means for normally distributed data using the Student *t*-test. We performed multivariate analysis to study the association between hospital type (tertiary vs. general hospital) and the use of HFNC and/or nCPAP, respondent type (consultant vs. nurse), preference of first-line modality and willingness to participate in future research, using the survey statistics module of Stata IC v13 (Stata Corporation, College Station, USA). The hospital was set as the primary sampling unit, and accounted for clustering of respondents within each hospital. Data analyses were performed using Stata and Microsoft Excel (Microsoft Corporation, USA).

Results

The survey was disseminated to 117 out of 171 eligible hospitals; responses were obtained from 97 hospitals (response rate: 83%). Survey responses were received from all 25 tertiary hospitals. The survey was distributed by regional PICU retrieval services to 8 out of 12 regions in England and Wales, reaching 92 general hospitals, of which 72 responded. Survey responses were provided by 159 individual respondents (mean: 1.6 responses per hospital). The majority of respondents were paediatric consultants (102/159, 64.2%) and the remainder were senior nurses.

Characteristics of the hospitals from which responses were obtained are shown in Table 1.

Availability of paediatric high dependency units (PHDU)

Most tertiary hospitals (88%) reported that they had a dedicated PHDU compared to only 12.5% of general hospitals, where children requiring high dependency level care were more likely to be cared for in dedicated PHDU beds located within the general ward (57%). 26 general hospitals (26.8%) reported no availability of PHDU.

Guidelines and protocols

No guidelines were used by 5 hospitals for the management of bronchiolitis. The remainder used local, regional and/or national guidelines. Overall, general hospitals were more likely to use guidelines than

Table 1 Characteristics of hospitals who responded to the survey ($n = 97$)

	Tertiary centre $n = 25$ (%)	General hospital $n = 72$ (%)
Hospital size[a]		
Very small (≤1500 admissions per year)	1 (4.0)	2 (2.8)
Small (1501–2500 admissions per year)	4 (16.0)	14 (19.4)
Medium (1501–5000 admissions per year)	9 (36.0)	34 (47.2)
Large (5001–6000 admissions per year)	3 (12.0)	9 (12.5)
Very large (>6000 admissions per year)	8 (32.0)	13 (18.1)
Care areas in hospital		
Dedicated paediatric high dependency unit	22 (88.0)	9 (12.5)
High dependency beds within paediatric ward	4 (16.0)	41 (56.9)
No paediatric high dependency beds	3 (12.0)	23 (31.9)
Dedicated paediatric intensive care beds	23 (92.0)	0 (0)
Dedicated paediatric emergency department	18 (72.0)	12 (16.7)
Bronchiolitis guideline used		
Local	20 (80.0)	62 (86.1)
Regional	3 (12.0)	13 (18.1)
National	2 (8.0)	13 (18.1)
No guideline	2 (8.0)	3 (4.2)
Availability of non-invasive respiratory support		
nCPAP	24 (96.0)	65 (90.3)
HFNC	20 (80.0)	51 (70.8)
Either HFNC or nCPAP	25 (100)	70 (97.2)
Both	19 (76.0)	46 (63.9)

[a]Classification based on number of paediatric inpatient admissions per year (as per the RCPCH Medical Workforce Census 2013)

tertiary hospitals. The majority of hospitals had local guidelines in place (82/97, 84.5%).

Hospital practice regarding non-invasive respiratory support in acute bronchiolitis

nCPAP

Twenty-four (96%) tertiary hospitals and 65 (90%) general hospitals reported being able to provide nCPAP. Of the 8 hospitals that did not use nCPAP, one commented that there was a lack of evidence to support its use and another that absence of adequate staff training prevented its use. nCPAP was delivered in a ward setting by 4 out of 25 (16%) tertiary hospitals and 41 out of 72 (56.9%) general hospitals, whereas it was more likely to be delivered in a PHDU or PICU setting in a tertiary centre.

Use of sedation to facilitate the provision of nCPAP was elicited from individual responders by asking them how often sedation was used: always, sometimes, rarely or never. Use of sedation was variable: 41/97 hospitals used sedation sometimes or routinely (42.3%) while 37/97 (38.1%) used it rarely. Nine hospitals reported never using sedation, while 9 hospitals did not submit information. Tertiary hospitals were more likely to use sedation sometimes or routinely than general hospitals (18/25, 72% versus 24/72, 33.3%, $p = 0.003$).

HFNC

Twenty (80%) of tertiary hospitals and 51 (70.8%) of general hospitals reported being able to provide HFNC (a further 9 hospitals were planning to implement the technology within the next 12 months). HFNC was delivered more frequently in the ward setting in general hospitals (38/72, 52.8% vs. 6/25, 24%), whereas it was more likely to be delivered in a HDU or PICU setting in a tertiary centre (20/25, 80% vs. 20/72, 27.8%).

We asked responders about hospital guidelines for maximal flow rates for HFNC in particular areas of their hospital. We used this as a reflection of safety concerns regarding introduction of this new technology. Not all responders commented, however, there is a trend towards higher flow rates being tolerated on paediatric wards and high dependency areas than in emergency departments of both tertiary and general hospitals (Table 2).

Either nCPAP or HFNC was available in all tertiary hospitals and in nearly all general hospitals (70/72, 97.2%), while two-thirds of the hospitals had access to both modalities (65/97, 67%).

Individual clinicians' practice regarding non-invasive respiratory support in acute bronchiolitis

Figure 1 illustrates oxygen requirement criteria that clinicians currently use to initiate nCPAP and HFNC in infants with acute bronchiolitis in tertiary hospitals (panel A) and general hospitals (panel B). Fig. 2 illustrates acidosis criteria that clinicians currently use to initiate nCPAP and HFNC in infants with acute bronchiolitis in tertiary hospitals (panel A) and general hospitals (panel B). A significant number of clinicians (see legends of Figs. 1 and 2) did not respond to these two questions, citing that they would not use specific oxygenation and acidosis criteria in isolation.

Figure 3 illustrates the clinical criteria of work of breathing, recurrent apnoeas and presence of high-risk co-morbid conditions (e.g., prematurity or cardiac disease) that influence the decision to initiate nCPAP and HFNC in tertiary hospitals (panel A) and general hospitals (panel B).

Clinician preferences for first-line modality

In response to a clinical vignette describing a 6-month old infant with acute bronchiolitis and respiratory distress, the majority of clinicians who had access to both nCPAP and HFNC (74/106, 69.8%) reported that they

Table 2 Maximal flow rates used locally for HFNC in tertiary and general hospitals

	Tertiary Hospitals ($n = 20$)			General Hospitals ($n = 51$)		
	1–5 L/min	6–10 L/min	>10 L/min	1–5 L/min	6–10 L/min	>10 L/min
Emergency Department	0	2 (10%)	0	2 (3%)	4 (7.8%)	7 (14%)
Paediatric Ward	0	5 (25%)	3 (15%)	3 (5.8%)	18 (35%)	18 (35%)
Paediatric High Dependency Ward	1 (5%)	6 (30%)	6 (30%)	5 (10%)	18 (35%)	13 (25%)

would start HFNC as the first-line treatment rather than nCPAP. When asked what they perceived the role of HFNC to be in clinical practice, many reported that they considered it as an alternative to nCPAP (78/106, 73.5%) or as a step up before nCPAP (84/106, 79.2%). A smaller proportion felt that it was also useful as a step-down therapy after discontinuation of nCPAP (63/106, 59.4%). There were no significant differences between tertiary hospitals and general hospitals in terms of clinician preference for first-line support mode.

Future research

When asked to rate the importance of various outcome measures to study in future research on a Likert scale (1: least important; 5: most important), clinicians rated reduction in the need for intubation and ventilation (mean score: 4.8 for general hospital respondents and 4.5 for tertiary centre respondents, $p = 0.01$) and avoiding transfer to another hospital (mean score: 4.7 for general hospitals and 4.0 for tertiary hospitals, $p < 0.001$) as the most important (Table 3). Half of all clinicians who responded were prepared to randomise children with acute bronchiolitis to either nCPAP or HFNC in a future clinical trial (80/159, 50.3%). An additional 42 clinicians (26.4%) would consider participation in an RCT, subject to the study design (free text comments indicated that the ability to crossover between treatment arms was an important consideration).

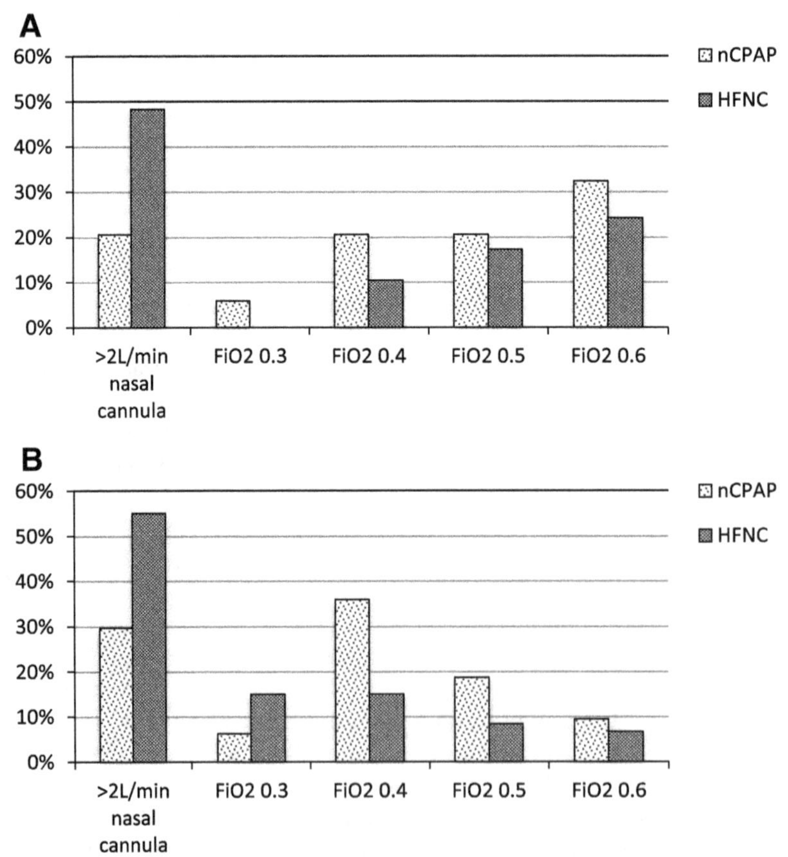

Fig. 1 Oxygen requirement threshold at which clinicians would start HFNC/nCPAP at tertiary hospitals (panel **a**) and general hospitals (panel **b**). Graphs show a breakdown of available responses: panel **a** – 34 (NCPAP) and 29 (HFNC) responses from 50 clinicians; panel **b** – 64 (nCPAP) and 60 (HFNC) responses from 109 clinicians

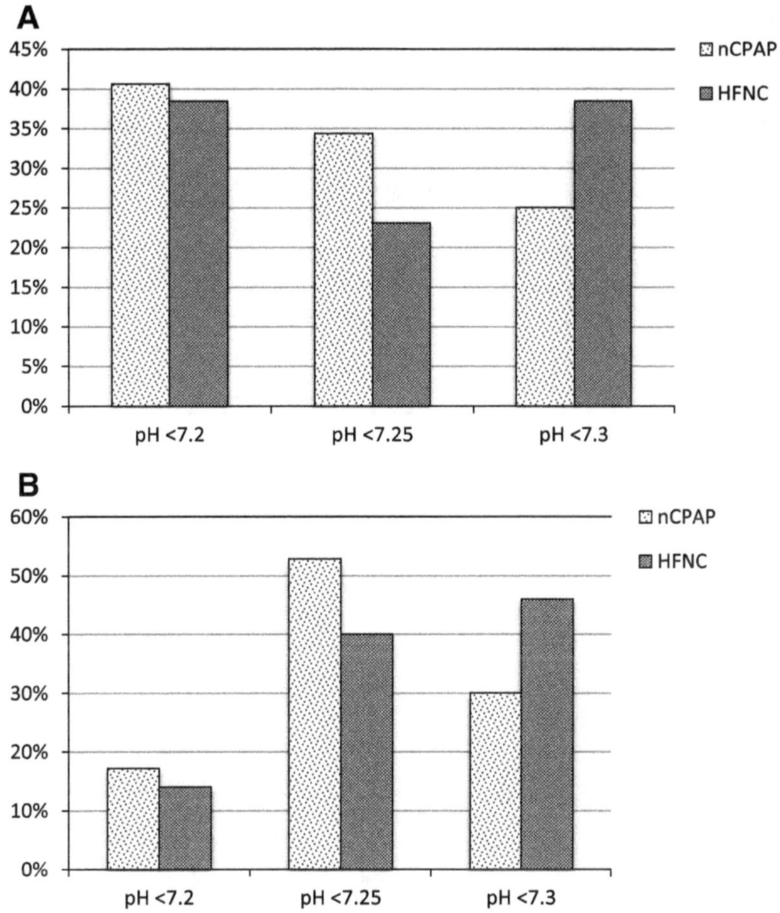

Fig. 2 Acidosis threshold at which clinicians would start nCPAP/HFNC at tertiary hospitals (panel **a**) and general hospitals (panel **b**). Graphs show a breakdown of available responses: panel **a** – 32 (NCPAP) and 26 (HFNC) responses from 50 clinicians; panel **b** – 70 (nCPAP) and 50 (HFNC) responses from 109 clinicians

A small proportion (9/159, 5.6%) reported that they were unwilling to participate in a trial due to their belief in the superiority of HFNC compared to nCPAP.

Multivariate analysis

Hospital type was not associated with the availability of HFNC either on its own, or availability of both support modalities, when adjusted for hospital size ($p = 0.28$ and $p = 0.17$ respectively). Respondent type was not associated with choosing HFNC as first-line treatment or with willingness to participate in a future trial, when adjusted for hospital type and size ($p = 0.65$ and $p = 0.89$ respectively).

Generalisability

In order to assess the generalisability of our findings, we compared the 54 general hospitals that were not surveyed with the 72 hospitals that were surveyed – there was no significant difference in the hospital size between the two groups ($p = 0.51$). Similarly, we compared the 72 general hospitals that responded to the survey with the 25 hospitals that did not respond – there was no significant difference in the hospital size ($p = 0.53$).

Discussion

Our national survey of hospitals reveals that the use of nCPAP and HFNC is widespread in young children with bronchiolitis. nCPAP appears to be used more frequently in high dependency and intensive care areas, while HFNC use is more frequent in paediatric wards. Clinicians appear to view HFNC and nCPAP as interchangeable modalities, but HFNC appears to be their preferred first-line support option.

nCPAP has been the traditional modality of respiratory support for bronchiolitis for over two decades [9]. It may help to maintain patency of small bronchioles, improve secretion clearance, gas exchange and reduce work of breathing [25]. Although small studies suggest a trend

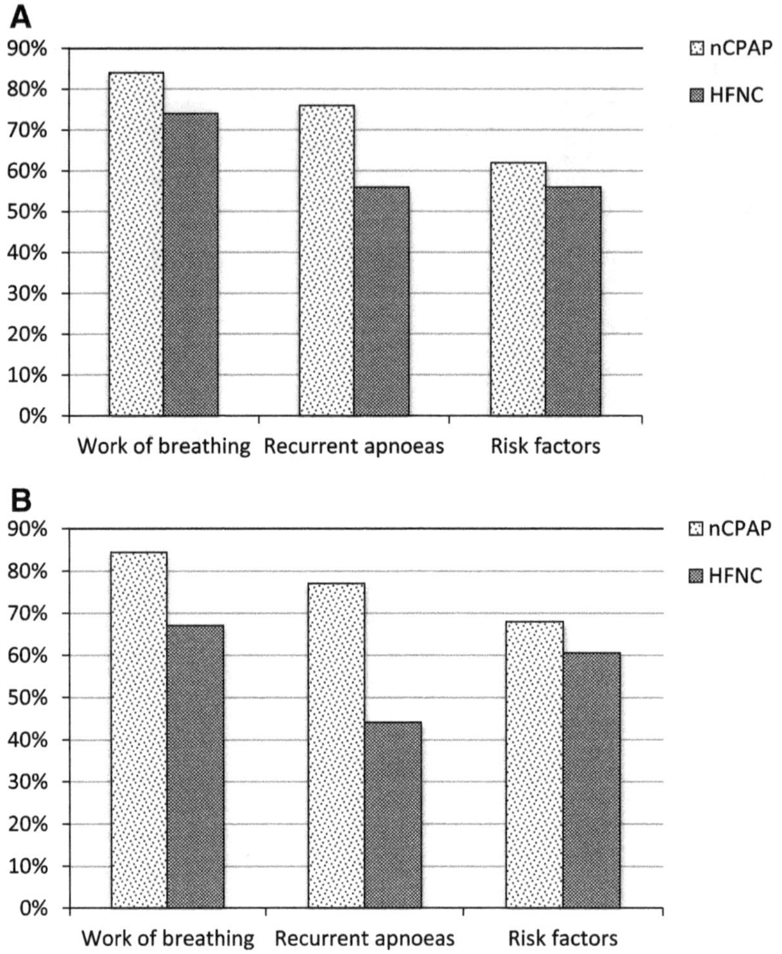

Fig. 3 Clinical factors that influence decision to start nCPAP/HFNC at tertiary hospitals (panel **a**) and general hospitals (panel **b**)

towards physiological improvement with early nCPAP use [12, 26], its impact on outcomes such as length of hospital stay and need for intubation and invasive ventilation have yet to be confirmed in large randomised controlled trials [27]. More recently, HFNC has increased in popularity [15]. HFNC delivers a gas mixture of oxygen/air, warmed to 34–37° Celsius with a relative humidity of almost 100%, at high flow rates. It reduces airway resistance, washes out end-expiratory gases and provides positive airway pressure, reducing work of breathing and improving in gas exchange [28–30]. It is also well tolerated [31].

Table 3 Patient outcomes viewed by clinicians as being important for study in future research (reported as a score, 1 indicating least important, 5 indicating very important)

	Tertiary hospitals (*n* = 50) Mean (SD) score	General hospitals (*n* = 109) Mean (SD) score
Reduction of rate of intubation and ventilation	4.5 (1.0)	4.8 (0.7)
Reduction in need for inter-hospital transfer	4.0 (1.2)	4.7 (0.7)
Reduction in length of stay	3.9 (1.0)	4.2 (0.8)
Reduction in complication rate	3.9 (1.2)	4.3 (0.9)
Improved patient tolerance	3.9 (1.1)	4.2 (0.9)
Reduced need for sedation	3.6 (1.2)	3.5 (1.2)
Parent/Carer Satisfaction	4.0 (0.9)	3.9 (1.1)

Our survey findings are similar to those of a recent survey of UK neonatal units –77% of neonatal units are using HFNC, mainly as an alternative to nCPAP [21]. Similar findings have been reported from Australia and New Zealand [32]. However, concerns regarding the safety of HFNC, and reports that it may delay timely access to invasive ventilation, do not support widespread adoption without ensuring an adequate level of clinical monitoring [17, 18].

Our survey results are important for several reasons. First, this is the first national survey of current practice in paediatrics relating to the use of non-invasive support for acute bronchiolitis. Both nCPAP and HFNC are available at most hospitals, but their use is variable and the clinical thresholds at which they are initiated are often different. Second, despite limited evidence, we have shown that HFNC appears to be the current preferred first-line support modality for infants with bronchiolitis. Third, despite enthusiasm for the use of HFNC, the majority of respondents were in clinical equipoise and were willing to participate in a future clinical trial, but a small proportion were not, a number that is only likely to rise in the face of increasing use and the absence of forthcoming evidence. Future studies should focus on clinical outcomes such as reduction in the need for intubation and ventilation and/or need for inter-hospital transfer.

Our survey had several strengths and limitations. We chose for practical purposes to send the survey link first to the regional retrieval services for onward dissemination, rather than directing it to each individual hospital. Even though the survey link was sent to all 12 PICU retrieval services, only 8 disseminated the survey to their network hospitals, thereby resulting in lower coverage than anticipated (54% of hospitals with inpatient paediatric facilities). However, since this was not a systematic process, it is unlikely to have resulted in significant bias. Indeed, we showed that hospitals that were not surveyed were similar to the ones that were surveyed, and that responders were similar to non-responders. The high survey response rate (83%) allows firm conclusions to be drawn regarding current practice. It is also worth highlighting that this was a self-reported questionnaire and as such, may not reflect actual practice, for which an audit of practice may be more useful. We also acknowledge that we studied a rapidly evolving field where clinical practice may already have changed since the survey was conducted.

Conclusions

Despite the paucity of supportive evidence, nCPAP and HFNC are routinely used to support infants with acute bronchiolitis. HFNC appears to be the preferred first-line modality although the indications for its use and clinical thresholds for its initiation are variable. There remains sufficient equipoise among clinicians to support a national randomised trial of non-invasive respiratory support in acute bronchiolitis.

Abbreviations

GH: General Hospital; HFNC: High Flow Nasal Cannula; nCPAP: Nasal continuous positive airway pressure; PHDU: Paediatric high dependency unit; PICU: Paediatric intensive care unit; RCT: Randomised controlled trial; RSV: Respiratory syncytial virus; TC: Tertiary centre

Acknowledgements

The Authors would like to thank Ms Rachel Winch, Workforce Projects Coordinator, Royal College of Paediatrics and Child Health and the Royal College of Paediatrics and Child Health for provision of data from the 2013 RCPCH Medical Workforce Census.

Funding

Not applicable.

Authors' contributions

PR conceptualised the study, reviewed and analysed the data, reviewed and revised the draft manuscript and approved the final manuscript submitted. HT designed the survey, carried out initial analyses, drafted the initial manuscript and approved the final manuscript submitted. RSA, JF, JP and AS piloted and distributed the survey. All authors read and approved the final manuscript.

Competing interests

The authors declare that they have no competing interests.

Author details

[1]Bristol Royal Hospital for Children, University Hospitals Bristol NHS Foundation Trust, Bristol, United Kingdom. [2]Great North Children's Hospital, The Newcastle upon Tyne Hospitals NHS Foundation Trust, Newcastle University, Newcastle upon Tyne, UK. [3]Institute of Cellular Medicine, Newcastle University, Newcastle upon Tyne, UK. [4]Country Durham and Darlington NHS Foundation trust, Darlington, UK. [5]Southampton Children's Hospital, Southampton, UK. [6]Institute of Child Health, University College London, GAP unit, Institute of Child Health, 30 Guilford Street, London WC1N 1EH, UK. [7]Children's Acute Transport Service, Great Ormond Street Hospital NHS Foundation Trust, London, UK.

References

1. Nagakumar P, Doull I. Current therapy for bronchiolitis. Arch Dis Child. 2012;97(9):827–30.
2. Henderson FW, Collier AM, Clyde Jr WA, Denny FW. Respiratory-syncytial-virus infections, reinfections and immunity. A prospective, longitudinal study in young children. N Engl J Med. 1979;300(10):530–4.
3. Zorc JJ, Hall CB. Bronchiolitis: recent evidence on diagnosis and management. Pediatrics. 2010;125(2):342–9.
4. Murray J, Bottle A, Sharland M, Modi N, Aylin P, Majeed A, et al. Risk factors for hospital admission with RSV bronchiolitis in England: a population-based birth cohort study. PLoS One. 2014;9(2):e89186.
5. Stockman LJ, Curns AT, Anderson LJ, Fischer-Langley G. Respiratory syncytial virus-associated hospitalizations among infants and young children in the United States, 1997–2006. Pediatr Infect Dis J. 2012;31(1):5–9.
6. Deshpande SA, Northern V. The clinical and health economic burden of respiratory syncytial virus disease among children under 2 years of age in a defined geographical area. Arch Dis Child. 2003;88(12):1065–9.
7. Mansbach JM, Piedra PA, Stevenson MD, Sullivan AF, Forgey TF, Clark S, et al. Prospective multicenter study of children with bronchiolitis requiring mechanical ventilation. Pediatrics. 2012;130(3):e492–500.
8. Lebel MH, Gauthier M, Lacroix J, Rousseau E, Buithieu M. Respiratory failure and mechanical ventilation in severe bronchiolitis. Arch Dis Child. 1989;64(10):1431–7.
9. Beasley JM, Jones SE. Continuous positive airway pressure in bronchiolitis. Br Med J (Clin Res Ed). 1981;283(6305):1506–8.
10. Javouhey E, Barats A, Richard N, Stamm D, Floret D. Non-invasive ventilation as primary ventilatory support for infants with severe bronchiolitis. Intensive Care Med. 2008;34(9):1608–14.
11. Yanez LJ, Yunge M, Emilfork M, Lapadula M, Alcantara A, Fernandez C, et al. A prospective, randomized, controlled trial of noninvasive ventilation in pediatric acute respiratory failure. Pediatr Crit Care Med. 2008;9(5):484–9.

12. Thia LP, McKenzie SA, Blyth TP, Minasian CC, Kozlowska WJ, Carr SB. Randomised controlled trial of nasal continuous positive airways pressure (CPAP) in bronchiolitis. Arch Dis Child. 2008;93(1):45–7.
13. Ducharme-Crevier L, Essouri S, Emeriaud G. Noninvasive ventilation in pediatric intensive care: from a promising to an established therapy, but for whom, when, why, and how? Pediatr Crit Care Med. 2015;16(5):481–2.
14. Oymar K, Bardsen K. Continuous positive airway pressure for bronchiolitis in a general paediatric ward; a feasibility study. BMC Pediatr. 2014;14:122.
15. Beggs S, Wong ZH, Kaul S, Ogden KJ, Walters JA. High-flow nasal cannula therapy for infants with bronchiolitis. Cochrane Database Syst Rev. 2014;1:CD009609.
16. Shetty S, Greenough A. Review finds insufficient evidence to support the routine use of heated, humidified high-flow nasal cannula use in neonates. Acta Paediatr. 2014;103(9):898–903.
17. Milesi C, Boubal M, Jacquot A, Baleine J, Durand S, Odena MP, et al. High-flow nasal cannula: recommendations for daily practice in pediatrics. Ann Intensive Care. 2014;4:29.
18. Hegde S, Prodhan P. Serious air leak syndrome complicating high-flow nasal cannula therapy: a report of 3 cases. Pediatrics. 2013;131(3):e939–44.
19. Baudin F, Gagnon S, Crulli B, Proulx F, Jouvet P, Emeriaud G. Modalities and complications associated with the use of high-flow nasal cannula: experience in a pediatric ICU. Respir Care. 2016;61(10):1305–10.
20. Crulli B, Loron G, Nishisaki A, Harrington K, Essouri S, Emeriaud G. Safety of paediatric tracheal intubation after non-invasive ventilation failure. Pediatr Pulmonol. 2016;51(2):165–72.
21. Ojha S, Gridley E, Dorling J. Use of heated humidified high-flow nasal cannula oxygen in neonates: a UK wide survey. Acta Paediatr. 2013;102(3):249–53.
22. Royal College of Paediatrics and Child Health. Medical Workforce Census 2013. London; 2014.
23. Royal College of Paediatrics and Child Health. High Dependency Care for Children - Time To Move On. London: Royal College of Paediatrics and Child Health; 2014.
24. Royal College of Nursing. Defining staffing levels for children and young people's services: RCN standards for clinical professionals and service managers. London: Royal College of Nursing; 2013.
25. Larrar S, Essouri S, Durand P, Chevret L, Haas V, Chabernaud JL, et al. Effects of nasal continuous positive airway pressure ventilation in infants with severe acute bronchiolitis. Arch Pediatr. 2006;13(11):1397–403.
26. Essouri S, Laurent M, Chevret L, Durand P, Ecochard E, Gajdos V, et al. Improved clinical and economic outcomes in severe bronchiolitis with pre-emptive nCPAP ventilatory strategy. Intensive Care Med. 2014;40(1):84–91.
27. Donlan M, Fontela PS, Puligandla PS. Use of continuous positive airway pressure (CPAP) in acute viral bronchiolitis: a systematic review. Pediatr Pulmonol. 2011;46(8):736–46.
28. Hough JL, Pham TM, Schibler A. Physiologic effect of high-flow nasal cannula in infants with bronchiolitis. Pediatr Crit Care Med. 2014;15(5):e214–9.
29. Pham TM, O'Malley L, Mayfield S, Martin S, Schibler A. The effect of high flow nasal cannula therapy on the work of breathing in infants with bronchiolitis. Pediatr Pulmonol. 2014;50:713–20.
30. Mayfield S, Bogossian F, O'Malley L, Schibler A. High-flow nasal cannula oxygen therapy for infants with bronchiolitis: pilot study. J Paediatr Child Health. 2014;50(5):373–8.
31. Klingenberg C, Pettersen M, Hansen EA, Gustavsen LJ, Dahl IA, Leknessund A, et al. Patient comfort during treatment with heated humidified high flow nasal cannulae versus nasal continuous positive airway pressure: a randomised cross-over trial. Arch Dis Child Fetal Neonatal Ed. 2014;99(2):F134–7.
32. Hough JL, Shearman AD, Jardine LA, Davies MW. Humidified high flow nasal cannulae: current practice in Australasian nurseries, a survey. J Paediatr Child Health. 2012;48(2):106–13.

Reduced *PRF1* enhancer methylation in children with a history of severe RSV bronchiolitis in infancy

Magdeldin Elgizouli[1], Chad Logan[2], Ruth Grychtol[3], Dietrich Rothenbacher[2], Alexandra Nieters[1*] and Andrea Heinzmann[3]

Abstract

Background: Acute lower respiratory tract infection is the commonest disease affecting children under five worldwide. Respiratory syncytial virus (RSV) is among the most common causative pathogens. Epidemiological data suggest an association between severe viral respiratory infections in infancy and increased incidence of childhood wheeze and asthma. DNA methylation is involved in immune cell differentiation and identity. It provides an avenue for environmental influences on the genome and therefore has potential as a marker for sustained effects of infectious insults. In this study we investigated the association between DNA methylation patterns in the perforin gene (*PRF1*) in childhood and a history of hospitalisation for severe RSV disease in the first two years of life.

Methods: In this retrospective study, we explored patterns of whole blood DNA methylation at a methylation sensitive region of the proximal *PRF1* enhancer in a group of children with a record of hospitalisation for severe RSV disease during infancy ($n = 43$) compared to healthy controls matched for age and sex with no similar hospitalisation history, no allergy and no persistent wheeze ($n = 43$). Univariate and bivariate conditional logistic regression analyses were conducted to test the association between *PRF1* enhancer methylation and record of hospitalisation for RSV disease.

Results: Children with a record of hospitalisation for severe RSV bronchiolitis demonstrated markedly lower levels of DNA methylation at two cytosine-phosphate-guanine dinucleotide (CpG) loci of the *PRF1* proximal enhancer, corresponding to a signal transducer and activator of transcription 5 (STAT5) responsive element, compared to controls, adjusted odds ratios of 0.82 (95% confidence interval [CI] 0.71, 0.94) and 0.73 (95% CI 0.58, 0.92) for each 1% increase in DNA methylation. Smoking in the household showed a significant influence on DNA methylation at the assayed positions.

Conclusions: Our findings support an association between childhood DNA methylation patterns in *PRF1* and a record of severe RSV infection in infancy. Longitudinal studies are required to establish the utility of *PRF1* methylation as a marker of severe RSV disease.

Keywords: Respiratory syncytial virus, Infant bronchiolitis, DNA methylation, Perforin, *PRF1*

* Correspondence: alexandra.nieters@uniklinik-freiburg.de
[1]Center for Chronic Immunodeficiency, Medical Center – University of Freiburg, Faculty of Medicine, University of Freiburg, Breisacherstr. 115 4, Freiburg D-79106, Germany
Full list of author information is available at the end of the article

Background

Acute lower respiratory tract infection (LRTI) is the leading cause of child mortality worldwide, the greater burden falling on developing countries [1]. On a global scale, respiratory syncytial virus (RSV) is the most common causative pathogen of LRTI in children under five years old and a major cause of hospital admission particularly in the first year of life. The incidence in infants is three times higher than overall incidence in children under five years of age [2].

Evidence is strong that viral respiratory infections in infancy are associated with increased risk of childhood wheezing, atopy and asthma [3], up to adolescence [4] and possibly early adulthood [5]. It is not entirely clear whether viral LRTIs including RSV are indeed a causal factor or simply indicate heightened susceptibility to asthma although considerable evidence supports a causal link [6].

DNA methylation, the commonest epigenetic alteration known to date, is crucial to processes of cellular differentiation and the establishment of cellular identity [7]. In contrast to genetic hardwire, genome-wide patterns of DNA methylation and other chromatin modifications do not persist throughout life but undergo specific changes at defined stages of development that contribute to lineage and tissue-specific gene expression [8]. As such, epigenetic modifications constitute a dynamic interface between genome and environment. Epigenetic modifications have been characterized in key effector and regulator genes as determinants of cell type and function in the immune system and modulators of immune response [9].

Epigenetic dysregulation is one potential mechanism which may mediate between adverse in utero and early life exposures such as severe infections and immunological functions in later life [10]. The interactions mediating the relationship between severe RSV bronchiolitis and adverse consequences in childhood are broadly understood to be immunological in nature [11] but are yet to be fully uncovered. Perforin is a potent cytolytic molecule of cytotoxic T cells and natural killer (NK) cells capable of non-specific lysis of virus-infected cells [12]. Perforin expression is under the control of interleukin (IL)-2, signalling through signal transducer and activator of transcription (STAT)-5 [13].

We previously reported higher methylation of specific cytosine-phosphate-guanine dinucleotide (CpG) positions corresponding to a STAT5 binding element in an enhancer region of *PRF1* in cord blood DNA of infants who subsequently developed frequent LRTI during their first year of life [14]. Considering the role perforin plays in the cellular immune response to virus infections, we hypothesised that severe RSV infection in infancy might be associated with alterations in *PRF1* methylation. Accordingly, we assayed DNA methylation at the two CpGs of the STAT5 element in the *PRF1* enhancer, in a cohort of children with a history of severe RSV bronchiolitis requiring hospitalisation during infancy compared to healthy children matched by sex and age at blood collection with no record of severe bronchiolitis, allergic disease or persistent wheeze.

Methods

Study subjects

Children with history of severe RSV disease were drawn from a cohort of children recruited at the University Children's Hospital and St Josef's Community Children Hospital in Freiburg, Germany, between September 1998 and March 2005 for the primary purpose of investigating genetic associations with severe RSV disease [15].

All children who were hospitalised for severe RSV disease in the first two years of life were considered eligible for inclusion in the cohort. Cases had symptoms of bronchiolitis at admission, such as wheezing and tachypnoea, and needed either supplementary oxygen and/or gavage feeding and/or intravenous fluids. Infection with RSV was confirmed by antigen test and/or polymerase chain reaction (PCR). Parents of all eligible patients were approached to enrol in the study and included upon informed consent.

Children with congenital heart defects, immunodeficiency, or chromosomal aberrations were excluded from the study. Information on treatment course was obtained from patients' hospital records regarding requirement for corticosteroid, antibiotic and oxygen therapy as well as a record of persistent wheeze. Indicators of family environment such as number of siblings and parents smoking in the house were obtained via standardized questionnaire filled in by the parents at time of blood draw. Blood samples were collected from study participants at a median of 3.25 years after hospitalisation (IQR 3.16–4.00). From a total baseline study population of 208 cases blood samples were obtained from 131 cases.

Healthy controls matched to cases by sex and approximate ages were recruited from healthy children seen at several paediatric practices in the same catchment area of Freiburg in southwestern Germany. Controls were recruited in the same time period as cases, 1998 to 2005, for the original purpose of the genetic association studies mentioned. Controls had no record of severe bronchiolitis in the first two years of life and were never diagnosed with persistent wheeze or allergic disease. Sex and age matching was not considered at time of recruitment but was undertaken for the purpose of this study. Controls were matched 1:1 on sex and the same age at blood sampling (plus or minus one year).

Blood samples were collected in ethylenediaminetetraacetic acid (EDTA) tubes processed, aliquoted and stored at −20 °C. Methylation assays were performed on genomic DNA derived from peripheral blood leukocyte samples of

43 children with a history of severe RSV disease and 43 healthy children with no history of severe RSV disease.

Collection of samples and study protocols were approved by the Ethics Commission of the Medical Centre, University of Freiburg. Written informed consent was obtained from parents of all participating children.

DNA extraction and bisulfite modification

Genomic DNA was manually extracted from peripheral blood leukocytes using the QIAamp® DNA Blood Midi Kit (Qiagen GmbH, Hilden, Germany) according to the manufacturer's protocol. DNA was stored at −20 °C before use. In preparation for pyrosequencing, 500 ng of DNA was bisulfite converted using the EZ DNA Methylation-Gold™ Kit (Zymo Research Corp, Irvine, CA, USA) according to the manufacturer's protocol. Non-methylated cytosines in this procedure are converted to uracil which is replaced in subsequent amplification by thymine while methylated cytosines are preserved unchanged.

Target cytosine dinucleotides

Cytosine methylation levels were measured in two CpG dinucleotides in the methylation sensitive region (MSR) of *PRF1* located 929 to 577 base pairs (bp) upstream of the transcription start site (TSS) and referred to as CpGs E1 and E2 as detailed previously [14]. Figure 1 shows the two CpGs investigated in the MSR of the *PRF1* proximal enhancer.

Bisulfite pyrosequencing

Quantification of cytosine percent methylation was performed by pyrosequencing of bilsulfite-converted DNA. Primers were designed with the PyroMark Assay Design Software v.2.0.1.15 (Qiagen GmbH, Hilden, Germany) to amplify the target region and purchased from Apara Biosciences GmbH (Denzlingen, Germany). Each assay included non-CpG cytosines as internal controls to verify efficient bisulfite conversion.

1.5 pmol each of the forward primer 5′-GAGTGGGA GAAGAGAGATG-3′ and the reverse biotinylated primer 5′-CCCCCAATACCCTATAAATCACTC-3′ were used to amplify the fragment of interest, sized 256 base pairs (bp), from an input amount of 0.5 µl bisulfite-converted DNA, 25 ng assuming complete recovery from bisulfite conversion, in a final reaction volume of 12.5 µl using the PyroMark PCR Kit (Qiagen GmbH, Hilden, Germany). PCR conditions were as follows 95 °C for 10 min; 50 cycles of 94 °C for 30 s, annealing for 30s, 72 °C for 30 s; and a final extension step at 72 °C for 10 min.

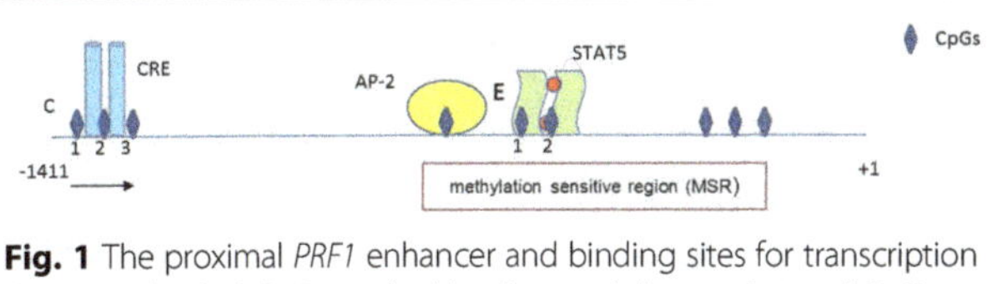

Fig. 1 The proximal *PRF1* enhancer and binding sites for transcription factors. Individual CpGs marked by diamond shapes. Assayed CpGs identified as E 1 and 2. CRE: cAMP responsive element; AP2: activating protein 2; STAT5: signal transducer and activator of transcription [14]

PCR products were rendered single stranded according to established protocol [16]. 3 pmol of the sequencing primer 5′-GTGAGGATAGTTAGTGG-3′ were used to perform the pyrosequencing reaction on the PyroMark Q96 MD apparatus (Qiagen GmbH, Hilden, Germany). The percentage methylation at each CpG was calculated using the PyroMark CpG Software v.1.0.11 build 14 (Qiagen GmbH, Hilden, Germany). The quantitative performance of the pyrosequencing assay was assessed by measuring methylation standards of known proportions of unmethylated (whole genome amplified) and fully methylated (*Sss-I* treated) genomic DNA and optimized by means of an annealing temperature gradient. Matched cases and controls were consistently assayed in the same batch. All samples were assayed in duplicates and the mean percentage of the two measurements calculated and used for statistical analyses.

Statistical analysis

Univariate analyses were conducted on each candidate gene locus to assess methylation results for normality and identify potential outliers. Methylation measurements greater than 3 standard deviations from the mean were considered as potential outliers. To identify potential confounding factors not accounted for by matching, age at sampling, gestational age (<37 weeks or ≥37 weeks), household smoking (yes or no), and whether or not the child had a sibling under 5 years of age (yes or no) were assessed for association with RSV case status and methylation levels using non-parametric testing methods (Chi-square, Fisher's exact, Spearman's coefficients and Kruskall-Wallis tests). Selection of potential confounders was based on a p-value ≤ 0.05. Household smoking was associated with both RSV case status and methylation levels and thus considered a potential confounding factor for adjustment in logistic regression models. Bivariate and adjusted conditional logistic regression models were used to calculate the odds ratio (OR) per 1% difference in methylation, 95% confidence interval (CI), and p-value for the association with case status at each candidate gene locus after adjustment for age at blood sampling and household smoking. In order to determine the effect of potential outliers on the results, a second bivariate analysis was performed restricted to pairs (case and matched control) containing no outlier values. All statistical analyses were performed using SAS 9.3 for Windows (SAS Institute, Cary, US).

Results

Study population

RSV cases and controls ($n = 86$) were 1:1 matched according to sex and approximate age at time of blood draw. Features of the RSV case-control population are presented in Table 1. Overall, children were predominantly male (65%). RSV cases had a median age of 3.3 years (interquartile range [IQR] 3.2, 4) while controls had a median age of 4 years (IQR 4.0, 5.0). The majority of children were born term, 81.1% of cases and 87.5% of controls. Cases had more often siblings and were more exposed to household smoking compared to controls (Table 1).

Among the cases 70% had a complicating bacterial infection requiring antibiotic medication, 30% received corticosteroid therapy and 10% already had a persistent wheeze before hospitalisation for RSV infection. Hospitalisation for severe RSV disease was associated with exposure to smoking in the household ($p = 0.02$) and having one or more siblings ($p = 0.02$).

Differential DNA methylation at the *PRF1* enhancer

Among all subjects, exposure to smoking in the household was associated with lower DNA methylation levels at E1 and E2 ($p = 0.003$, 0.004) but no associations were observed for gestational age, sex, or sibling status. Among RSV cases only (for whom more robust data was available), a diagnosis of persistent wheeze prior to hospitalisation for RSV disease was associated with lower DNA methylation levels in E1 ($p = 0.04$). None of the other clinical characteristics explored showed a statistically significant association with DNA methylation at the *PRF1* loci except maternal asthma ($p = 0.04$ with E2) (Table 2). When cases and controls were combined, exposure to smoking in the household was associated with lower DNA methylation levels at E1 and E2 ($p = 0.003$, 0.004) but no associations for gestational age, sex, and sibling status remained non-significant (Table 3).

Median DNA methylation levels of 69.5% (IQR 62.5, 74.5) and 65.0% (IQR 62.0, 70.0) were observed at CpGs E1 and E2 (illustrated in Fig. 1) in children hospitalised for RSV disease compared to 79.0% (IQR 75.0, 84.0) and 75.0% (IQR 72.0, 79.0) in controls ($p < 0.001$). Logistic regression analysis adjusted for exposure to smoking in the household demonstrated OR of 0.82 (95% CI 0.71, 0.94) and 0.73 (95% CI 0.58, 0.92) for E1 and E2 respectively for each 1% increase in methylation in association with case status (Table 4).

In an additional sensitivity analysis, adjustment for age at blood draw was performed to account for the loose age matching between cases and controls. Adjustment for age at blood sampling alone did not alter the point estimates. The small sample size however did not allow adjustment for both household smoking exposure and age at blood sampling.

Discussion

We investigated the whole blood DNA methylation pattern of two CpG sites in the proximal enhancer of the immune effector gene *PRF1* in a group of children with a history of hospitalisation for RSV disease in infancy compared to healthy children of matched sex and approximate age at blood sampling. In cases with RSV history we found markedly lower levels of DNA methylation at two loci of the *PRF1* proximal enhancer. In addition, infants who were admitted for RSV disease were predominantly male, had one sibling or more, and were more likely to come from a household where an adult smoked.

Table 1 Characteristics of children with history of hospitalisation for RSV bronchiolitis and healthy controls

	RSV-cases		Controls		*p*-value*
	n	% or median (p25, p75)	n	% or median (p25, p75)	
Age at blood sampling (years)	43	3.3 (3.2, 4.0)	43	4.0 (4.0, 5.0)	<.001
Gender					1
Female	15	34.9%	15	34.9%	
Male	28	65.1%	28	65.1%	
Gestational age					0.53
≥37 weeks	30	81.1%	28	87.5%	
<37 weeks	7	18.9%	4	12.5%	
Sibling status					0.02
None	2	5.7%	9	29%	
≥1	33	94.3%	22	71%	
Smoking in household					0.02
No	19	47.5%	24	75%	
Yes	21	52.5%	8	25%	

**p*-value calculated as either chi-square, Fisher's exact, or Kruskal-Wallis test

Table 2 Differential *PRF1* enhancer methylation according to clinical features of RSV bronchiolitis among cases only

Characteristics	DNA methylation levels at the *PRF1* enhancer					
	CpG E1			CpG E2		
	n	median (p25, p75) or Spearman's coefficient	*p*-value*	n	median (p25, p75) or Spearman's coefficient	*p*-value*
Age at hospitalisation (years)	38	−014	0.42	38	−016	0.33
Age at blood sampling	43	0.08	0.61	43	0.10	0.54
Gender			0.79			0.30
Female	15	68.0 (62.5, 73.5)		15	67.0 (63.0, 70.0)	
Male	28	69.5 (61.0, 74.5)		28	64.8 (59.3, 70.0)	
Gestational age			0.32			0.98
≥37 weeks	30	68.3 (63.0, 73.5)		30	64.8 (62.0, 68.5)	
<37 weeks	7	62.0 (36.0, 73.5)		7	65.5 (36.0, 72.0)	
Sibling status			0.62			0.57
None	2	55.3 (36.0, 74.5)		2	53.0 36.0, 70.0)	
≥1	33	69.5 (63.0, 74.5)		33	65.5 (63.0, 71.5)	
Smoking in the household			0.08			0.14
No	19	72.0 (66.0, 74.0)		19	67.0 (63.5, 72.0)	
Yes	21	65.5 (61.0, 70.0)		21	64.0 (61.5, 68.5)	
Previous wheeze			0.04			0.13
No	36	69.5 (63.8, 74.5)		36	65.5 (62.5, 71.0)	
Yes	4	62.3 (43.5, 64.3)		4	63.3 (42.0, 64.5)	
Parent allergic disease			0.50			0.23
No	20	69.5 (63.0, 75.0)		20	67.0 (63.5, 71.8)	
Yes	20	68.8 (62.3, 72.8)		20	64.0 (61.8, 69.3)	
Paternal asthma			0.07			0.19
No	37	69.5 (63.0, 74.5)		37	65.0 (63.0, 70.5)	
Yes	3	62.0 (25.0, 66.0)		3	63.5 (21.0, 65.5)	
Maternal asthma			0.32			0.04
No	37	69.5 (63.0, 74.5)		37	65.5 (63.0, 70.5)	
Yes	3	66.0 (25.0, 70.0)		3	61.5 (21.0, 63.5)	
Days of oxygen supplementation	40	−0.05	0.74	40	−0.11	0.51
Antibiotic therapy			0.62			0.65
No	12	69.5 (46.8, 74.5)		12	65.0 (46.5, 71.8)	
Yes	28	69.5 (63.8, 74.0)		28	65.0 (63.5, 69.5)	
Corticosteroid therapy			0.38			0.32
No	28	67.8 (61.8, 74.0)		28	64.8 (61.5, 70.3)	
Yes	12	71.3 (65.0, 74.0)		12	66.5 (64.0, 71.0)	

Differences in the total number of observations are due to missing data
n number of observations, *p25* 25th percentile, *p75* 75th percentile
**p*-value for categorical variables calculated using Kruskal-Wallis test

Holberg and colleagues reported a significant association of male sex with severe RSV infection in the first three months of life in the Tucson Children's Respiratory Study [17], an association confirmed in multiple other studies [18]. Having a sibling has been repeatedly reported as a risk factor for RSV induced LRTI in infancy [19]. The association with passive exposure to cigarette smoke is less consistent [18] but appears strong in combination with prematurity [20]. Infants exposed to postnatal maternal smoking suffer a more severe course of RSV disease with lower oxygen saturation during hospitalisation than the non-exposed [21]. In a large-scale surveillance of US children under five years spanning four years Hall and co-workers identified only age under

Table 3 Differential *PRF1* enhancer methylation according to characteristics of RSV bronchiolitis among all subjects (cases and controls combined)

Characteristics	DNA methylation levels at the *PRF1* enhancer					
	CpG E1			CpG E2		
	n	median (p25, p75)	*p*-value*	n	median (p25, p75)	*p*-value*
Gender			0.06			0.09
Female	30	74.8 (66.0, 83.0)		30	73.3 (67.0, 78.5)	
Male	56	74.0 (60.0, 78.8)		56	70.8 (64.3, 74.5)	
Gestational age			0.26			0.61
≥37 weeks	58	74.5 (67.5, 80.0)		58	70.8 (64.0, 75.0)	
<37 weeks	11	73.5 (55, 75.5)		11	70.0 (55.0, 73.5)	
Sibling status			0.34			0.25
None	11	75.5 (74.5, 84.5)		11	73.0 (70.0, 78.5)	
≥1	55	74.5 (66.0, 80.0)		55	71.5 (64.0, 75.0)	
Smoking in the household			0.003			0.004
No	43	75.5 (70.0, 83.2)		43	72.0 (67.0, 78.5)	
Yes	29	69.5 (62.5, 76.0)		29	68.0 (63.0, 72.5)	

Differences in the total number of observations are due to missing data
n number of observations, *p25* 25th percentile, *p75* 75th percentile
**p*-value calculated using Kruskal-Wallis test

six months and history of prematurity as independent risk factors for RSV hospitalisation [22]. The discrepancy may be related to the wider age definition in the latter study.

From the variables available for this analysis only exposure to smoking in the household showed an association with DNA methylation at the *PRF1* enhancer. Smoking is a potent environmental modulator of genome-wide DNA methylation including in utero, when methylation patterns are analysed in cord blood [23]. The association we observed between reduced DNA methylation at the *PRF1* enhancer in whole blood three to four years after hospitalisation for severe RSV disease during infancy remained significant after adjustment for smoking exposure. A separate analysis adjusted for age was performed to address the loose age matching in the study population but showed no significant difference in estimates.

The two CpGs assayed are located in a segment of the *PRF1* enhancer characterised as a methylation sensitive segment. Methylation of the *PRF1* MSR results in suppression of *PRF1* while demethylation is associated with heightened expression in T cells [24]. Our analysis was performed on DNA derived from whole blood, and we cannot with the available measurements rule out a confounding effect of cell subtype composition on our measurements. Hence, our results might reflect an expansion of the perforin-positive lymphocyte population rather than a true demethylation event in otherwise *PRF1*-methylated cells or more likely a combination of both. Perforin is normally expressed in almost all NK cells, NKT cells, γα T cells and around 20–30% of cytotoxic T cells and is broadly considered a marker of effector CD8+ T cell activation [25].

Table 4 Crude and adjusted model results for association between *PRF1* enhancer methylation and previous RSV bronchiolitis

PRF1 CpG position	Model Crude		Adjusted[a]	
	Odds Ratio (95% CI)[†]	*p*-value	Odds Ratio (95% CI)[†]	*p*-value
E1	0.81 (0.71, 0.92)	<0.001	0.82 (0.71, 0.94)	0.010
E2	0.67 (0.52, 0.87)	0.003	0.73 (0.58, 0.92)	0.009

[a]adjusted for household smoking
[†]Odds ratio for risk of case status based on a 1% increase in PRF1 methylation level and case status

CD8+ T cell proliferation and differentiation from naïve to effector and memory T cells in response to virus infection is associated with distinct epigenetic profiles corresponding to cell-specific transcriptional programmes [26]. We previously reported a prospective association between increased methylation at the *PRF1* enhancer MSR in cord blood and LRTI in the first year of life suggesting a reduced T cell/perforin reaction [14]. A robust cell-mediated cytotoxic response is necessary for viral clearance of RSV infection [27] but failure to effectively regulate this reaction might contribute to T cell mediated lung injury [28].

Accordingly, the reduced DNA methylation we observe in this retrospective study in contrast to the increased DNA methylation at the same locus in our prospective study of cord blood *PRF1* methylation and LRTI risk in the first year of life might reflect the differing requirements for a cytotoxic T cell response in these two situations. A robust cytotoxic response is needed to protect against respiratory viral infection, and reduced *PRF1* expression in newborns as indicated by higher DNA methylation is associated with increased risk of LRTI. On the other hand, increased expression of *PRF1* as indicated by reduction in DNA methylation, is associated with a record of severe RSV infection, and might contribute to lung damage. For instance, Arnold et al. reported an increase in perforin-positive peripheral blood lymphocytes in both intrinsic and allergic asthma [29].

Within the group of children with a history of RSV hospitalisation, we observed a greater reduction of whole blood DNA methylation at the *PRF1* enhancer in a subgroup who had a persistent wheeze before hospitalisation. Accordingly, we assayed the same locus in a separate group of asthmatic children and could observe intermediate levels of DNA methylation when compared to the higher levels in controls and lower levels in children with a history of hospitalisation for RSV disease (data not shown). Our analysis of asthmatic children (6 years old) is hampered by the lack of exact age-matched healthy controls which may have resulted in spurious results.

The cross-sectional design of this study does not allow for conclusions regarding temporal changes in DNA methylation. Only a longitudinal analysis would establish whether the reduced DNA methylation levels we observed are restored as the affected children grow. Therefore, further research may be warranted to establish causality. Childhood is a period of intense age-related changes in peripheral blood DNA methylation with a three to four-fold higher rate of change compared to adulthood [30].

Recurrent wheezing is a common complication of severe RSV bronchiolitis in infancy Meta-analysis of longitudinal studies however suggests that the heightened risk of wheeze and/or asthma is abolished by the fifth year of follow up [31]. DNA methylation is discussed as a mechanism of gene-environment interplay in the pathogenesis of asthma [32]. Several candidate gene and genome-wide association studies have so far documented differential DNA methylation patterns in asthma patients, including in T cells [33] and airway epithelial cells [34].

When looking at the results, the following limitations should be considered: Due to difficulty in obtaining a larger number of sex and age matched controls our study consisted of only 86 subjects. We had only limited additional data on our subjects to test for potential confounding. Though we were able to rule out confounding by two important factors previously associated with severe RSV infection (presence of smoking in the household and additional siblings in the household), the limited sample size did not allow for a thorough investigation of potential confounders. We could not completely rule out the possibility that the association we observed was due to chance selection of discordant subjects. Finally, due to the retrospective nature of the case-control design and measurement of only blood DNA methylation at one point in time, it remains unclear whether methylation levels were affected already prior to RSV infection. To further explore our preliminary findings a longitudinal analysis of a larger cohort with the possibility of isolating lymphocyte subtypes backed by sufficient epidemiological exposure data would be required.

Conclusions

We observed a reduction in blood DNA methylation of the *PRF1* proximal enhancer in children in association with previous hospitalisation for severe RSV bronchiolitis during infancy. This pattern of differential DNA methylation is worthy of investigation as a candidate marker for complications of severe RSV infection particularly persistent wheeze and childhood asthma. Our findings underscore the importance of considering the temporal dimension when studying DNA methylation patterns. Furthermore, they highlight the need for well-matched adequately powered longitudinal studies of epigenome-wide DNA methylation which, when supplemented with further epidemiological data, may improve our understanding of the dynamics of gene-environment interaction in the pathogenesis of disease.

Abbreviations

Bp: Base pair; CI: Confidence interval; CpG: Cytosine-phosphate-guanine; IQR: Interquartile range; LRTI: Lower respiratory tract infection; MSR: Methylation sensitive region; NK: Natural killer; OR: Odds ratio; PRF: Perforin; RSV: Respiratory syncytial virus; STAT5: Signal transducer and activator of transcription 5; TSS: Transcription start site

Acknowledgements

We thank Livia Maccioni for her assistance in final revision of the manuscript for submission.

Funding

This study was supported by the German Federal Ministry of Education and Research (BMBF 01EO1303). ME was funded by a grant of the German Academic Exchange Service (DAAD A/10/90132). The article processing charge was funded by the German Research Foundation (DFG) and the Albert Ludwigs University Freiburg in the funding programme Open Access Publishing.

Authors' contributions

ME performed the laboratory work, wrote the manuscript and participated in design of the study. CL performed the statistical analysis and helped draft the manuscript. RG contributed to collection of clinical data and interpretation of results. DR participated in design of the study and critically revised the manuscript. AH provided biological samples and clinical data. AN and AH conceived and designed the study and participated in revision. All authors read and approved the final manuscript.

Competing interests
The authors declare that they have no competing interests.

Author details
[1]Center for Chronic Immunodeficiency, Medical Center – University of Freiburg, Faculty of Medicine, University of Freiburg, Breisacherstr. 115 4, Freiburg D-79106, Germany. [2]Institute of Epidemiology and Medical Biometry, Ulm University, Ulm, Germany. [3]Department of Pediatrics and Adolescent Medicine, Medical Center – University of Freiburg, Faculty of Medicine, University of Freiburg, Freiburg, Germany.

References
1. Nair H, Simoes EA, Rudan I, Gessner BD, Azziz-Baumgartner E, Zhang JS, Feikin DR, Mackenzie GA, Moisi JC, Roca A, et al. Global and regional burden of hospital admissions for severe acute lower respiratory infections in young children in 2010: a systematic analysis. Lancet. 2013;381(9875):1380–90.
2. Nair H, Nokes DJ, Gessner BD, Dherani M, Madhi SA, Singleton RJ, O'Brien KL, Roca A, Wright PF, Bruce N, et al. Global burden of acute lower respiratory infections due to respiratory syncytial virus in young children: a systematic review and meta-analysis. Lancet. 2010;375(9725):1545–55.
3. James KM, Gebretsadik T, Escobar GJ, Wu P, Carroll KN, Li SX, Walsh EM, Mitchel EF, Sloan C, Hartert TV. Risk of childhood asthma following infant bronchiolitis during the respiratory syncytial virus season. J Allergy Clin Immunol. 2013;132(1):227–9.
4. Sigurs N, Gustafsson PM, Bjarnason R, Lundberg F, Schmidt S, Sigurbergsson F, Kjellman B. Severe respiratory syncytial virus bronchiolitis in infancy and asthma and allergy at age 13. Am J Respir Crit Care Med. 2005;171(2):137–41.
5. Sigurs N, Aljassim F, Kjellman B, Robinson PD, Sigurbergsson F, Bjarnason R, Gustafsson PM. Asthma and allergy patterns over 18 years after severe RSV bronchiolitis in the first year of life. Thorax. 2010;65(12):1045–52.
6. Feldman AS, He Y, Moore ML, Hershenson MB, Hartert TV. Toward primary prevention of asthma. Reviewing the evidence for early-life respiratory viral infections as modifiable risk factors to prevent childhood asthma. Am J Respir Crit Care Med. 2015;191(1):34–44.
7. Ji H, Ehrlich LI, Seita J, Murakami P, Doi A, Lindau P, Lee H, Aryee MJ, Irizarry RA, Kim K, et al. Comprehensive methylome map of lineage commitment from haematopoietic progenitors. Nature. 2010;467(7313):338–42.
8. Cantone I, Fisher AG. Epigenetic programming and reprogramming during development. Nat Struct Mol Biol. 2013;20(3):282–9.
9. Obata Y, Furusawa Y, Hase K. Epigenetic modifications of the immune system in health and disease. Immunol Cell Biol. 2015;93(3):226–32.
10. Waterland RA, Michels KB. Epigenetic epidemiology of the developmental origins hypothesis. Annu Rev Nutr. 2007;27:363–88.
11. Legg JP, Hussain IR, Warner JA, Johnston SL, Warner JO. Type 1 and type 2 cytokine imbalance in acute respiratory syncytial virus bronchiolitis. Am J Respir Crit Care Med. 2003;168(6):633–9.
12. Hoves S, Trapani JA, Voskoboinik I. The battlefield of perforin/granzyme cell death pathways. J Leukoc Biol. 2010;87(2):237–43.
13. Zhang J, Scordi I, Smyth MJ, Lichtenheld MG. Interleukin 2 receptor signaling regulates the perforin gene through signal transducer and activator of transcription (Stat) 5 activation of two enhancers. J Exp Med. 1999;190(9):1297–308.
14. Elgizouli M, Logan C, Nieters A, Brenner H, Rothenbacher D. Cord blood PRF1 methylation patterns and risk of lower respiratory tract infections in infants: findings from the Ulm Birth Cohort. Medicine. 2015;94(1):e332.
15. Puthothu B, Krueger M, Forster J, Heinze J, Weckmann M, Heinzmann A. Interleukin (IL)-18 polymorphism 133C/G is associated with severe respiratory syncytial virus infection. Pediatr Infect Dis J. 2007;26(12):1094–8.
16. Tost J, Gut IG. DNA methylation analysis by pyrosequencing. Nat Protoc. 2007;2(9):2265–75.
17. Holberg CJ, Wright AL, Martinez FD, Ray CG, Taussig LM, Lebowitz MD. Risk factors for respiratory syncytial virus-associated lower respiratory illnesses in the first year of life. Am J Epidemiol. 1991;133(11):1135–51.
18. Simoes EA. Environmental and demographic risk factors for respiratory syncytial virus lower respiratory tract disease. J Pediatr. 2003;143(5 Suppl):S118–26.
19. Rossi GA, Medici MC, Arcangeletti MC, Lanari M, Merolla R, Paparatti UD, Silvestri M, Pistorio A, Chezzi C. Risk factors for severe RSV-induced lower respiratory tract infection over four consecutive epidemics. Eur J Pediatr. 2007;166(12):1267–72.
20. Blanken MO, Rovers MM, Molenaar JM, Winkler-Seinstra PL, Meijer A, Kimpen JL, Bont L. Respiratory syncytial virus and recurrent wheeze in healthy preterm infants. N Engl J Med. 2013;368(19):1791–9.
21. Bradley JP, Bacharier LB, Bonfiglio J, Schechtman KB, Strunk R, Storch G, Castro M. Severity of respiratory syncytial virus bronchiolitis is affected by cigarette smoke exposure and atopy. Pediatrics. 2005;115(1):e7–14.
22. Hall CB, Weinberg GA, Iwane MK, Blumkin AK, Edwards KM, Staat MA, Auinger P, Griffin MR, Poehling KA, Erdman D, et al. The burden of respiratory syncytial virus infection in young children. N Engl J Med. 2009;360(6):588–98.
23. Richmond RC, Simpkin AJ, Woodward G, Gaunt TR, Lyttleton O, McArdle WL, Ring SM, Smith AD, Timpson NJ, Tilling K, et al. Prenatal exposure to maternal smoking and offspring DNA methylation across the lifecourse: findings from the Avon Longitudinal Study of Parents and Children (ALSPAC). Hum Mol Genet. 2015;24(8):2201–17.
24. Lu Q, Wu A, Ray D, Deng C, Attwood J, Hanash S, Pipkin M, Lichtenheld M, Richardson B. DNA methylation and chromatin structure regulate T cell perforin gene expression. J Immunol. 2003;170(10):5124–32.
25. Bade B, Boettcher HE, Lohrmann J, Hink-Schauer C, Bratke K, Jenne DE, Virchow Jr JC, Luttmann W. Differential expression of the granzymes A, K and M and perforin in human peripheral blood lymphocytes. Int Immunol. 2005;17(11):1419–28.
26. Russ BE, Olshanksy M, Smallwood HS, Li J, Denton AE, Prier JE, Stock AT, Croom HA, Cullen JG, Nguyen ML, et al. Distinct epigenetic signatures delineate transcriptional programs during virus-specific CD8(+) T cell differentiation. Immunity. 2014;41(5):853–65.
27. Isaacs D, Bangham CR, McMichael AJ. Cell-mediated cytotoxic response to respiratory syncytial virus in infants with bronchiolitis. Lancet. 1987;2(8562):769–71.
28. Bruder D, Srikiatkhachorn A, Enelow RI. Cellular immunity and lung injury in respiratory virus infection. Viral Immunol. 2006;19(2):147–55.
29. Arnold V, Balkow S, Staats R, Matthys H, Luttmann W, Virchow Jr JC. Increase in perforin-positive peripheral blood lymphocytes in extrinsic and intrinsic asthma. Am J Respir Crit Care Med. 2000;161(1):182–6.
30. Alisch RS, Barwick BG, Chopra P, Myrick LK, Satten GA, Conneely KN, Warren ST. Age-associated DNA methylation in pediatric populations. Genome Res. 2012;22(4):623–32.
31. Kneyber MCJ, Steyerberg EW, de Groot R, Moll HA. Long-term effects of respiratory syncytial virus (RSV) bronchiolitis in infants and young children: a quantitative review. Acta Paediatr. 2000;89(6):654–60.
32. de Planell-Saguer M, Lovinsky-Desir S, Miller RL. Epigenetic regulation: the interface between prenatal and early-life exposure and asthma susceptibility. Environ Mol Mutagen. 2014;55(3):231–43.
33. Runyon RS, Cachola LM, Rajeshuni N, Hunter T, Garcia M, Ahn R, Lurmann F, Krasnow R, Jack LM, Miller RL, et al. Asthma discordance in twins is linked to epigenetic modifications of T cells. PLoS One. 2012;7(11):e48796.
34. Stefanowicz D, Hackett TL, Garmaroudi FS, Gunther OP, Neumann S, Sutanto EN, Ling KM, Kobor MS, Kicic A, Stick SM, et al. DNA methylation profiles of airway epithelial cells and PBMCs from healthy, atopic and asthmatic children. PLoS One. 2012;7(9):e44213.

12

Simultaneous detection of respiratory syncytial virus and human metapneumovirus by one-step multiplex real-time RT-PCR in patients with respiratory symptoms

Huey-Ling You[1,2†], Shun-Jen Chang[3†], Hong-Ren Yu[4], Chia-Chin Li[1], Chang-Han Chen[5,6,7] and Wei-Ting Liao[8,9*]

Abstract

Background: Both respiratory syncytial virus (RSV) and human metapneumovirus (hMPV) are important viral pathogens causing respiratory tract infection (RTI) in the pediatric population. However, the clinical manifestations of RSV and hMPV infections are similar. Therefore, a reliable and rapid diagnostic tool is needed for diagnostic performance.

Methods: In order to optimize diagnosis efficiency of RTI, the aim of this study is to establish a rapid and advanced method for simultaneous detecting RSV and hMPV in nasopharyngeal aspirates specimens from patients. We designed a one-step triplex real-time RT-PCR (qRT-PCR) protocol using TaqMan probes for detecting RSV and hMPV. The plasmid clones containing RSV nucleoprotein gene and hMPV fusion gene were established as reference standards. We used virus culture supernatants from 86 known pediatric RTI patient to test the specificity and sensitivity of our assay. Then we used total 222 nasopharyngeal aspirates specimens from pediatric patients hospitalized with respiratory symptoms to evaluate our assay.

Results: Our one-step triplex qRT-PCR assay showed 100% sensitivity and specificity in testing RSV and hMPV in 86 known virus culture supernatants, with excellent linearity ($R^2 > 0.99$) and reliable reproducibility (CV lower than 1.04%). This assay has a wide dynamic range 10^2-10^9copies/reaction (limit of detection; LOD = 100 copies/reaction). A total of 222 patients hospitalized with respiratory symptoms were enrolled for clinical evaluation. In these samples, our qRT-PCR assay detected 68 RSV positive and 18 hMPV positive cases. However, standard virus culture only detected 8 RSV positive cases and 0 hMPV cases. Based on this improved triplex qRT-PCR assay, we found that RSV infection was associated with severe inflammation by chest X-ray and occurrence of pneumonia which were not observed previously.

Conclusions: In summary, we have developed a highly specific and sensitive one-step triplex qRT-PCR assay to detect hMPV and RSV simultaneously. This assay offers a valuable tool for routine diagnosis.

Keywords: RSV, hMPV, Real-time RT-PCR, Respiratory tract infection

* Correspondence: wtliao@kmu.edu.tw
[†]Equal contributors
[8]Department of Biotechnology, College of Life Science, Kaohsiung Medical University, No. 100 Shih-Chuan 1st Road, Kaohsiung 807, Taiwan
[9]Department of Biological Sciences, National Sun Yat-Sen University, Kaohsiung, Taiwan
Full list of author information is available at the end of the article

Background

Acute respiratory tract infection (RTI) is estimated to be the second important cause of death throughout the world among children less than 5 years old [1]. Both respiratory syncytial virus (RSV) and human metapneumovirus (hMPV) are important viral pathogens inducing RTI [2–4]. RSV and hMPV are non-segmented, negative-strand, enveloped RNA viruses. Both of them are classified within the Pneumovirinae subfamily of the Paramyxoviridae family. RSV is implicated in the majority of respiratory tract infection, which accounts for 60–80% of the bronchiolitis cases in children below 12 months of age [5]. Recently, it has been demonstrated that hMPV also causes acute respiratory tract infections, similar to RSV [1, 6]. hMPV was first identified in 2001 from a pediatric patient with respiratory diseases in the Netherlands [7]. hMPV causes a wide spectrum of disease ranging from mild upper RTI to more severe lower RTI such as bronchiolitis or pneumonia. Second to RSV, hMPV causes bronchiolitis and accounts for 5–15% of child hospitalizations for RTI [8, 9].

Both RSV and hMPV infections induce disruption of respiratory epithelial architecture, sloughing of epithelial cells, loss of cilation and acute pulmonary inflammation characterized by alveolitis, interstitial inflammation and peribronchiolitis [7, 9]. Following, acute otitis media is the most common complication of RTI due to RSV or hMPV [8]. At present, the initial clinical manifestations of RSV are indistinguishable from those of hMPV [10–12]. One possible reference to distinguish RSV and hMPV infections is based on the epidemiological data. The median age of hMPV-positive hospitalized patients is 6-12 months, which is significantly higher than that of RSV (2-3 months) [13].

RSV and hMPV do not appear to be significantly associated with asymptomatic carriage in the respiratory tract of healthy persons. However, the diagnosis efficiency for these 2 virus infection is low using the classical virus culture methods. Both viruses are labile in the environment and are susceptible to drying [14]. For viral culture, RSV can growth in the HEp-2, A549, or Vero cells and usually takes 3–5 days to revealing characteristic syncytial cytopathic pattern [7, 15–17]. In contrast, hMPV can growth in the LLC-MK2 cells. The growth of hMPV is slow and often requires several blind passages before any cytopathic effect (CPE) is apparent, particularly following primary isolation, which often takes more than 10 days [18]. These lengthy viral culture processes, in part, limited the opportunity for optimal initial diagnosis and the following therapeutic adjustment for RTI patient. Therefore, a reliable and rapid diagnostic tool is needed. Rapid and accurate laboratory diagnosis of viral RTI is crucial for optimal clinical management, diminishes unnecessary use of antibiotics, and allows for use of antivirals when appropriate.

Objectives

The aim of this study is to design and assess the diagnostic performance of clinical specimens for the simultaneous identification of RSV and hMPV by using one-step triplex qRT-PCR assay with TaqMan probes. To this aim, we first performed our primer and probe design. Then we used cultured viruses to evaluate the specificity of our primers using qRT-PCR. Finally, we used this established qRT-PCR assay to detect the viral load in nasopharyngeal aspirates.

Methods

Primers and probe design

The primers and probes for RSV, hMPV and GAPDH were designed by Primer 3 website (http://bioinfo.ut.ee/primer3-0.4.0/primer3/). We selected RSV nucleoprotein gene conserved regions as a target for our RSV primer and probe designs. For hMPV, we selected hMPV fusion protein gene conserved regions as a target for our primer and probe designs. The target sequence of our primer and probe designs was showed in Table 1. The

Table 1 Design of the one-step triplex qRT-PCR assays for the detection of RSV, hMPV and Internal Control

Virus	Target gene	Name of primer or probe	Sequence (5′ → 3′)	Position
RSV	Nucleoprotein	RSV-F	TGATACACTSAACAAAGATCAACTTCTG	27–54[a]
		RSV-R	TCTCCTGTGCTMCGTTGRAT	73–92[a]
		RSV-probe	VIC-CATCCAGCAAATACAC-MGBNFQ	56–71[a]
hMPV	Fusion protein	hMPV-F	TCAGAATGCAGGGTCAACTGTT	156–177[b]
		hMPV-R	GACATGGTCTCCTCTTGTTTCACA	199–222[b]
		hMPV-probe	FAM-CAAGCTTCCCGTTCTCAGCC-MGBNFQ	179–197[b]
Internal Control	GAPDH	GAPDH-F	GAAGGTGAAGGTCGGAGTC	108–126[c]
		GAPDH-R	GAAGATGGTGATGGGATTTC	314–333[c]
		GAPDH-probe	NED-CAAGCTTCCCGTTCTCAGCC-MGBNFQ	285–304[c]

[a]GenBank Accession no. DQ780565.1
[b]GenBank Accession no. AY295956.1
[c]GenBank Accession no. NM_002046

specificity of these primer and probe sequences were tested by the BLAST algorithm.

To rapidly and accurately quantify the RSV and hMPV in nasopharyngeal aspirates, we combined 3 single qRT-PCR, amplifying RSV, hMPV and GAPDH (internal control), in a one-tube reaction. For this one-tube reaction, the probe for RSV was labeled with the dye VIC dye at its 5′ end and minor groove binder (MGB) at its 3′end. The probe for hMPV was labeled with the reporter 6-carboxyfluorescein (FAM) dye at its 5′ end and MGB at its 3′ end. The probe for GAPDH was labeled with NED dye at its 5′ end and MGB at its 3′ end. RSV, hMPV and GAPDH amplification signals were separately detected by the VIC, FAM and NED channels by multi-channel qRT-PCR detection system. The primers for direct sequencing as described following: hMPV-F: 5′-CAACT GTTTACTACCCAAATGA-3′, hMPV-R: 5′-ATAGGG TGTCTTCCTGTGC-3′; RSV-F: 5′-TTAACCAGCAAA GTGTTAGAYCTCAA-3′, RSV-R: 5′-CTGRTCATTTG TTATRGGCATATCATTG-3′.

Virus culture and immunofluorescence assay

In brief, sterile beads were added to the samples, vortexed and processed routinely followed by centrifuged at 2000 rpm for 7 min. Specimens were then decontaminated by adding a 10% antibiotic mixture (Gibco, N.Y.USA) and incubating for 1 h at 4 °C. A volume of 200 μL of sample was inoculated into each of the following cell lines: MRC-5, HEp2, RD, MDCK, and LLCMK2 (ATCC, Manassas, VA, USA). One μΛ of maintenance medium (minimal essential medium with 1% fetal bovine serum) (Gibco, N.Y.USA) was added to each cell line and incubated at 37 °C for 14 days. The CPE was observed every other working day by inverted light microscopy (Olympus, Japan). After CPE appeared, cell smears were prepared and fixed in chilled acetone at −20 °C for 10 min and then tested by fluorescein-conjugated monoclonal antibody in a direct immunofluorescence assay (D^3 Ultra 8™ DFA Respiratory Virus Screening & ID Kit, Diagnostic Hybrids, USA). Stained cell smears were examined in a fluorescence microscope at 400× magnification (Olympus, Japan). Un-inoculated cell smear was used as negative control.

Reference standard

To establish reference standards for RSV and hMPV viral load, we established 2 plasmid clones containing RSV nucleoprotein gene sequence and hMPV fusion protein gene sequence. These plasmids were amplified and cloned into a pCR® 2.1-TOPO® cloning vector using a TOPO TA cloning kit for sequencing (Invitrogen, Carlsbad, CA). Sequencing of the cloned insert established the fidelity of the sequence. Plasmid DNA containing each fragment sequence was purified, linearized by restriction enzyme digestion. The concentration of DNA was measured at least four times by a spectrophotometer (IMPLEN NanoPhotometer™, CA, USA), and the numbers of copies per μL were calculated using the mean values and the following formula: $[(g/\mu L\ DNA)/(length \times 660)] \times 6.022 \times 10^{23}$, where the length is the number of nucleotides. Tenfold dilutions equivalent to 10^2 to 10^9 copies/reaction of plasmid were used to determine the limit of detection (LOD) of the one-step triplex qRT-PCR assay.

Sample collection

This study included infants (<24 months) and young children (<6 years old) admitted to the pediatric department of Kaohsiung Chang Gung Memorial Hospital. Children and infants were eligible if identified as having one or more of the following symptoms: difficulty in breathing, nasal discharge, blocked nose, cough, or fast breathing for age. Nasopharyngeal aspirates were prospectively collected from November, 2010 to August, 2011. Informed consent was signed from the parent/guardian of each child. The nasopharyngeal aspirates (NPAs) were sent for virus isolation and identification. The RSV and hMPV were identified by using two methods in each individual sample. One was one-step triplex qRT-PCR, the other was immunofluorescence approach to confirm the virus etiology after CPE formation. Ethical approval for the study was obtained from the Chang Gung Memorial Hospital Ethics Committee (99-2746B).

Nucleic acid extraction and triplex RT-PCR (qRT-PCR)

RNA was extracted from the supernatants of cultured viruses or nasopharyngeal aspirates by QIAamp viral RNA mini kit (Qiagen, Valencia, CA, USA) according to the manufactures instructions. All the RNA extraction procedure was conducted at BSL-2 laboratory. The qRT-PCR of a final concentration of 12.5 μL Master Mix and 0.625 μL Enzyme Mix (TaqManR RNA-to-CT™ *1-Step* Kit, Applied Biosystems), 400 nM each primer; 200 nM each probe, plus 7 μL of target RNA and was made up to a volume of 25 μL with nuclease free water (Promega Corp. Madison, USA). The reactions were incubated at 48 °C for 30 min, followed by 95 °C for 15 s (inactivation reverse transcriptase/activation Taq polymerase), 40 cycles of 95 °C for 15 s (denaturation), and 54 °C for 1 min (annealing). RT-PCR assays were performed on an ABI 7500-fast (Applied Biosystem). If Ct >40 with lower concentration of virus, the amount of specimens was augmented for increasing the concentration of RNA and following One-step RT-PCR and direct sequencing.

Statistic analysis

The sensitivity and specificity of triplex qRT-PCR results were analyzed by the receiver operating characteristic

(ROC) method by SPSS software (SPSS statistical package version 17, SPSS Inc., Chicago, IL). The linearity and reproducibility for RSV and hMPV triplex qRT-PCR were analyzed by and linear regression and absolute quantification analysis (StepOnePlus software v2.3) provided by ABI 7500-fast PCR machine. Demographic data was analyzed by Student's "t" test and chi-square using SPSS software. A p-value < 0.05 was considered significant.

Results

Assay specificity

A total of 86 virus culture stocks were used in specificity testing. The different virus etiology including RSV ($n = 20$), hMPV ($n = 23$), adenovirus ($n = 10$), enterovirus ($n = 8$), influenza A ($n = 4$), influenza B ($n = 4$), CMV ($n = 5$), HSV-1 ($n = 3$), parainfluenza type 1 ($n = 3$), parainfluenza type 2 ($n = 3$) and parainfluenza type 3($n = 3$). No positive result was obtained for non-RSV or non-hMPV. We also used DEPC water as a negative control. The internal control and positive-control reactions were positive. Results showed that this one-step triplex qRT-PCR assay was specific and did not cross among RSV, hMPV and internal control GAPHD, with each other. Primer pair RSVF/RSVR and probe RSV-probe reacted only with RSV samples, whereas primers hMPVF/hMPVR and probe hMPV-probe allowed for the specific detection of hMPV isolates. The sensitivity and specificity of the one-step triplex qRT-PCR assay were both 100% when testing known viral stocks (Table 2).

Assay linearity

Linearity of the one-step triplex qRT-PCR assay was determined using serial 10-fold dilutions of RSV and hMPV standard in viral transport medium (VTM) at the following concentrations:10^2, 10^3, 10^4, 10^5, 10^6, 10^7, $10^8$and 10^9 copies/reaction. The extracted DNA was then analyzed by the triplex qRT-PCR assay. Three replicates were tested in a single run at each concentration. The relationship between the observed values and true concentrations of analyses was examined through linear regression. The limit of detection (LOD) of the triplex qRT-PCR assay was 100 copies/reaction. Linear regression analysis of the Ct values against the log10 RSV and hMPV plasmid concentration yielded $R^2 = 0.998$ (Fig. 1a) and 0.992 (Fig. 1b), respectively. The detail statistic results were showed in Table 3.

Assay precision

Precision was estimated by performing the one-step triplex qRT-PCR assay twice per day (each run separated by a minimum of 2 h) over 2 days, by the same technician using the same equipment and reagent lot numbers. The intra-assay variation was assessed by testing 2 samples with different viral loads (10^8 and 10^2 copies/reaction) 3 times in a single run, while the inter-assay variation was assessed by testing the same samples 3 times in 2 separate runs. In our assay, the coefficient of variation (CV,

Table 2 Analytical sensitivity and specificity of triplex qRT-PCR assay in 86 known virus culture supernatants

Virus Culture Stocks	Cultural Results No.(n)	Triplex qRT-PCR Results (n)	
		RSV+	hMPV+
RSV	20	20	0
hMPV	23	0	23
Adenovirus	10	0	0
Enterovirus	8	0	0
Influenza A virus	4	0	0
Influenza B virus	4	0	0
CMV	5	0	0
HSV-1	3	0	0
Parainfluenza virus 1	3	0	0
Parainfluenza virus 2	3	0	0
Parainfluenza virus 3	3	0	0
Total	86		

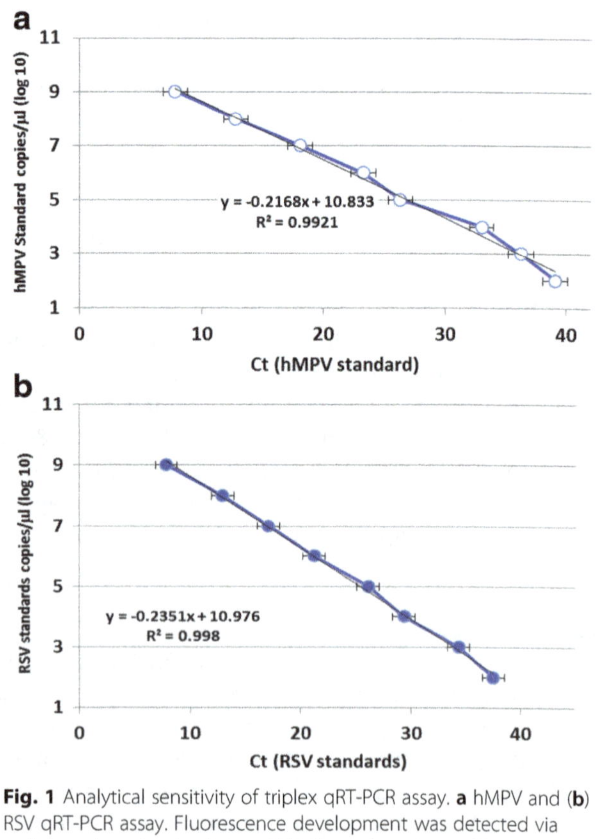

Fig. 1 Analytical sensitivity of triplex qRT-PCR assay. **a** hMPV and (**b**) RSV qRT-PCR assay. Fluorescence development was detected via real-time detection in triplex qRT-PCR run by using a dilution range of 10^9–10^2 DNA molecules/reaction of the hMPV and RSV molecular standards (Graph generated by ESE quant tube scanner studio software)

Table 3 The linearity data for RSV and hMPV triplex qRT-PCR

Target	Slope	Intercept	r^2	Linear range (copies/reaction)	LOD[a] (copies/ reaction)
hMPV	−4.57	45.19	0.992	10^2–10^9	100
RSV	−3.91	44.85	0.998	10^2–10^9	100

[a]Limit of detection

express imprecision) was lower than 5%. The intra-assay CV ranged from 0.10 to 0.47%, while the inter-assay CV ranged from 0.23 to 1.04% (Table 4).

Clinical evaluation

A total of 222 pediatric patients hospitalized with respiratory symptoms were enrolled from November 2010 through August 2011. Study patients were 61% male and 39% female with a mean age of 0.91 years old (ranges from32 days to 14 years old). The admitting diagnoses of these infants were bronchiolitis (58%), brochopneumonia (24%), and pneumonia (18%). Our one-step triplex qRT-PCR results showed that the viral load of the RSV or hMPV-positive samples from clinical specimens varied over a wide range, presenting threshold between Ct 21 and 44 (21 and 44 cycles). As a result, 68 specimens (30.6%) were found RSV positive, 18 specimens (8.1%) were found hMPV positive by our one-step triplex qRT-PCR. However, standard virus culture only detected 8 RSV positive cases (3.6%) and 0 hMPV cases (0%) (Table 5). In detecting RSV, the major distribution of threshold cycles ranged between Ct 21 and 25 (1,035,656 copies/ reaction ~77,992 copies/reaction). In detecting hMPV, the major distribution of threshold cycles ranged between Ct 31 and 35 (8395 copies/ reaction ~476 copies/ reaction) (Fig. 2).

qRT-PCR RSV positive patients were associated with increased severe inflammation and pneumonia

The demographic data based on RSV/hMPV one-step triplex qRT-PCR detection in 222 infants hospitalized with respiratory symptoms showed that male patients have higher percentages in RSV or hMPV infection. RSV

Table 4 Reproducibility of the triplex qRT-PCR assay

	Target	Conc. (copies/ reaction)	Number of determinations	Mean Ct	SD	CV (%)
Intra-assay	hMPV	10^8	3	13.90	0.033	0.24
		10^2	3	35.69	0.170	0.47
	RSV	10^8	3	15.80	0.015	0.10
		10^2	3	39.10	0.112	0.29
Inter-assay	hMPV	10^8	6	13.89	0.032	0.23
		10^2	6	36.46	0.863	0.91
	RSV	10^8	6	16.18	0.430	1.04
		10^2	6	38.98	0.225	0.58

Table 5 Comparing of triplex qRT-PCR assay and virus culture in nasopharyngeal aspirates from 222 patients hospitalized with respiratory symptoms

Virus Culture Stocks	Cultural Results No.(n)	Triplex qRT-PCR Results (n)	
		RSV+	hMPV+
RSV	8	8	0
hMPV	0	0	0
Adenovirus	16	0	0
Enterovirus	8	0	0
Influenza A virus	1	0	0
Influenza B virus	1	0	0
CMV	3	0	0
Parainfluenza virus 1	3	0	0
Parainfluenza virus 2	1	0	0
Parainfluenza virus 3	13	0	0
[a]NVI	168	60	18
Total	222	68	18

[a]*NVI* Non virus identified using virus culture

and hMPV infection cases were significantly associated with severe lung inflammation based on chest X-Ray index. Complication of pneumonia was observed in more than 90% of RSV or hMPV infection patient (Table 6). In addition, we found that RSV or hMPV infection is not associated with C-reactive protein level, indicating the importance of making definite diagnosis in early intervention of RSV and hMPV associated adverse effects, such as severe inflammation and pneumonia.

Discussion

In this study, we established a rapid and internally controlled triplex qRT-PCR assay that can identify RSV and

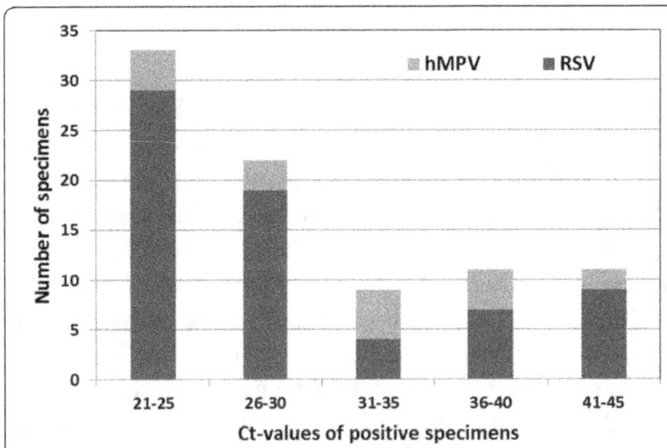

Fig. 2 Ct values distribution of RSV and hMPV positive clinical specimens. Our one-step triplex qRT-PCR results showed that the viral load of the RSV or hMPV-positive samples from clinical specimens varied over a wide range, presenting threshold cycles between 21 and 44. RSV has a maximum occurrence detected between Ct 21 and 25, but hMPV has a maximum occurrence between Ct 31 and 35

Table 6 Demographic and clinical characteristics from 222 patients hospitalized with respiratory symptoms

	Triplex qRT-PCR Results			*P*-value
	Negative (*n* = 136)	RSV+ (*n* = 68)	hMPV+ (*n* = 18)	
Gender (%)				
F	62(45.6)	22(32.4)	3(16.7)	0.030*
M	74(54.4)	46(67.6)	15(83.3)	
Age (years-old)				
	1.38 ± 1.89	1.15 ± 1.22	1.00 ± 1.29	0.119
CXR index (%)				
N/A	27(19.9)	3(4.4)	4(22.2)	0.008*
Mild inflammation	43(31.6	18(26.5)	4(22.2)	
Severe inflammation	66(48.5)	47(69.1)	10(55.6)	
ICU treatment (%)				
No	77(56.6)	47(69.1)	12(66.7)	0.118
Yes	59(43.4)	21(30.9)	6(33.3)	
Pneumonia (%)				
No	95(69.9)	6(8.8)	1(5.6)	0.001*
Yes	41(30.1)	62(91.2)	17(94.4)	
Hypersomina (%)				
No	131(96.3)	65(95.6)	18(100)	0.621
Yes	5(3.7)	3(4.4)	0(0)	
Intubation (%)				
No	134(98.5)	67(98.5)	17(94.4)	0.599
Yes	2(1.5)	1(1.5)	1(5.6)	
CRP index (%)				
N/A	8(5.9)	3(4.4)	0(0)	0.938
< 5	62(45.6)	34(50.5)	6(33.3)	
Positive	66(48.5)	31(45.6)	12(66.7)	

N/A not available, *CXR index* Chest X-Ray index, *ICU* Intensive care unit, *CRP* C-reactive protein
$^{*}P < 0.05$

hMPV virus in one reaction mixtures. The validation parameters described here were in accordance with procedural and statistical methods as recommended in the Validation of Analytical Procedures (Clinical and laboratory standard institute, CLSI 2009). The development of fluorescent methods and instruments that allow real-time monitoring of the amplification process is considered an important step for molecular biology [19]. Real-time RT-PCR has become a well-established procedure in terms of rapid detection of nucleic acid targets. Incorporation of housekeeping genes as internal control is important to exclude false negative results due to incomplete RNA extraction or inhibition of PCR. The optimized assays reported here, allow specific and sensitive detection of RSV and hMPV, as well as of an internal amplification control. Furthermore, this method can be multiplexed using different fluorogenic dyes for the three probes.

In this current study, we determined the copy numbers of RSV and hMPV and internal control (GAPDH) at the same time in one test sample. The procedures of RNA extraction and reagent preparation and efficiency of instruments could be monitor by triplex qRT-PCR in one sample. Furthermore, this approach also reduced the results of "false-negative" and cost down. However, some groups detected target virus and internal control by using duplex qRT-PCR that may increase the time-consuming [20].

This triplex qRT-PCR provides several clinical advantages. First, this method saves the time for diagnostic performance, compared to virus culture. Second, our method increased the accuracy of RSV and hMPV detection. The rapid and accurate RSV and hMPV detection may help for early intervention of the related clinical events or complications, such as severe lung inflammation and pneumonia.

Conclusion

Altogether, the three sets of primer/probe in the one-step triplex qRT-PCR assay presented in this study is a specific and sensitive diagnostic tool to rapid screening for the detection of RSV and hMPV RNA. It is useful method in routine laboratory diagnostics.

Abbreviations

CPE: Cytopathic effect; hMPV: Human metapneumovirus; LOD: Limit of detection; NPAs: Nasopharyngeal aspirates; RSV: Respiratory syncytial virus; RTI: Respiratory tract infection

Acknowledgements

We thank the staff members of the department of laboratory medicine of Kaohsiung Chang Gung Memorial Hospital for their assistance in virus identification.

Funding

This study was supported by funding from grants CMRPG891371 from Chang Gung Memorial Hospital, Taiwan. This work was supported in part by Taiwan Ministry of Science and Technology grants (MOST 104-2320-B-182A-010 and MOST 105-2320-B-182A-016), Chang Gung Memorial Hospital (CMRPG8B1251-3, CMRPG8C0591-2, and CMRPG8E1471-2), and Kaohsiung Medical University (Aim for the Top Universities Grant, grant No. KMU-TP104E23).

Authors' contributions

HLY and WTL: Experimental design and manuscript draft. HLY and HRU: Manipulation of experiment and sample collection. CCL and SJC and CHC: Statistic analysis and manuscript draft partly. All authors were read and approved the manuscript.

Competing interests

The authors declare that they have no conflicts of interest to report.

Author details
[1]Departments of Laboratory Medicine, Kaohsiung Chang Gung Memorial Hospital, Kaohsiung, Taiwan. [2]Department of Medical Laboratory Sciences and Biotechnology, Fooyin University, Kaohsiung, Taiwan. [3]Department of Kinesiology, Health and Leisure Studies, National University of Kaohsiung, Kaohsiung, Taiwan. [4]Department of Pediatrics, Kaohsiung Chang Gung Memorial Hospital and Chang Gung University College of Medicine, Kaohsiung, Taiwan. [5]Institute for Translational Research in Biomedicine, Kaohsiung Chang Gung Memorial Hospital, Kaohsiung, Taiwan. [6]Institute for Translational Research in Biomedicine, Kaohsiung Chang Gung Memorial Hospital, Kaohsiung, Taiwan. [7]Department of Applied Chemistry, and Graduate Institute of Biomedicine and Biomedical Technology, National Chi Nan University, Nanto, Taiwan. [8]Department of Biotechnology, College of Life Science, Kaohsiung Medical University, No. 100 Shih-Chuan 1st Road, Kaohsiung 807, Taiwan. [9]Department of Biological Sciences, National Sun Yat-Sen University, Kaohsiung, Taiwan.

References

1. Paget SP, Andresen DN, Kesson AM, Egan JR. Comparison of human metapneumovirus and respiratory syncytial virus in children admitted to a paediatric intensive care unit. J Paediatr Child Health. 2011;47(10):737–41.
2. Berkley JA, Munywoki P, Ngama M, Kazungu S, Abwao J, Bett A, Lassauniere R, Kresfelder T, Cane PA, Venter M, et al. Viral etiology of severe pneumonia among Kenyan infants and children. JAMA. 2010;303(20):2051–7.
3. Nair H, Nokes DJ, Gessner BD, Dherani M, Madhi SA, Singleton RJ, O'Brien KL, Roca A, Wright PF, Bruce N, et al. Global burden of acute lower respiratory infections due to respiratory syncytial virus in young children: a systematic review and meta-analysis. Lancet. 2010;375(9725):1545–55.
4. Forgie IM, O'Neill KP, Lloyd-Evans N, Leinonen M, Campbell H, Whittle HC, Greenwood BM. Etiology of acute lower respiratory tract infections in Gambian children: I. Acute lower respiratory tract infections in infants presenting at the hospital. Pediatr Infect Dis J. 1991;10(1):33–41.
5. Nagakumar P, Doull I. Current therapy for bronchiolitis. Arch Dis Child. 2012; 97(9):827–30.
6. Manoha C, Espinosa S, Aho SL, Huet F, Pothier P. Epidemiological and clinical features of hMPV, RSV and RVs infections in young children. J Clin Virol. 2007;38(3):221–6.
7. van den Hoogen BG, de Jong JC, Groen J, Kuiken T, de Groot R, Fouchier RA, Osterhaus AD. A newly discovered human pneumovirus isolated from young children with respiratory tract disease. Nat Med. 2001;7(6):719–24.
8. Papenburg J, Boivin G. The distinguishing features of human metapneumovirus and respiratory syncytial virus. Rev Med Virol. 2010; 20(4):245–60.
9. van den Hoogen BG, Osterhaus DM, Fouchier RA. Clinical impact and diagnosis of human metapneumovirus infection. Pediatr Infect Dis J. 2004; 23(1 Suppl):S25–32.
10. Schildgen V, van den Hoogen B, Fouchier R, Tripp RA, Alvarez R, Manoha C, Williams J, Schildgen O. Human Metapneumovirus: lessons learned over the first decade. Clin Microbiol Rev. 2011;24(4):734–54.
11. Louie JK, Schnurr DP, Pan CY, Kiang D, Carter C, Tougaw S, Ventura J, Norman A, Belmusto V, Rosenberg J, et al. A summer outbreak of human metapneumovirus infection in a long-term-care facility. J Infect Dis. 2007; 196(5):705–8.
12. Wilkesmann A, Schildgen O, Eis-Hubinger AM, Geikowski T, Glatzel T, Lentze MJ, Bode U, Simon A. Human metapneumovirus infections cause similar symptoms and clinical severity as respiratory syncytial virus infections. Eur J Pediatr. 2006;165(7):467–75.
13. Kahn JS. Epidemiology of human metapneumovirus. Clin Microbiol Rev. 2006;19(3):546–57.
14. Muller A, Tillmann RL, Muller A, Simon A, Schildgen O. Stability of human metapneumovirus and human coronavirus NL63 on medical instruments and in the patient environment. J Hosp Infect. 2008;69(4):406–8.
15. Peret TC, Boivin G, Li Y, Couillard M, Humphrey C, Osterhaus AD, Erdman DD, Anderson LJ. Characterization of human metapneumoviruses isolated from patients in North America. J Infect Dis. 2002;185(11):1660–3.
16. Boivin G, Abed Y, Pelletier G, Ruel L, Moisan D, Cote S, Peret TC, Erdman DD, Anderson LJ. Virological features and clinical manifestations associated with human metapneumovirus: a new paramyxovirus responsible for acute respiratory-tract infections in all age groups. J Infect Dis. 2002;186(9):1330–4.
17. Williams JV, Harris PA, Tollefson SJ, Halburnt-Rush LL, Pingsterhaus JM, Edwards KM, Wright PF, Crowe Jr JE. Human metapneumovirus and lower respiratory tract disease in otherwise healthy infants and children. N Engl J Med. 2004;350(5):443–50.
18. Zhang Y, Wei Y, Li J, Li J. Development and optimization of a direct plaque assay for human and avian metapneumoviruses. J Virol Methods. 2012; 185(1):61–8.
19. Holland PM, Abramson RD, Watson R, Gelfand DH. Detection of specific polymerase chain reaction product by utilizing the 5'——3' exonuclease activity of Thermus aquaticus DNA polymerase. Proc Natl Acad Sci U S A. 1991;88(16):7276–80.
20. Jokela P, Piiparinen H, Luiro K, Lappalainen M. Detection of human metapneumovirus and respiratory syncytial virus by duplex real-time RT-PCR assay in comparison with direct fluorescent assay. Clin Microbiol Infect. 2010;16(10):1568–73.

13

Interstitial pneumonia pattern on day 7 chest radiograph predicts bronchopulmonary dysplasia in preterm infants

Hye-Rim Kim[1,4,5†], Ji Young Kim[2†], Bo La Yun[2], Byoungkook Lee[3], Chang Won Choi[4,5*] and Beyong Il Kim[4,5]

Abstract

Background: Early identification of infants at higher risk of developing bronchopulmonary dysplasia (BPD) may enable a targeted approach to reduce BPD. We aimed to evaluate the hypothesis that the interstitial pneumonia pattern on the day 7 chest radiograph predicts BPD or death before 36 weeks postmenstrual age (PMA).

Methods: A retrospective cohort study was performed on 336 preterm infants (birth weight < 1500 g and gestational age < 32 postmenstrual weeks) who were admitted to a single tertiary academic center between January 2008 and December 2014. Day 7 chest radiographs were independently reviewed by two pediatric radiologists who were unaware of the clinical information regarding each individual infant.

Results: Data from 304 infants who survived more than 7 days after birth were collected. The interstitial pneumonia pattern on the day 7 chest radiograph was independently associated with BPD or death before 36 weeks PMA (odds ratio [OR] 4.0, 95% confidence interval [CI] 1.1–14.4). The interstitial pneumonia pattern on the day 7 chest radiograph predicted BPD or death with a specificity of 98%. Histologic chorioamnionitis was a preceding factor that was independently associated with the interstitial pneumonia pattern on the day 7 chest radiograph (OR 3.7, 95% CI 1.3–10.3).

Conclusions: The interstitial pneumonia pattern on the day 7 chest radiograph has a high specificity for predicting BPD or death and can be utilized to select high-risk preterm infants who will benefit from potentially preventive interventions against BPD.

Keywords: Bronchopulmonary dysplasia, Chest radiograph, Predictor, Interstitial pneumonia

Background

Bronchopulmonary dysplasia (BPD) is a major cause of mortality and morbidity in preterm infants [1]. Neonatal care has improved dramatically over recent decades, and antenatal corticosteroid treatment, surfactant replacement therapy and more sophisticated assisted ventilation have greatly reduced the severity of respiratory morbidity and mortality. Nonetheless, the incidence of BPD has not decreased [2–5]. Approximately 20 to 40% of very low birth weight (VLBW, birth weight < 1500 g) infants and 12 to 13% of preterm infants born before 32 weeks postmenstrual age (PMA) are affected by BPD [6, 7].

Identification of perinatal or early postnatal predictors of BPD may enable us to implement potentially preventive strategies before BPD has been established. Numerous studies have attempted to identify predictors for BPD. Scoring systems for predicting BPD that include gestational age, birth weight, gender, patent ductus arteriosus (PDA), sepsis and mechanical ventilation in regression models have been presented [8]. Laughon et al. [9] developed a predictive model using data from the NICHD Neonatal Research Network Benchmarking

* Correspondence: choicw@snu.ac.kr
†Equal contributors
[4]Department of Pediatrics, Seoul National University College of Medicine, Seoul, Republic of Korea
[5]Department of Pediatrics, Seoul National University Bundang Hospital, 82 Gumi-ro 173 Beon-gil, Bundang-gu, Seongnam 13620, Republic of Korea
Full list of author information is available at the end of the article

Trial. This model incorporated gestational age, birth weight, race, ethnicity, gender, respiratory support and fractional concentration of inspired oxygen (FiO_2) on postnatal days 7, 14, 21 and 28.

Several studies included chest radiographs as a component of the prediction scoring system for BPD. Chest radiographs are a daily routine examination that is part of intensive care for preterm infants, especially during the early postnatal period. In a study, the day 7 chest radiographs with cystic elements or interstitial changes were associated with oxygen dependency at day 28 [10]. Greenough et al. [11] suggested that the day 7 chest radiographs with interstitial shadows or cystic elements predict BPD or death before discharge. Similarly, in our experience, interstitial pneumonia patterns on chest radiographs around the end of the first week of life typically heralded later development of BPD. Furthermore, interstitial pneumonia patterns on the day 7 chest radiographs seem to be associated with histologic chorioamnionitis. The purpose of the present study was to evaluate whether interstitial pneumonia patterns on the day 7 chest radiographs can predict BPD or death and are associated with histologic chorioamnionitis.

Methods

Subjects and data collection

This study included all VLBW (<1500 g) infants who were born before 32 gestational weeks and admitted to the neonatal intensive care unit (NICU) at Seoul National University Bundang Hospital between January 2008 and December 2014. Infants who were transferred to other hospitals before 36 weeks PMA and those who died within 7 days of birth were excluded.

Antenatal, perinatal, and neonatal data were retrospectively collected from the original medical records of the infants included in this study. The primary outcome was BPD or death before 36 weeks PMA. BPD was defined as the need for supplemental oxygen or assisted ventilation, including nasal continuous positive airway pressure at 36 weeks PMA [12]. Histologic chorioamnionitis was diagnosed by the presence of neutrophils infiltrating any of the amnion, choriodecidua, umbilical cord, or chorionic plate according to the grading system suggested by Salafia et al. [13]. Respiratory distress syndrome (RDS) was defined by the presence of respiratory distress, as indicated by an increased oxygen requirement (fractional concentration of inspired oxygen ≥0.4) and compatible chest radiologic findings. PDA was diagnosed with echocardiography, and symptomatic PDA was defined as hemodynamically significant PDA requiring medical or surgical closure. Early-onset sepsis was defined as blood culture-proven bacterial sepsis that occurred before 7 days of life while late-onset after 7 days of life.

Radiologic evaluation for interstitial pneumonia patterns

Chest radiographs obtained on day 7 of life were individually reviewed by two pediatric radiologists (Kim JY, Yun BL) who were unaware of the clinical information regarding each individual infant. Interstitial changes on the day 7 chest radiographs were independently graded by each radiologist with a single grading system (Table 1). Of the total subject preterm infants, chest radiograph images were not obtained from four infants on day 7 of life. As an alternative, chest radiographs on day 6 of life were reviewed for three infants, and a chest radiograph on day 8 of life was reviewed for one infant. Grade 3 and 4 interstitial changes were defined as interstitial pneumonia patterns (Fig. 1).

Statistical analysis

In the univariate analysis, comparisons between groups were performed using the t-test for normally distributed continuous variables, the Mann-Whitney U test for non-normally distributed variables, and the chi-square test for comparison of categorical variables. Multivariate analysis was performed by logistic regression and adjusted odds ratios (OR), and 95% confidence intervals (CI) were calculated. The inter-observer reliability between the two radiologists was tested using kappa (κ) statistics.

Statistical analyses were performed using the IBM SPSS Statistics software package, version 22.0 (IBM, Armonk, NY). Statistical significance was defined as $p < 0.05$.

Ethical statement

The Seoul National University Bundang Hospital Institutional Review Board (IRB) approved the collection and use of the clinical information for research purposes before the investigation was started and waived the requirement for informed consent (IRB No. B1512–328-105).

Results

Clinical characteristics of the subjects

During the study period, 336 VLBW infants were born before 32 gestational weeks and admitted to our NICU. Among them, 32 infants were excluded: 25 infants who died before 7 days of life and 7 infants who were transferred to other hospitals before 36 weeks PMA. In total, 304 infants were included in the analyses (Fig. 2).

Clinical characteristics of the 304 infants are presented in Additional file 1. The mean gestational age was 28

Table 1 Chest radiograph grading system for interstitial changes

Grade	Descriptor
1	No demonstrable abnormality
2	Granular infiltration
3	Diffuse streaky interstitial infiltration
4	Diffuse coarse reticular infiltration

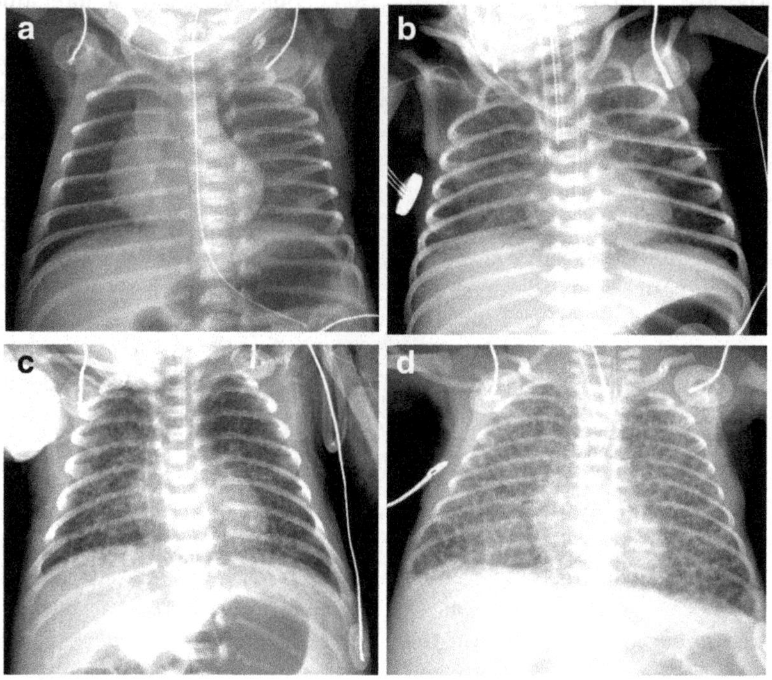

Fig. 1 Chest radiographs representing each grade. **a** No demonstrable abnormality (grade 1). **b** Granular infiltration (grade 2). **c** Diffuse streaky interstitial thickening (grade 3). **d** Diffuse coarse interstitial thickening (grade 4)

$^{+2}$ weeks (range: 23^{+1}–31^{+6} weeks), and the mean birth weight was 1032 g (range: 420–1495 g). The male-to-female ratio of the subjects was 1:1.

Factors associated with bronchopulmonary dysplasia or death

Of the 304 infants, 123 (40.5%) infants developed BPD or died before 36 weeks PMA: 110 infants developed BPD; 13 infants died before 36 weeks PMA. Lower birth weight and gestational age, RDS, symptomatic PDA, invasive ventilation on day 7 of life, and the interstitial pneumonia pattern on the day 7 chest radiograph, which was our primary concern, were factors significantly associated with BPD or death before 36 weeks PMA (Table 2). Multivariate analysis with these significant associated factors included in the logistic regression model revealed that lower birth weight, invasive ventilation on day 7 of life, and the interstitial pneumonia pattern on the day 7 chest radiograph were independently associated with BPD or death before 36 weeks PMA. The adjusted OR and its 95% CI of the interstitial pneumonia pattern on the day 7 chest radiograph for BPD or death before 36 weeks PMA were 4.0 and 1.1–14.4, respectively (Fig. 3). The sensitivity, specificity, positive predictive value, and negative predictive value of the interstitial

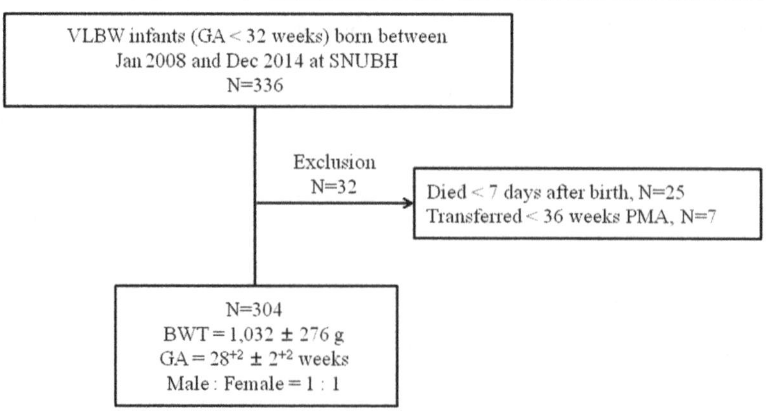

Fig. 2 Study subject. VLBW = very low birth weight; GA = gestational age; SNUBH = Seoul National University Bundang Hospital; PMA = postmenstrual age; BWT = birth weight

Table 2 Demographic and perinatal characteristics of infants with bronchopulmonary dysplasia or death before 36 weeks postmenstrual age

	No BPD or death N = 181	BPD or death N = 123	P
Birth weight (g), mean ± SD	1161 ± 227	842 ± 228	<0.001
Gestational age (weeks), mean ± SD	$29^{+1} \pm 1^{+5}$	$26^{+6} \pm 1^{+6}$	<0.001
Male (%)	86 (47.5)	69 (56.1)	0.142
Caesarean section (%)	136 (75.1)	80 (65.0)	0.071
Multiple gestation (%)	54 (29.8)	40 (32.5)	0.616
Antenatal steroid (%)	165 (91.2)	106 (86.2)	0.191
Premature rupture of membrane (%)	80 (44.2)	54 (43.9)	1.000
Preeclampsia (%)	49 (27.1)	29 (23.6)	0.507
Histologic chorioamnionitis (%)	86 (47.5)	59 (48.0)	1.000
Respiratory distress syndrome (%)	101 (55.8)	107 (87.0)	<0.001
Symptomatic patent ductus arteriosus (%)	74 (40.9)	91 (74.0)	<0.001
Early-onset neonatal sepsis (%)	1 (0.6)	2 (1.6)	0.568
Invasive ventilation on day 7 of life (%)	16 (8.8)	74 (60.2)	<0.001
Interstitial pneumonia patterns on day 7 chest radiographs (%)	4 (2.2)	31 (25.2)	<0.001

BPD bronchopulmonary dysplasia, *SD* standard deviation

pneumonia pattern on the day 7 chest radiograph for BPD or death before 36 weeks PMA were 25%, 98%, 89% and 66%, respectively. The specificity and positive predictive value of the interstitial pneumonia pattern on the day 7 chest radiograph for BPD or death was higher than those of birth weight (cut-off value of 1000 g), gestational age (cut-off value of 28 weeks), and invasive ventilation on day 7 of life (Table 3). Comorbidities and outcomes of infants with BPD or death before 36 weeks PMA were presented in Additional file 1.

Interstitial pneumonia pattern on the day 7 chest radiograph

Of the 304 infants, 35 (11.5%) infants exhibited the interstitial pneumonia pattern on the day 7 chest radiographs. Agreement between the two radiologists in grading interstitial changes on the day 7 chest radiographs had good inter-observer reproducibility (r = 0.940, p < 0.001). Especially for grade 3 and 4 interstitial changes, which were used to define the interstitial pneumonia pattern, the agreement between the two radiologists was 100%.

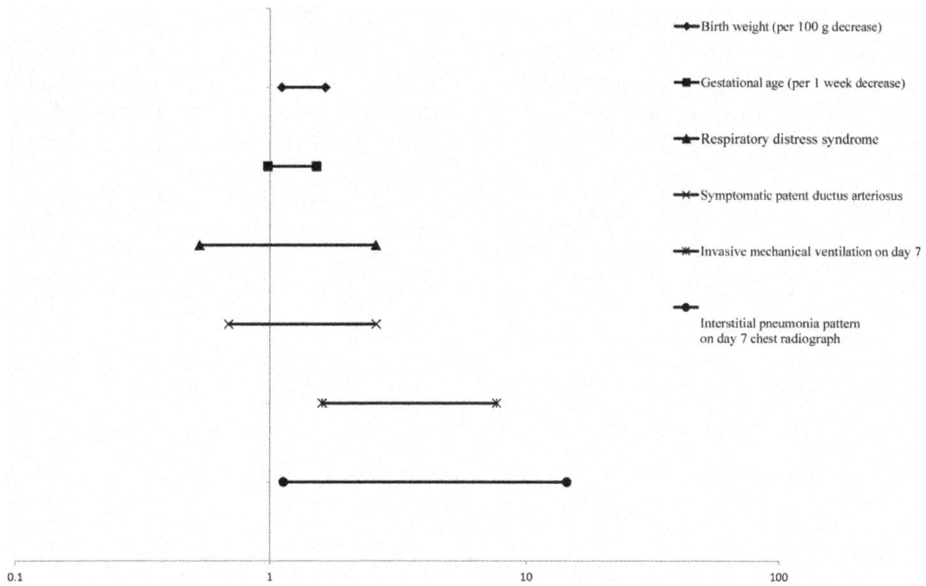

Fig. 3 Multivariate modeling with adjusted odds ratios for BPD or death before 36 weeks postmenstrual age

Table 3 Predictive characteristics of interstitial pneumonia patterns on day 7 chest radiographs and other associated factors for BPD or death before 36 weeks postmenstrual age

	Cut-off value[a]	Sensitivity	Specificity	PPV	NPV
Birth weight	1000 g	66%	84%	74%	75%
Gestational age	28 weeks	80%	72%	66%	84%
Invasive ventilation on day 7 of life	-	60%	91%	82%	77%
Interstitial pneumonia patterns on day 7 chest radiographs	-	25%	98%	89%	66%

PPV positive predictive value, *NPV* negative predictive value
[a] Derived from receiver operating characteristic curve

Factors associated with the interstitial pneumonia pattern on the day 7 chest radiograph

Lower birth weight and gestational age, RDS, premature rupture of membrane, and histologic chorioamnionitis were factors significantly associated with the interstitial pneumonia pattern on the day 7 chest radiograph (Table 4). Multivariate analysis with these significantly associated factors included in the logistic regression model revealed that lower birth weight and gestational age and histological chorioamnionitis were independently associated with the interstitial pneumonia pattern on the day 7 chest radiograph. The adjusted OR and its 95% CI of histologic chorioamnionitis for the interstitial pneumonia pattern on the day 7 chest radiograph were 3.7 and 1.3–10.3, respectively (Fig. 4).

Discussion

To date, not a few studies have suggested chest radiograph scoring systems to predict BPD [10, 11, 14–19]. However, the currently described scoring systems are often too complex for clinicians to use at the bedside [10, 11, 14] or are applied to chest radiographs taken at 3–4 weeks of age when BPD is already being established [15]. High-resolution chest computed tomography (CT) has been used in recent studies to evaluate the severity of BPD in older-aged infants [20]. However, it is difficult to apply chest CT in practice to newborn preterm infants for the early prediction of BPD. By contrast, our chest radiograph grading system is very simple in that it only evaluates interstitial changes and consists of only four grades. The ease and clarity of our grading system are supported by the fact that there was a high degree of agreement in the grading results between the two radiologists. Our grading system also uses chest radiographs taken on day 7 of life, which is a time point when whether the preterm infants will progress to BPD or not cannot be judged easily. In this regard, our chest radiograph grading system for the prediction of BPD has advantages over other scoring systems using chest radiographs and is expected to be readily available to clinicians at the bedside.

The present study showed that the interstitial pneumonia pattern on the day 7 chest radiograph was significantly associated with BPD or death before 36 weeks PMA and predicted BPD or death with 98% specificity in VLBW infants who were born before 32 weeks PMA. Accordingly, the interstitial pneumonia pattern on the day 7 chest radiograph can help clinicians identify high-risk group of infants for BPD or death at a relative early postnatal age.

Early identification of high-risk infants for BPD is crucial to implement potentially preventive or early therapeutic interventions for BPD. Aggressive application of non-invasive ventilation, more restrictive use of oxygen, and postnatal corticosteroids or novel therapies that are currently being evaluated, including stem cells, would be more effective when implemented as early as possible before structural damage is solidified [21–26]. The previously suggested prediction models for BPD include birth weight, gestational age, gender, and duration of oxygen

Table 4 The perinatal factors associated with interstitial pneumonia patterns on day 7 chest radiographs

	No interstitial pneumonia patterns on day 7 *N* = 269	Interstitial pneumonia patterns on day 7 *N* = 35	*P*
Birth weight (g), mean ± SD	1062 ± 267	793 ± 220	<0.001
Gestational age (weeks), mean ± SD	$28^{+3} \pm 1^{+6}$	$25^{+6} \pm 1^{+4}$	<0.001
Male (%)	138 (51.3)	17 (48.6)	0.858
Caesarean section (%)	194 (72.1)	22 (62.9)	0.321
Multiple gestation (%)	84 (31.2)	10 (28.6)	0.847
Antenatal steroid (%)	242 (90.0)	29 (82.9)	0.243
Premature rupture of membrane (%)	113 (42.0)	21 (60.0)	0.048
Preeclampsia (%)	72 (26.8)	6 (17.1)	0.303
Histologic chorioamnionitis (%)	118 (43.9)	27 (77.1)	<0.001

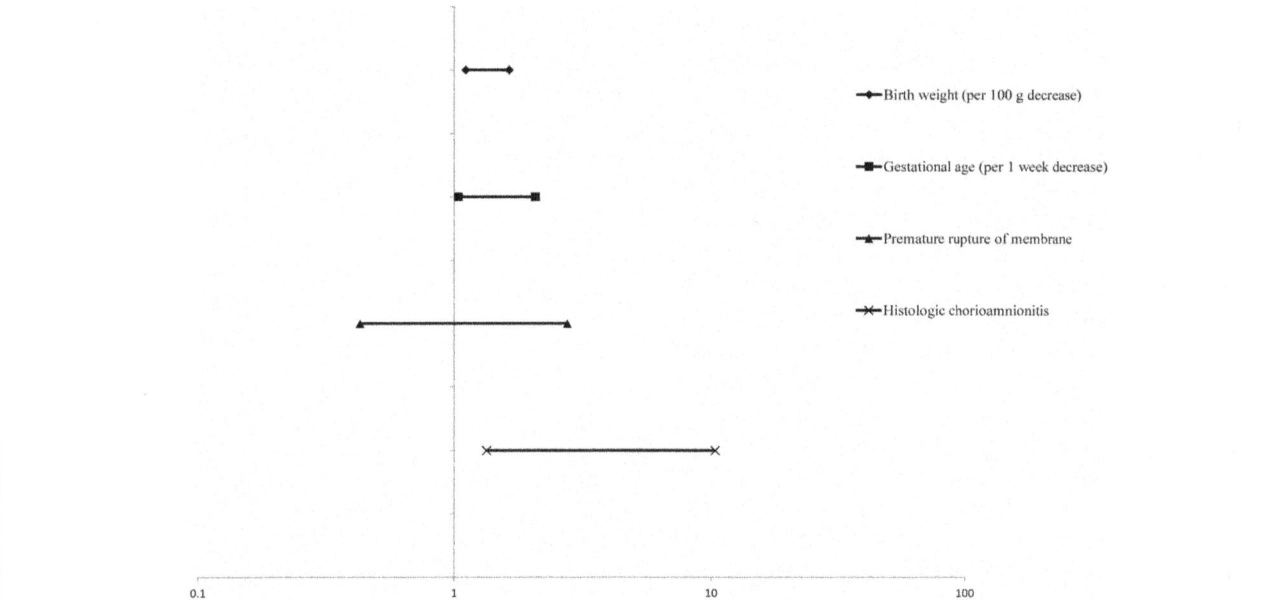

Fig. 4 Multivariate modeling with adjusted odds ratios for the interstitial pneumonia pattern on the day 7 chest radiograph

therapy and mechanical ventilation as the major risk factors [8, 9, 27–29]. Similarly, birth weight, gestational age, and invasivel ventilation on day 7 of life were significant risk factors for BPD or death in our study, and their effects on BPD or death were adjusted during the multivariate analysis step.

As mentioned above, chest radiographs have also been tested for predictors for BPD [10, 11, 14–19]. Several chest radiographic scoring systems have been suggested as prediction tools for BPD. Yuksel et al. showed that radiographic appearance at 7 days of life reached 71% sensitivity and 88% specificity in predicting BPD [10]. Chest radiographs were scored according to the volume of the thorax, presence of opacification, haziness, interstitial changes and cystic elements. Greenough et al. [11] suggested that chest radiographs at 7 days of life can be used to predict BPD or death before discharge. They found that the development of BPD can be predicted by the presence of interstitial shadows or fibrosis, whereas death can be predicted by the presence of cysts. In our study, we focused on the interstitial changes alone in evaluating chest radiographs. The interstitial changes on the day 7 chest radiographs were easily noticeable, and a high degree of agreement between observers was obtained [16]. Furthermore, interstitial changes on chest radiograph are less influenced by inflation status, which will be variable in the preterm infants. Interstitial changes on chest radiograph indicate lung injury, including airway and pulmonary vascular damages and interstitial edema [17]. The presence of interstitial changes on chest radiograph is significantly associated with BPD [10, 11, 18] or adverse respiratory outcomes [19]. Cystic changes on chest radiograph are also associated with BPD or death [11]. However, we did not evaluate cystic changes in this study because cystic changes on chest radiographs were more difficult to distinguish from other diseases, such as infection, sequelae of pulmonary hemorrhage, and pulmonary interstitial emphysema [16]. In addition, cystic changes on chest radiograph represent chronic pathological changes and appear later [17].

Of note, interstitial changes appear from as early as the first several days of life. By day 7 of life, interstitial changes became obvious in preterm infants with the interstitial pneumonia patterns on their chest radiographs. With regard to predicting BPD using chest radiographic findings, the subjectivity of the reviewers and lack of inter-observer agreement have been reported to be problematic [30]. In the present study, we used a simple chest radiographic grading system that exclusively assessed interstitial changes, and good inter-observer reproducibility was obtained between two radiologists. Taken together, the interstitial pneumonia pattern on the day 7 chest radiograph may be an early and objective predictor of BPD or death that can be utilized to select preterm infants at high risk of BPD or death as early as possible.

Whereas the interstitial pneumonia pattern on the day 7 chest radiograph was associated with future BPD or death, it was also associated with histologic chorioamnionitis in the past. The association of the interstitial pneumonia pattern on the day 7 chest radiograph with previous histologic chorioamnionitis remained significant after adjustment for birth weight, gestational age, and premature rupture of membrane. Several studies have demonstrated that chorioamnionitis or intrauterine infection can disrupt lung development by inducing fetal pulmonary inflammatory responses [31–35]. A meta-analysis also demonstrated that histologic chorioamnionitis is significantly associated with the increased incidence of BPD [36]. In this regard, the interstitial pneumonia pattern on the day 7 chest radiographs might correspond to a phase in the pathophysiology of pulmonary inflammation that starts with chorioamnionitis and leads to a later diagnosis of BPD. The most frequently discovered microorganism in the amniotic fluid of pregnant woman with histologic chorioamnionitis is *Ureaplasma urealyticum*, which is a proven cause of fetal and neonatal pneumonia [37]. Thus, the interstitial pneumonia pattern on the day 7 chest radiograph may be a reflection of interstitial pneumonia caused by microorganisms, including *Ureaplasma urealyticum*. However, interstitial thickening due to interstitial hypercellularity and focal deposition of elastin and collagen are common pathologic changes revealed in the evolving BPD [38]. The interstitial pneumonia pattern may also be a reflection of these pathologic changes. At this point, it is not clear whether the interstitial pneumonia pattern is a reflection of interstitial pneumonia caused by microorganisms or a reflection of early pathologic changes observed in evolving BPD.

The main limitation of the present study is the retrospective design from a single center. Further prospective studies are required to validate our results. In addition, further research is needed to clarify the underlying pathology reflected by the interstitial pneumonia pattern on the chest radiograph in preterm infants who later develop BPD.

Conclusions

The findings of this study suggest that the interstitial pneumonia pattern on the day 7 chest radiograph predicts BPD or death before 36 weeks PMA. Chest radiographs are used in daily clinical practice, and the interstitial pneumonia pattern on the day 7 chest radiograph is easy to identify. Furthermore, the interstitial pneumonia pattern on the day 7 day chest radiograph has a high specificity for predicting BPD or death and can be utilized to select high-risk preterm infants who will benefit most from potentially preventive interventions against BPD.

Abbreviations

BPD: Bronchopulmonary dysplasia; NICU: Neonatal intensive care unit; PDA: Patent ductus arteriosus; PMA: Postmenstrual age; RDS: Respiratory distress syndrome; VLBW: Very low birth weight

Acknowledgements

None.

Funding

This study was supported by the Basic Research Program through the National Research Foundation of Korea funded by the Ministry of Education (NRF-2015R1D1A1A09059577).

Authors' contributions

HR Kim and JY Kim conceptualized and designed the study, and wrote the first draft of the manuscripts. JY Kim and BL Yun performed radiologic evaluation. BK Lee carried out the clinical data collection and data analysis. CW Choi conceptualized and designed the study and reviewed and revised the manuscripts. BI Kim provided suggestions with regard to the content and concept of the manuscript. All authors read and approved the final manuscript.

Competing interests

The authors declare that they have no competing interests.

Author details

[1]Department of Pediatrics, Bundang CHA Medical Center, CHA University, Seongnam, Republic of Korea. [2]Department of Radiology, Seoul National University Bundang Hospital, Seongnam, Republic of Korea. [3]Department of Pediatrics, Wonju Severance Christian Hospital, Wonju, Republic of Korea. [4]Department of Pediatrics, Seoul National University College of Medicine, Seoul, Republic of Korea. [5]Department of Pediatrics, Seoul National University Bundang Hospital, 82 Gumi-ro 173 Beon-gil, Bundang-gu, Seongnam 13620, Republic of Korea.

References

1. Jobe AH. The new bronchopulmonary dysplasia. Curr Opin Pediatr. 2011;23:167–72.
2. Smith VC, Zupancic JA, McCormick MC, Croen LA, Greene J, Escobar GJ, et al. Trends in severe bronchopulmonary dysplasia rates between 1994 and 2002. J Pediatr. 2005;146:469–73.
3. Manktelow BN, Draper ES, Annamalai S, Field D. Factors affecting the incidence of chronic lung disease of prematurity in 1987, 1992, and 1997. Arch Dis Child Fetal Neonatal Ed. 2001;85(1):F33–5.
4. Lemons JA, Bauer CR, Oh W, Korones SB, Papile LA, Stoll BJ, et al. Very low birth weight outcomes of the National Institute of Child Health and Human Development neonatal research network, January 1995 through December 1996. Pediatrics. 2001;107(1):e1.
5. Shah PS, Sankaran K, Aziz K, Allen AC, Seshia M, Ohlsson A, et al. Outcomes of preterm infants <29 weeks gestation over 10-year period in Canada: a cause for concern? J Perinatol. 2012;32(2):132–8.
6. Ambalavanan N, Walsh M, Bobashev G, Das A, Levine B, Carlo WA, et al. Intercenter differences in bronchopulmonary dysplasia or death among very low birth weight infants. Pediatrics. 2011;127:106–16.
7. Klinger G, Sirota L, Lusky A, Reichman B. Bronchopulmonary dysplasia in very low birth weight infants is associated with prolonged hospital stay. J Pediatr. 2006;26(10):640–4.
8. Trembath A, Laughon MM. Predictors of bronchopulmonary dysplasia. Clin Perinatol. 2012;39(3):585–601.
9. Laughon MM, Langer JC, Bose CL, Smith PB, Ambalavanan N, Kennedy KA, et al. Prediction of bronchopulmonary dysplasia by postnatal age in extremely premature infants. Am J Respir Crit Care Med. 2011;183:1715–22.
10. Yuksel B, Greenough A, Karani J. Prediction of chronic lung disease from the chest radiograph appearance at seven days of age. Acta Paediatr. 1993;82:944–7.
11. Greenough A, Thomas M, Dimitriou G, Williams O, Johnson A, Limb E, et al. Prediction of outcome from the chest radiograph appearance on day 7 of very prematurely born infants. Eur J Pediatr. 2004;163(1):14–8.
12. Shennan AT, Dunn MS, Ohlsson A, Lennox K, Hopkins EM. Abnormal pulmonary outcomes in premature infants: prediction from oxygen requirement in the neonatal period. Pediatrics. 1988;82:527–32.
13. Salafia CM, Weigl C, Silberman L. The prevalence and distribution of acute placental inflammation in uncomplicated term pregnancies. Obstet Gynecol. 1989;73:383–9.

14. Edwards DK. Radiology of hyaline membrane disease, transient tachypnea of the newborn, and bronchopulmonary dysplasia. Lung development: biological and clinical perspectives: Academic; 1982. p. 47–89.
15. Toce SS, Farrell PM, Leavitt LA, Samuels DP, Edwards DK. Clinical and roentgenographic scoring systems for assessing bronchopulmonary dysplasia. Am J Dis Child. 1984;138:581–5.
16. Hyödynmaa E, Korhonen P, Ahonen S, Luukkaala T, Tammela O. Frequency and clinical correlates of radiographic patterns of bronchopulmonary dysplasia in very low birth weight infants by term age. Eur J Pediatr. 2012;171:95–102.
17. Swischuk LE, Shetty BP, John SD. The lungs in immature infants: how important is surfactant therapy in preventing chronic lung problems? Pediatr Radiol. 1996;26:508–11.
18. Greenough A, Kavvadia V, Johnson A, Calvert S, Peacock J, Karani J. A simple chest radiograph score to predict chronic lung disease in prematurely born infants. Br J Radiol. 1999;72:530–3.
19. Yuksel B, Greenough A, Karani J, Page A. Chest radiograph scoring system for use in preterm infants. Br J Radiol. 1991;64:1015–8.
20. Wilson AC. What does imaging of the chest tell us about bronchopulmonary dysplasia? Pediat Respir Rev. 2010;11:158–61.
21. Schmolzer GM, Kumar M, Pichler G, Aziz K, O'Reilly M, Cheung PY. Non-invasive versus invasive respiratory support in preterm infants at birth: systematic review and meta-analysis. BMJ. 2013;347:f5980.
22. SUPPORT Study Group of the Eunice Kennedy Shriver NICHD Neonatal Research Network, Carlo WA, Finer NN, Walsh MC, Rich W, Gantz MG, Laptook AR, et al. Target ranges of oxygen saturation in extremely preterm infants. N Engl J Med. 2010;362(21):1959–69.
23. Doyle LW, Ehrenkranz RA, Halliday HL. Early (< 8 days) postnatal corticosteroids for preventing chronic lung disease in preterm infants. Cochrane Database Syst Rev. 2014;5:CD001146.
24. Doyle LW, Ehrenkranz RA, Halliday HL. Late (> 7 days) postnatal corticosteroids for chronic lung disease in preterm infants. Cochrane Database Syst Rev. 2014;5:CD001145.
25. Chang YS, Ahn SY, Yoo HS, Sung SI, Choi SJ, Oh WI, et al. Mesenchymal stem cells for bronchopulmonary dysplasia: phase I dose-escalation clinical trial. J Pediatr. 2014;164:966–72.
26. Park WS. Stem cells for the prevention of bronchopulmonary dysplasia. In: Bhandari V, editor. Bronchopulmonary dysplasia. Philadelphia: Humana Press; 2016. p. 299–314.
27. Rojas MA, Gonzalez A, Bancalari E, Claure N, Poole C, Silva-Neto G. Changing trends in the epidemiology and pathogenesis of neonatal chronic lung disease. J Pediatr. 1995;126:605–10.
28. Marshall DD, Kotelchuck M, Young TE, Bose CL, Kruyer L, O'Shea TM. Risk factors for chronic lung disease in the surfactant era: a North Carolina population-based study of very low birth weight infants. North Carolina Neonatologists Association. Pediatrics. 1999;104:1345–50.
29. Oh W, Poindexter BB, Perritt R, Lemons JA, Bauer CR, Ehrenkranz RA, et al. Association between fluid intake and weight loss during the first ten days of life and risk of bronchopulmonary dysplasia in extremely low birth weight infants. J Pediatr. 2005;147:786–90.
30. Moya MP, Bisset GS, Auten RL, Miller C, Hollingworth C, Frush DP. Reliability of CXR for the diagnosis of bronchopulmonary dysplasia. Pediatr Radiol. 2001;31:339–42.
31. Speer CP. Chorioamnionitis, postnatal factors and proinflammatory response in the pathogenetic sequence of bronchopulmonary dysplasia. Neonatology. 2009;95(4):353–61.
32. Viscardi RM. Perinatal inflammation and lung injury. Semin Fetal Neonatal Med. 2012;17(1):30–5.
33. Kramer BW, Kallapur S, Newnham J, Jobe AH. Prenatal inflammation and lung development. Semin Fetal and Neonatal Med. 2009;14:2–7.
34. Kim DH, Choi CW, Kim EK, Kim HS, Kim BI, Choi JH, et al. Association of increased pulmonary interleukin-6 with the priming effect of intra-amniotic lipopolysaccharide on hyperoxic lung injury in a rat model of bronchopulmonary dysplasia. Neonatology. 2010;98(1):23–32.
35. Choi CW, Lee J, Oh JY, Lee SH, Lee HJ, Kim BI. Protective effect of chorioamnionitis on the development of bronchopulmonary dysplasia triggered by postnatal systemic inflammation in neonatal rats. Pediatr Res. 2015;79(2):287–94.
36. Hartling L, Liang Y, Lacaze-Masmonteil T. Chorioamnionitis as a risk factor for bronchopulmonary dysplasia: a systematic review and meta-analysis. Arch Dis Child Fetal Neonatal Ed. 2012;97:F8–17.
37. Hardy RD, Ramilo O. Mycoplasmal infections. In: Remington JS, Klein JO, Wilson CB, Nizet V, Maldonado YA, eds. Infectious Diseases of the Fetus and Newborn Infant, 7th edn. Philadelphia: Elsevier. 2011:607–20.
38. Coalson JJ, Winter VT, Siler-Khodr T, Yoder BA. Neonatal chronic lung disease in extremely immature baboons. Am J Respir Crit Care Med. 1999; 160:1333–46.

14

Low birth weight contributed to increased serum IL-6 levels in infantile respiratory syncytial virus infection

Yuan-Jian Sheng[1], Shan-Shan Xu[2], Xue-Jing Li[1], Jin-Ling Liu[1], Xi-Ling Wu[1] and Xue-Feng Xu[1*]

Abstract

Background: To evaluate the role of serum cytokines in the pathogenesis of respiratory syncytial virus (RSV) infection in infants with low birth weight (LBW).

Methods: A prospective observational study was performed, and hospitalized children with lower respiratory tract infection (LRTI) were recruited. Three hundred fifty-eight patients < 1 year met the inclusion criteria: 116 patients had only RSV infection (RSV group); 242 patients had no RSV or other specific pathogen (non-RSV group). Serum interleukin-2 (IL-2), IL-4, IL-6, IL-10, tumor necrosis factor-α (TNF-α), and interferon-γ (IFN-γ) were detected through flow cytometry.

Results: No significant differences in serum IL-2, 4, 6, 10, and IFN-γ levels were observed between the RSV and non-RSV groups. For RSV infected infants with or without wheezing, delivery mode had no obvious effect on the changes of serum cytokine levels. However, the level of IL-6 in the RSV-infected infants with LBW was significantly higher than that in infants with normal birth weight.

Conclusions: Serum IL-6 level was significantly increased in RSV infected infants with LBW. It is likely that the specific serum cytokine pattern will contribute to our understanding of the pathogenesis of RSV infections, especially in RSV-infected infants with LBW.

Keywords: Cytokine, Infant, Lower respiratory tract infection, Low birth weight, Respiratory syncytial virus

Background

Lower respiratory tract infection (LRTI) is the leading cause of global child mortality. Respiratory syncytial virus (RSV) is believed to be the most important viral pathogen causing LRTI in young children. Furthermore, the incidence for severe LRTI was highest in infants aged 0–11 months [1]. RSV is not only the leading pathogen of LRTI including pneumonia and bronchiolitis, but is also closely associated with the development of asthma [2]. A number of clinical epidemiology studies have revealed that there is a strong association between RSV bronchiolitis in infancy and the development of wheezing or asthma in later childhood. About 40% of children after severe RSV bronchiolitis subsequently develop asthma [2, 3]. Despite the importance of RSV as a respiratory pathogen, the underlying mechanisms of the development of subsequent wheezing and asthma following primary RSV infection remain unclear.

RSV infection may increase the susceptibility to developing allergic immune responses by breaking immune tolerance to allergens early in life through regulatory T cells [4]. Moreover, RSV-induced neurogenic inflammation appears to potentiate neural pathways that favor bronchoconstriction and mucus production [5]. Interestingly, studies have shown that infection with RSV also results in a significant increase in proinflammatory cytokines such as interleukin (IL)-1, IL-6, IL-8, interferon (IFN)-γ, and tumor necrosis factor (TNF)-α, contributing to development of recurrent wheezing or asthma [3]. Our previous study has shown that low birth weight (LBW) or intrauterine growth retardation significantly increases the risk of childhood asthma. Children with

* Correspondence: xuxuefeng@zju.edu.cn
[1]Department of Respiratory Medicine, The Children's Hospital, Zhejiang University School of Medicine, Hangzhou 310052, China
Full list of author information is available at the end of the article

LBW have an approximately 16% higher risk of asthma compared with those with normal birth weight (NBW) [6]. Another study by Rossi et al. further revealed that LBW was not only associated with the increased risk of asthma or wheezing, but also with RSV infection severity [7].

Although we recognize the significant role of low birth weight in infantile RSV-induced LRTI or wheezing, the mechanism of this phenomenon remains unknown. In view of the potential role of cytokines, we hypothesized that LBW induces a specific cytokine profile in infantile bronchiolitis or wheezing induced by RSV infection, leading to more significant manifestations related to asthma. The present study aims to evaluate the possible role of cytokines in the pathogenesis of RSV infection in infants with LBW.

Methods

Data collection

In this prospective observational study, hospitalized children with lower respiratory tract infections (LRTI) from the Respiratory Department of the Children's Hospital of Zhejiang University School of Medicine between January 2013 and December 2014 were recruited. LRTI, including bronchiolitis and pneumonia, has been defined as equivalent to clinical pneumonia, which is characterized by acute onset cough or difficulty breathing with fast breathing for age [8]. Inclusion criteria were hospital admission, LRTI, age <1 year and positive respiratory immunofluorescence detection for RSV [9]. Patients with severe illness and non-severe illness were distinguished by the need for intensive care. Wheezing is defined as a continuous high-pitched sound with musical quality emitting from the chest during expiration [10]. Wheezing symptoms were assessed by at least two clinicians from our study team or the treating physicians (during the weekend). Records on admission age, birth weight, gender, diagnosis, viral pathogen detection, bacterial culture results, laboratory test, length of stay and other relevant medical conditions were collected. Those patients with chronic lung diseases, congenital heart disease, cerebral palsy or tumor were excluded.

Identification of respiratory virus in nasopharyngeal aspirates (NPA)

Samples of nasopharyngeal aspirates (NPA) were obtained from the nasopharynx through catheters after instilling 5 ml of sterile physiologic saline solution into mucus traps at the time of hospitalization. Respiratory immunofluorescence detection via NPA for respiratory syncytial virus (RSV), influenza virus A and B, parainfluenza virus, and adenovirus were carried out. Serum at the time of admission was collected for *M. pneumoniae* antibody measurements: IgM and IgG to *M. pneumoniae* were tested by means of an enzyme-linked immunosorbent assay (ELISA) according to the manufacturer's instructions. *M. pneumoniae* DNA in NPA specimens was detected by fluorescence quantitative real-time PCR. Meanwhile, sputum cultures were also performed.

Cytokine measurement

Peripheral blood samples were collected at the time of admission. The blood sample was transferred to a serum separating tube and centrifuged at 1000 g at room temperature for 20 min after clotting. The serum was carefully harvested and the measurement of the cytokines was performed by flow cytometry immediately, or the serum was temporarily stored at 2–8 °C until analysis. Concentrations of IL-2, IL-4, IL-6, IL-10, TNF-α, and IFN-γ were quantitatively determined with use of the cytometric bead array (CBA) kit (CBA Human Th1/Th2 Cytokine Kit II; BD Biosciences, San Jose, California) as described previously [11]. The minimal and maximum limits of detection for all cytokines were 1 and 5000 pg/mL, respectively.

Statistics

Statistical analysis was performed using descriptive statistics such as frequency and percentage, mean and standard error of mean (SEM). The continuous variables between two groups were compared by Student's t-test. A general linear model was used to assess multiple potential confounders. All data were analyzed with PASW Statistics 18 software (SPSS Inc. Chicago, US). A *P*-value of less than 0.05 was considered to be statistically significant.

Results

Clinical characteristics

In the present study, 358 children with LRTI < 1 year met the inclusion criteria; 116 patients had only RSV infection (RSV group); 242 patients had no RSV or other specific pathogen infections (non-RSV group). No significant differences in birth weight, days of hospitalization, WBC counts, percentage of neutrophils and eosinophils were observed between the two groups of patients (Table 1). There were also no significant differences in birth weight, days of hospitalization, WBC counts, percentage of neutrophils and eosinophils between LBW (birth weight < 3.0 kg) and NBW (birth weight ≥ 3.0 kg) groups (Table 1). The mean age of the RSV group was significantly lower than that of the non-RSV group (Table 1). In RSV patients, the age of the LBW group was also significantly lower than that of the NBW group (Table 1). The values of C reactive protein (CRP) and procalcitonin (PCT) in both groups were within the normal reference ranges.

Table 1 Clinical characteristics of patients

Groups	Age (year)	Birth weight (kg)	Days of hospitalization	WBC (10^9/L)	N%	EOS%	CRP (mg/L)	PCT (ng/L)
Pathogens								
RSV (116)	0.29 ± 0.02**	3.24 ± 0.05	7.06 ± 0.47	10.22 ± 0.89	29.52 ± 1.42	1.74 ± 0.14	4.93 ± 0.97	0.16 ± 0.02
non-RSV (242)	0.60 ± 0.02	3.29 ± 0.03	8.69 ± 0.35	9.19 ± 0.17	33.78 ± 1.10	2.19 ± 0.17	4.96 ± 0.46	0.11 ± 0.01
Birth weight								
LBW (89)	0.50 ± 0.04	–	7.66 ± 0.58	9.20 ± 0.27	34.61 ± 1.93	2.00 ± 0.20	5.69 ± 0.79	0.13 ± 0.02
NBW (269)	0.50 ± 0.02	–	8.32 ± 0.32	9.63 ± 0.40	31.67 ± 0.98	2.01 ± 0.15	4.71 ± 0.52	0.12 ± 0.01
RSV patients								
LBW (32)	0.21 ± 0.03**	–	6.72 ± 0.91	8.56 ± 0.42	29.25 ± 1.90	2.03 ± 0.27	4.72 ± 1.06	0.16 ± 0.04
NBW (84)	0.33 ± 0.03	–	7.19 ± 0.56	10.85 ± 1.22	29.62 ± 1.82	1.63 ± 0.17	5.01 ± 1.23	0.16 ± 0.03

Continuous variables are represented by mean ± standard error of mean (SEM). $^{**}P < 0.01$ for comparison with non-RSV group or NBW group. *WBC* white blood cell, *EOS* eosinophils, *CRP* C reactive protein, *PCT* procalcitonin, *RSV* respiratory syncytial virus, *LBW* Low birth weight, *NBW* normal birth weight

Serum cytokine responses in relation to LRTI

In these patients with LRTI, serum IL-2 and IFN-γ levels in both the RSV and non-RSV groups were within the normal reference ranges (shown in Table 2). Although serum IL-4 and IL-10 levels were increased, there were no significantly statistical differences between the two groups. Serum IL-6 levels in the RSV group were similar to those in the non-RSV group. Compared with the increased average serum TNF-α level in the non-RSV group, average serum TNF-α level of the RSV group was within the normal reference range. A significantly statistical difference was observed between the groups ($P = 0.024$).

Serum cytokine levels in RSV patients

Serum cytokine levels of RSV-infected patients in different subgroups are shown in Table 3. Compared with RSV-infected infants with birth weight ≥ 3.0 kg (NBW), the level of IL-6 in RSV-infected infants with birth weight < 3.0 kg (LBW) was significantly increased. The general linear model revealed that body weight at admission, days of hospitalization, gender, delivery mode, and wheezing were not obviously associated with IL-6 levels. Only low birth weight ($P = 0.035$) was strongly correlated with changes of serum IL-6 levels. Although average serum TNF-α level in RSV-infected infants with LBW was higher than that in infants with NBW, there was no statistical difference between them. No significant differences in other cytokines were observed between birth weight subgroups. Likewise, for RSV infected infants, delivery mode and wheezing mode had no significant effects on the serum cytokine levels (Table 3).

Serum cytokine levels in RSV infants with wheezing

Serum cytokine levels of RSV-infected infants with wheezing in different subgroups are shown in Table 4. For RSV infected infants with wheezing, delivery mode had no obvious effect on the serum cytokine levels. Although average IL-6 level in the RSV-infected infants with wheezing and LBW was higher than that in infants with wheezing and NBW, there was no statistical difference between them. Average serum TNF-α level in the infants with wheezing and LBW was higher than that in infants with NBW, but there was also no statistical difference between them. No significant differences in other cytokines were observed between birth weight subgroups (Table 4).

Discussion

Respiratory syncytial virus (RSV) is the leading viral cause of acute LRTI worldwide, and the most important viral pathogen in infancy, especially among young infants less than 6 months [12]. A large number of studies have established a link between infantile RSV infection and wheezing or asthma [2]. Moreover, the increased evidence indicates that cytokines are strongly correlated with the pathogenic mechanism of RSV-induced wheezing or asthma attacks [13–17].

IL-6 is an important proinflammatory cytokine, promoting Th2 cell differentiation and simultaneously inhibiting Th1 cell polarization. TNF-α is another important proinflammatory cytokine that is involved in both acute and chronic inflammatory responses. IL-6 and TNF-α mRNA and protein levels in bronchoalveolar lavage fluid

Table 2 Serum cytokine levels (pg/mL) among various groups

	No.	IL-2 (SEM)	IL-4 (SEM)	IL-6 (SEM)	IL-10 (SEM)	TNF-α (SEM)	IFN-γ (SEM)
Reference value		1.1–9.8	0.1–3.0	1.7–16.6	2.6–4.9	0.1–5.2	1.6–17.3
RSV group	116	3.98 (0.15)	3.25 (0.07)	54.06 (12.89)	9.87 (1.06)	*3.86 (1.24)	11.85 (1.08)
non-RSV group	242	3.51 (0.10)	3.31 (0.06)	60.30 (9.04)	8.21 (0.69)	9.81 (1.79)	15.54 (1.54)

In all subjects, $^{*}P = 0.024$, as compared with non-RSV group. *RSV* respiratory syncytial virus, *IL* interleukin, *SEM* standard error of mean

Table 3 Serum cytokine levels (pg/mL) among RSV patients

	No.	IL-2 (SEM)	IL-4 (SEM)	IL-6 (SEM)	IL-10 (SEM)	TNF-α (SEM)	IFN-γ (SEM)
Reference value		1.1–9.8	0.1–3.0	1.7–16.6	2.6–4.9	0.1–5.2	1.6–17.3
Birth weight							
< 3.0 kg	32	3.90 (0.23)	3.53 (0.16)	*107.26 (34.23)	10.06 (1.23)	8.07 (4.44)	11.12 (1.03)
≥ 3.0 kg	84	4.01 (0.19)	3.14 (0.08)	33.79 (11.55)	9.79 (1.39)	2.26 0.12)	12.13 (1.45)
Delivery mode							
Vaginal delivery	64	3.99 (0.20)	3.31 (0.09)	67.66 (19.04)	9.01 (1.28)	3.06 (0.67)	11.85 (1.11)
Caesarean section	52	3.97 (0.23)	3.18 (0.11)	37.32 (16.59)	10.92 (1.75)	4.84 (2.64)	11.86 (2.00)
Wheezing							
No wheezing	31	3.83 (0.35)	3.04 (0.16)	42.49 (19.14)	11.94 (3.40)	2.33 (0.22)	10.22 (1.46)
With wheezing	85	4.03 (0.16)	3.32 (0.08)	58.28 (16.19)	9.12 (0.75)	4.41 (1.69)	12.45 (1.38)

*$P < 0.05$, as compared with RSV patients with birth weight ≥ 3.0 kg. *IL* interleukin, *SEM* standard error of mean

in term infants with RSV bronchiolitis were greater than the control group. However, in preterm infants with RSV bronchiolitis, IL-6 and TNF-α proteins significantly decreased [15]. The decrease in IL-6 and TNF-α protein levels in preterm infants may be correlated with the prolonged clinical course seen in those RSV patients [15]. Another study by Oda et al. demonstrated that serum IL-6 levels from patients with RSV infection were high compared with a control group, but there was no statistical significance [18]. Unlike local cytokine expression, our study indicated that systemic IL-6 levels in the RSV group were also high (greater than normal reference value), but there was no statistical significance compared with the non-RSV group. However, average serum TNF-α level from the RSV group was significantly lower than from the non-RSV group. It is likely that the decreased local or systemic TNF-α levels contributed to the prolonged clinical course and wheezing seen in those infants with RSV infection. Similar to other studies [13, 19, 20], no obvious changes in serum IL-2, 4, 10 and IFN-γ levels were observed in the present study.

A large number of studies have confirmed a link between infantile RSV infection and the development of wheezing or asthma in later childhood [2]. Moreover, individuals with LBW were more inclined to develop severe RSV infection, resulting in an increased risk of wheezing or asthma [6, 7]. The potential mechanism might be explained in part by the fact that serum cytokine concentrations in infants with RSV infection were strongly related to birth weight, not to delivery mode. IL-6 high patients had significantly worse lung function and more frequent asthma exacerbations than IL-6 low patients [21]. Circulating IL-6 is elevated in asthmatic patients and in bronchoalveolar lavage fluid of patients in whom asthma is clinically active. IL-6 levels probably reflect an activated state of the lung, and may have a role as a biomarker for asthma [22]. In the present study, increased serum IL-6 levels in infants with LBW might also play an important role in RSV induced wheezing or asthma. Although average serum IL-6 in RSV patients with wheezing was higher than in those without wheezing, there was no significant difference between them. This phenomenon further indicated that only LBW was likely to cause obvious increases in serum IL-6 levels in infants with RSV infection. In general, IL-6 is moderately increased in virus infections, lower than in *Mycoplasma pneumoniae* and bacterial infections [11, 23]. The present study also confirmed this trend. It has been previously documented that the levels of pro-inflammatory cytokines such as IL-6 were consistently higher in RSV patients at hospital admission, discharge, and 1 month after discharge than control levels. There was a trend towards greater IL-6 production in RSV infection, but not IFN-γ production [13]. These cytokines

Table 4 Serum cytokine levels (pg/mL) among RSV patients with wheezing

	No.	IL-2 (SEM)	IL-4 (SEM)	IL-6 (SEM)	IL-10 (SEM)	TNF-α (SEM)	IFN-γ (SEM)
Reference value		1.1–9.8	0.1–3.0	1.7–16.6	2.6–4.9	0.1–5.2	1.6–17.3
Birth weight							
< 3.0 kg	22	4.04 (0.26)	3.68 (0.19)	117.08 (44.04)	10.87 (1.48)	10.61 (6.43)	11.86 (1.35)
≥ 3.0 kg	63	4.03 (0.20)	3.20 (0.08)	37.75 (14.95)	8.50 (0.86)	2.25 (0.14)	12.66 (1.80)
Delivery mode							
Vaginal delivery	44	4.04 (0.20)	3.37 (0.11)	70.56 (24.55)	8.37 (1.03)	3.33 (0.97)	12.17 (1.28)
Caesarean section	41	4.03 (0.26)	3.27 (0.12)	45.10 (20.91)	9.91 (1.08)	5.58 (3.35)	12.75 (2.52)

IL interleukin, *SEM* standard error of mean

recruit inflammatory and immunocompetent cells into the sites of airway inflammation. Therefore, it is likely that the increased IL-6 response in RSV patients with wheezing would provide a substratum for the development of subsequent asthma, resulting in more significant changes related to asthma, especially in children with LBW.

Additionally, a previous study by Rusconi et al. showed that the adjusted risk ratio for development of asthma was 1.33 for elective cesarean delivery compared with spontaneous vaginal delivery [24]. However, Werner et al. found no support for the hypothesis that children delivered by caesarean section have an increased risk of asthma during the first 15–18 years of life [25]. Furthermore, delivery by caesarean section was not clearly associated with hospitalizations for asthma and other wheezing disorders up to 12 years of age compared to vaginal delivery [26]. In view of the potential role of delivery mode in the development of asthma or other wheezing diseases, we also evaluated the possible role of delivery mode in cytokine changes during infantile RSV infections. No obvious changes in serum cytokines were observed between the caesarean section and vaginal delivery groups. Therefore, the present study cannot confirm the correlation between delivery mode and cytokine changes in infantile RSV infections.

Nevertheless, our study has some limitations. Besides the six cytokines in this study, other inflammatory cytokines were reported to be related to pathogenesis of RSV infection, such as IL-5, 13, and 17 [3]. We investigated the above six cytokines only because of the availability of the commercial CBA kit consisting of the six cytokines: IL-2, 4, 6, 10, TNF-α, and IFN-γ. Secondly, because commercial respiratory immunofluorescence kit via NPA in our hospital only detected respiratory syncytial virus (RSV), influenza virus A and B, parainfluenza virus, and adenovirus, not including rhinovirus, we did not perform rhinovirus testing in the present study. It is likely that the RSV-rhinovirus co-infection is the most common co-infection, or Non-RSV infected patients might have rhinovirus infection. Thirdly, although all the samples were collected on admission, we are not certain if they were collected at the same stage of infection. Finally, this study mainly focused on a certain period of hospitalization; long term follow-up study was not performed. Therefore, larger prospective studies are necessary to explore the potential role of serum cytokines in RSV patients with LBW.

Conclusions

In conclusion, our study demonstrated that serum IL-6 level was significantly increased in RSV infected infants with LBW, regardless of wheezing status. It is likely that specific serum cytokine patterns may contribute to the development of wheezing or asthma later in life in RSV-infected individuals, especially in RSV-infected infants with LBW.

Abbreviation

CRP: C reactive protein; IFN: Interferon; LBW: Low birth weight; LRTI: Lower respiratory tract infection; NBW: Normal birth weight; NPA: Nasopharyngeal aspirates; PCT: Procalcitonin; RSV: Respiratory syncytial virus; TNF: Tumor necrosis factor

Acknowledgements

We thank Dr. Sun for her help. We also thank Dr. Elizabeth L. Kramer from Cincinnati Children's Hospital Medical Center for reviewing this manuscript. We also thank the Zhejiang Key Laboratory for Diagnosis and Therapy of Neonatal Diseases and the Key Laboratory of Reproductive Genetics Ministry of Education for their assistance.

Funding

This work was supported by grants from the National Natural Science Foundation of China (No. 81270723), Project of Zhejiang Provincial Department of Education (Y201431434), and Zheng Shu Medical Elite Scholarship Fund. The study sponsors had no involvement in the design of the study, collection, analysis, interpretation of data, and the writing of manuscript.

Authors' contributions

XFX, YJS, and SSX conceptualize the analysis, XJL, JLL, XLW collected and cleaned the data, XFX, YJS, JLL, and XLW performed data analysis. XFX, YJS, SSX, and XJL prepared the manuscript. XFX, YJS, and XLW provided revision of the final manuscript. XFX had full access to all of the data in the study and takes responsibility for the integrity of the data and the accuracy of the data analysis. All authors read and approved the manuscript.

Competing interests

The authors declare that they have no competing interests.

Author details

[1]Department of Respiratory Medicine, The Children's Hospital, Zhejiang University School of Medicine, Hangzhou 310052, China. [2]Department of Neonatology, The Children's Hospital, Zhejiang University School of Medicine, Hangzhou 310052, People's Republic of China.

References

1. Nair H, Simões EAF, Rudan I, Gessner BD, Azziz-Baumgartner E, Zhang JSF, Feikin DR, Mackenzie GA, Moïïsi JC, Roca A, et al. Global and regional burden of hospital admissions for severe acute lower respiratory infections in young children in 2010: a systematic analysis. Lancet. 2013;381(9875):1380–90.
2. Knudson CJ, Varga SM. The relationship between respiratory syncytial virus and asthma. Vet Pathol. 2015;52(1):97–106.

3. Zeng R, Li C, Li N, Wei L, Cui Y. The role of cytokines and chemokines in severe respiratory syncytial virus infection and subsequent asthma. Cytokine. 2011;53(1):1–7.
4. Krishnamoorthy N, Khare A, Oriss TB, Raundhal M, Morse C, Yarlagadda M, Wenzel SE, Moore ML, Peebles RS Jr, Ray A, et al. Early infection with respiratory syncytial virus impairs regulatory T cell function and increases susceptibility to allergic asthma. Nat Med. 2012;18(10):1525–30.
5. Rossi GA, Colin AA. Infantile respiratory syncytial virus and human rhinovirus infections: respective role in inception and persistence of wheezing. Eur Respir J. 2015;45(3):774–89.
6. XF X, Li YJ, Sheng YJ, Liu JL, Tang LF, Chen ZM. Effect of low birth weight on childhood asthma: a meta-analysis. BMC Pediatr. 2014;14(1):275.
7. Rossi GA, Medici MC, Arcangeletti MC, Lanari M, Merolla R, Paparatti UD, Silvestri M, Pistorio A, Chezzi C, Osservatorio RSV Study Group. Risk factors for severe RSV-induced lower respiratory tract infection over four consecutive epidemics. Eur J Pediatr. 2007;166(12):1267–72.
8. Nair H, Nokes DJ, Gessner BD, Dherani M, Madhi SA, Singleton RJ, O'Brien KL, Roca A, Wright PF, Bruce N, et al. Global burden of acute lower respiratory infections due to respiratory syncytial virus in young children: a systematic review and meta-analysis. Lancet. 2010;375(9725): 1545–55.
9. Bont L, Heijnen CJ, Kavelaars A, van Aalderen WM, Brus F, Draaisma JT, Geelen SM, van Vught HJ, Kimpen JL. Peripheral blood cytokine responses and disease severity in respiratory syncytial virus bronchiolitis. Eur Respir J. 1999;14(1):144–9.
10. Brand PL, Baraldi E, Bisgaard H, Boner AL, Castro-Rodriguez JA, Custovic A, de Blic J, de Jongste JC, Eber E, Everard ML, et al. Definition, assessment and treatment of wheezing disorders in preschool children: an evidence-based approach. Eur Respir J. 2008;32(4):1096–110.
11. Xu XF, Li XJ, Liu JL, Wu L, Chen ZM. Serum cytokine profile contributes to discriminating M. pneumoniae pneumonia in children. Cytokine. 2016;86:73–8.
12. Rodríguez-Martínez CE, Rodríguez DA, Nino G. Respiratory syncytial virus, adenoviruses, and mixed acute lower respiratory infections in children in a developing country. J Med Virol. 2015;87(5):774–81.
13. JW O, Lee HB, Park IK, Kang JO. Interleukin-6, interleukin-8, interleukin-11, and interferon-gamma levels in nasopharyngeal aspirates from wheezing children with respiratory syncytial virus or influenza A virus infection. Pediatr Allergy Immunol. 2002;13(5):350–6.
14. Mobbs KJ, Smyth RL, O'Hea U, Ashby D, Ritson P, Hart CA. Cytokines in severe respiratory syncytial virus bronchiolitis. Pediatr Pulmonol. 2002;33(6):449–52.
15. McNamara PS, Flanagan BF, Selby AM, Hart CA, Smyth RL. Pro- and anti-inflammatory responses in respiratory syncytial virus bronchiolitis. Eur Respir J. 2004;23(1):106–12.
16. Legg JP, Hussain IR, Warner JA, Johnston SL, Warner JO. Type 1 and type 2 cytokine imbalance in acute respiratory syncytial virus bronchiolitis. Am J Respir Crit Care Med. 2003;168(6):633–9.
17. Brown PM, Schneeberger DL, Piedimonte G. Biomarkers of respiratory syncytial virus (RSV) infection: specific neurotrophin and cytokine levels provide increased accuracy in predicting disease severity. Paediatr Respir Rev. 2015; 16(4):232–40.
18. Oshansky CM, Zhang W, Moore E, Tripp RA. The host response and molecular pathogenesis associated with respiratory syncytial virus infection. Future Microbiol. 2009;4(3):279–97.
19. Oda K, Yamamoto Y. Serum interferon-gamma, interleukin-4, and interleukin-6 in infants with adenovirus and respiratory syncytial virus infection. Pediatr Int. 2008;50(1):92–4.
20. Garcia C, Soriano-Fallas A, Lozano J, Leos N, Gomez AM, Ramilo O, Mejias A. Decreased innate immune cytokine responses correlate with disease severity in children with respiratory syncytial virus and human rhinovirus bronchiolitis. Pediatr Infect Dis J. 2012;31(1):86–9.
21. Peters MC, McGrath KW, Hawkins GA, Hastie AT, Levy BD, Israel E, Phillips BR, Mauger DT, Comhair SA, Erzurum SC, et al. Plasma interleukin-6 concentrations, metabolic dysfunction, and asthma severity: a cross-sectional analysis of two cohorts. Lancet Respir Med. 2016;4(7):574–84.
22. Poynter ME, Irvin CG. Interleukin-6 as a biomarker for asthma: hype or is there something else? Eur Respir J. 2016;48(4):979–81.
23. Menendez R, Sahuquillo-Arce JM, Reyes S, Martinez R, Polverino E, Cilloniz C, Cordoba JG, Montull B, Torres A. Cytokine activation patterns and biomarkers are influenced by microorganisms in community-acquired pneumonia. Chest. 2012;141(6):1537–45.
24. Rusconi F, Zugna D, Annesi-Maesano I, Baiz N, Barros H, Correia S, Duijts L, Forastiere F, Inskip H, Kelleher CC, et al. Mode of delivery and asthma at school age in 9 European birth cohorts. Am J Epidemiol. 2017;185(6):465–73.
25. Werner A, Ramlau-Hansen CH, Jeppesen SK, Thulstrup AM, Olsen J. Caesarean delivery and risk of developing asthma in the offspring. Acta Paediatr. 2007;96(4):595–6.
26. Leung JY, Li AM, Leung GM, Schooling CM. Mode of delivery and childhood hospitalizations for asthma and other wheezing disorders. Clin Exp Allergy. 2015;45(6):1109–17.

15

Nutritional status, exclusive breastfeeding and management of acute respiratory illness and diarrhea in the first 6 months of life in infants from two regions of Indonesia

V. Oktaria[1,2,3*], K. J. Lee[2,3], J. E. Bines[2,3], E. Watts[3], C. D. Satria[1], J. Atthobari[1,4], H. Nirwati[1,5], C. D. Kirkwood[3,6], Y. Soenarto[1] and M. H. Danchin[2,3]

Abstract

Background: Infant morbidity and mortality rates remain high in Indonesia, with acute respiratory illnesses (ARI) and diarrhea the leading two health problems in children under 5 years. We aimed to describe the nutritional status, feeding practice and case management of ARI and diarrhea of infants from two regions of Indonesia during the first 6 months of life.

Methods: This study was an observational study conducted in parallel to an immunogenicity and efficacy trial of an oral rotavirus vaccine (RV3-BB) in the Klaten and Yogyakarta regions, Indonesia. Mothers were interviewed at 3 time points: within the first 6 days of their infant's life, and at 8–10 and 22–24 weeks of age. Questions asked included pregnancy history, infant nutritional status, feeding status and health of infants within up to 2 weeks prior to the assessment.

Results: Between February 2013 and January 2014, 233 mother-infant pairs were recruited. 60% (136/223) of infants were exclusively breastfed (EBF) until 6 months of age with the strongest support for EBF reported by mothers themselves 70% (101/223) and 25% (36/223) from their partners. At 6 months, 6% (14/223) of infants were underweight and severely underweight; 4% (8/ 223) wasted and severely wasted; and 12% (28/223) were stunted and severely stunted. Non-recommended medication use was high, with 54% (21/39) of infants with reported cough within 2 weeks of an assessment receiving cough medication, 70% (27 /39) an antihistamine, 26% (10/39) a mucolytic and 15% (6 /39) an oral bronchodilator. At age 22–24 week, infants with reported diarrhea within 2 weeks of an assessment had low use of oral rehydration solutions (ORS) (3/21;14%) and zinc therapy (2/ 21;10%).

Conclusion: In this unique observational study, breastfeeding rates of 60% at 6 months were below the Indonesian national target of >75%. Adherence to WHO guidelines for management of ARI and diarrhea was poor, with high use of non-recommended cough medications and oral bronchodilators in the first 6 months of life and low use of ORS and zinc therapy. Ongoing education of primary health care workers and parents regarding management of common illness is needed in Indonesia.

Keywords: Nutritional status, Case-management, Indonesian infants, Breastfeeding, Acute respiratory illness

* Correspondence: vicka.oktaria@ugm.ac.id
[1]Pediatrics Research Office, Child Health Department, Faculty of Medicine, Universitas Gadjah Mada/ DR Sardjito Hospital, Yogyakarta, Indonesia
[2]Department of Pediatrics, Faculty of Medicine, Dentistry and Health Sciences, The University of Melbourne, Melbourne, Australia
Full list of author information is available at the end of the article

Background

Despite the improvement in the health status of Indonesian infants in the last two decades, mortality rates remain high, estimated at 24.5 deaths per 1000 live births in 2013 [1, 2]. Acute respiratory illnesses (ARI) and diarrhea are the leading causes of mortality in Indonesian children under 5 years of age [3] and were the main targets of the fourth millennium development goal (MDG) to reduce child mortality by two thirds by 2015 [3]. Globally, Indonesia has amongst the highest incidence of ARI, with approximately 6 million new ARI cases per year in children under 5 years estimated in 2008 [4]. In 2013, the prevalence of ARI and diarrhea was 0.24 and 3.5% respectively as reported in the 2013 Indonesia Basic Health Research (IBHS), [6] a national cross-sectional survey to capture the health problems in 33 provinces in Indonesia ($n = 1,027,763$) such as any episodes of ARI and diarrhea in the 4 and 2 weeks prior to the survey and case management of diarrhea with Oral Rehydration Solution (ORS) and zinc. The IBHS also reported that malnutrition was common, with 6.8% of children under 5 years of age defined as wasted, 5.3% as severely wasted, 19.2% as stunted and 18% as severely stunted in 2013 [5, 6]. Importantly, macronutrient deficiencies have been associated with an increased risk of developing ARI and diarrhea, [7] with a 4-fold increase in ARI-related deaths in severely malnourished children compared to children with normal nutritional status [8, 9].

Identifying effective disease prevention and management strategies in Indonesia remains an important goal to decrease the morbidity and mortality rate from ARI and diarrhea. The World Health Organization (WHO) and The United Nations Children's Emergency Fund (UNICEF) recommend exclusive breastfeeding (EBF) for 6 months, continued breastfeeding up to 2 years of age and improvement of case management in health facilities for protection, prevention and treatment of pneumonia and diarrhea [11]. Similarly, the Indonesian government recommends EBF for the first 6 months to improve nutritional status and to provide additional protection against ARI and diarrhea [7–9, 12–15] but the national coverage of EBF was reported by the Ministry of Health to be only 54% at 6 months in 2013 [5]. Furthermore, the routine national immunisation program covers BCG, hepatitis B, polio, DPT, HiB and measles vaccines, with with rotavirus and pneumococcal vaccines currently limited to the private sector [10].

One of challenges of case management in health facilities in developing countries is poor adherence to available guidelines to manage ARI and diarrhea [16, 17], resulting in inaccurate assessment of the signs and symptoms which contribute to incorrect diagnosis, inappropriate treatment [16–18] and poor outcomes [19, 20]. In Indonesia, the current available guidelines for ARI case management from the Indonesian Pediatric society and WHO are symptomatic relief and maintenance of adequate oral hydration for the treatment of Upper Respiratory Tract Infections (URTI) and antibiotics for pneumonia [21, 22]. However, current case management practice, such as the prescription of medications and how the WHO and local pediatric recommendations were followed for ARI and diarrhea in South East Asia, including Indonesia, is not well described.

We aimed to describe the nutritional status, feeding practice and case management of ARI and diarrhea of infants enrolled in a rotavirus vaccine clinical trial during the first 6 months of life in the Klaten and Jogjakarta regions in Indonesia. In particular this study focuses on the rate of EBF, the infants' nutritional status assessed at three time-point visits and the medication prescribed for ARI and diarrhea. We hypothesized that [1] poor nutritional status would be common in infants, [2] rates of EBF would be high and that [3] the management of acute ARI and diarrhea would not be consistent with the available guidelines in Indonesia.

Methods

We conducted an observational study, in parallel to a clinical trial of an oral rotavirus vaccine (RV3-BB) in the Klaten and Yogyakarta regions, Indonesia.

Study location and population

This study was conducted at the 11 study sites involved in the Phase IIb RV3-BB Rotavirus Vaccine Clinical Trial from 14th February 2013 and 8th January 2014, including nine Primary Health Care Centers and two hospitals, in Klaten (rural, Central Java province) and Sleman (semi-urban, Yogyakarta province). Selection of these Primary Health Care Centers was to provide information from rural and semi-urban villages. Both the Klaten and Sleman regions are located in the Java, the most densely populated island in Indonesia. The Klaten region is situated in central java, on the border between the central java and Yogyakarta provinces. The region is divided into 26 districts with a population of just over 1.2 million people [23]. Sleman, is situated in Yogyakarta province and is more urbanized, with a population of 1,167,481 people in 2015 [24]. In 2010, the proportion of famillies living in poverty in Klaten was slightly higher compared to Sleman, (17.5% vs. 10.7%) with the national level at 13.3% [25–27].

Recruitment to this study

This study recruited participants from those who had given consent to participate in a Phase IIb Vaccine Clinical Trial of the RV3-BB. The main vaccine trial randomised 1649 participants to receive either vaccine or placebo, with follow-up to 18 months of age to assess vaccine efficacy. To fulfill one of the trial's secondary objectives immune response was assessed in a predetermined subgroup of 282 of the trial participants. The Phase IIb vaccine trial is trial was registered within the Australian New Zealand Clinical Trial Registry (https://www.anzctr.org.au, trial registration ID ACTRN12612001282875).

After delivery, potential trial participants attended either the hospital or Primary Health Care Center at 0–5 days of age for trial eligibility assessment prior to the administration of the first dose of investigational product. The main inclusion criteria for the trial were full term infants in good health with a birth weight between 2.5-4 kg inclusive. The main exclusion criteria included any medical, psychiatric, or social conditions of a parent/guardian that in the opinion of the investigator would prevent the neonate's parent(s)/guardian(s) from giving proper informed consent or from complying with the study protocol; neonates with known or suspected suppressed immune systems, bleeding diathesis, or those who had received blood products or other investigational products; neonates with an HIV positive mother; infants in whom the Expanded Program on Immunization vaccines were contraindicated; and moderate or severe illness 48 h preceding randomisation. Once participants were deemed eligible to enter the immunogenicity study, mothers were invited to participate in and provide consent for our study. The study involved two components:

1. Face-to-face interviews to collect information on nutritional status, feeding practice and case management of ARI and diarrhea; as well as.
2. Collection of breast-milk samples for analysis of the correlation of maternal antibodies with vaccine take (analyses ongoing; data not presented).

Our study commenced a month after 49 participants had already been recruited in the immunogenicity study. Of the remaining 233 participants, we invited each mother to provide consent for our study. We approached the remaining 233 trial participants. In total 233 out of 282 mothers in the immunogenicity study of the trial were enrolled in this study.

Data collection

Case report forms (CRFs)

Separate study specific CRFs were designed to capture the required data at each of the three follow-up assessment time-points in this study through face-to-face interview with the mother. The time-points for the three visits (0–5 days, 8–10 and 22–24 weeks of age) were in alignment with the visits for the trial's investigational product (IP) dosing, which occurred at the hospitals or primary health care centers.

Information on the antenatal period, including the mother's background and weight gain during pregnancy, monthly family income, living environment, health and pregnancy as well as the baby's health status after delivery were collected at the initial interview. The second and third interviews focused on the baby's nutrition, feeding status and health, including medications prescribed for ARI or diarrhea, as recalled by the parents within the preceding 2 weeks. Infant's weight and length were recorded during visits at the vaccination clinic or sought from medical records when face-to face visits were unsuccessful within 2 weeks window time of scheduled meeting. Additional data were obtained from medical records held at the local Primary health care clinics (PHCs) when any illness necessitating a clinical visit within the preceding 2 weeks was reported by mothers. Phone interviews were performed when face-to-face interviews at clinics were not possible and home visits were attempted if parent(s) were un-contactable by phone.

Clinical definitions

Socio economic status was captured using monthly family income and defined as low if income was < IDR 1,000,000 (< USD 75), medium for income between IDR 1,000,000 to IDR 5,000,000 (USD 75–375) and high for income > IDR 5,000,000 (more than USD 375) per month. EBF was defined as infants who were exclusively breast fed at the time of the assessment with no additional food or formula. Strongest support of EBF was defined as who was reported by the mother to provide the strongest support to continue EBF and the option was herself, the father or any relative or friend. Mothers were asked for reasons if they had stopped breastfeeding before the assessment.

Infant nutritional status was determined by height and weight and was classified according to WHO definitions, where <2 standard deviations (SD) below the mean for weight for age (underweight), low height/length for age (stunted), and low weight for height/length (wasted), were classified as moderate acute malnutrition - MAM; and <3 SDs below the mean for low weight for age (severely underweight), low height/length for age (severely stunted), and low weight for height/length (severely wasted) were classified as severe acute malnutrition (SAM). Weight for length > 1 SD and ≤2 SD above the mean was classified as possible risk of overweight, > 2 SD and ≤3 SD above the mean was classified as overweight and weight for length > 3 SD above the mean was classified as obese. Any respiratory symptom, such as runny nose and wheezing, associated with cough with or without fever was defined as "ARI with cough". "ARI without cough" was defined as any respiratory symptom as above without cough, with or without the presence of fever. Diarrhea was defined as three or more stools in a 24-h period that were looser than normal.

Ethics

Ethics approval for the Phase IIb rotavirus vaccine trial and this study was obtained from the Faculty of Medicine, University of Gadjah Mada in Indonesia (KE/ FK/ 465/EC and KE/FK/788/EC) and Royal Children Hospital, Melbourne, Australia (HREC No. 32060 and 34212).

Data analysis

The demographic characteristics, environmental factors, health of the pregnancy and delivery details of the study population are presented as means ± SDs or medians and interquartile ranges (IQR) for non-normal data (continuous variables), and numbers and proportions for categorical variables. Nutrition, feeding status and health of the infant are presented at the 3 time-points (0–6 days after birth, 8–10 weeks and 22–24 weeks of age). The EBF prevalence as well as management of ARI and diarrhea in those who report an episode of ARI/diarrhea in the preceding 2 weeks are presented as proportions. STATA version 11.0 was used to perform all data analyses.

Results

In total, 233 out of 282 (83%) participants in the trial's immunogenicity sub study were enrolled in this study between February 2013 and January 2014. The majority of participants were from rural Klaten (188/233; 81%) and semi-urban Sleman (45/233;19%).

Maternal demographics

The median (IQR) for maternal age was 29 (range: 24–34) years, with the majority of mothers from rural regions (81%) (Table 1). The majority of mothers were predominantly unemployed (157/233; 67%), of low socio-economic status (188/233; 81%), with high school as the highest education level attained. Regular daily intake of any iron supplements during pregnancy was high (226/233; 97%). Calcium supplementation was also high (171/233; 77%), with only 57% (126/233) of mothers drinking fortified milk (calcium, iron, folic acid and vitamins) and only 45% (99/223) took vitamin C tablets during pregnancy. Most mothers had a normal delivery (186/233; 80%), with few caesarean deliveries (33/233; 14%) and a low reported complication rate (13/233; 6%).

Infant's nutritional status

The majority of infants had a normal weight for age and length for age at all three time points. However, despite all babies having a birth weight of >2.5 kg at birth, at 8–10 and 22–24 weeks of age, 5% of infants had weight for age and weight for length for age < –2SD (Table 2). At birth, 8–10 and 22–24 weeks of age, 5% (11/233), 5% (11/228), and 9% (21/223), of infants were stunted and 2% (4/233), 3% (6/228) and 3% (7/223), of infants were severely stunted respectively. The proportions that were overweight and obese at birth, at 8–10 and 22–24 weeks of age were less than 5% but the proportion of infants who were at risk of overweight (weight for length > 1 SD and ≤2 SD) was 20% (44/233), 18% (41/228), and 16% (37/223), respectively. The majority of infants with normal anthropometric status at birth also had normal anthropometric status at 22–24 weeks of age (Table 3). Most infants (222/223; 99%) were not receiving any nutritional supplements, such as iron, from birth to 6 months. At 8–10 weeks, 80% (183/228) of mothers were still EBF, which dropped to 60% (136/223) by 6 months.

Table 1 Demographic Characteristics of parents at the time of delivery

	Total *N* = 233
Mothers age (years), median (IQR)	29 (24–34)
Mother's highest education, N (%)	
Middle school or less	82 (35)
High school	128 (55)
University	22 (9)
Other	1 (0)
Mother's Occupation, N (%)	
Unemployed	157 (67)
Part-time employment	15 (6)
Casual employment	19 (8)
Full-time employment	42 (18)
Family Income per month, N (%)	
Low (< 75 USD)	188 (81)
Middle (75–375 USD)	36 (16)
High (> 375 USD	1 (0)

Among those who breastfed their infants, mothers reported that the strongest support for EBF was reported to be from the mothers themselves 70% (101/223) and 25% (36/223) from their partners (Table 4). The most common reason for discontinuing EBF at 6 months was mothers needing to return to work (18/223; 25%), followed by inadequate breast milk supply (12/223; 16%) and lack of maternal confidence that breast milk was adequate nutrition (12/223; 16%). Most mothers were feeding (breast milk and/or formula) their infants very frequently, with 69% (158/223) feeding their child over 10 times a day by 22–24 weeks of age.

Table 2 Infants' growth and nutritional status

Characteristic	At birth n = 233	8–10 weeks $n = 228$[a]	22–24 weeks $n = 223$[b]
Weight (grams), mean (SD)	3098 (320)	5120 (703)	7100 (916)
Length (cms), median (IQR)	48 (47–49)	57 (56–58)	65 (63–67)
Weight for age[c] N (%)			
Normal	232 (99)	211(93)	209 (94)
Under nutrition	0 (0)	17(7)	14 (6)
Underweight (MAM)	0 (0)	12 (5)	13 (6)
Severely underweight (SAM)	0 (0)	5 (2)	1 (1)
Length for age[d], N (%)			
Normal	215 (94)	211 (93)	195 (87)
Under nutrition	15 (7)	17 (8)	28 (12)
Stunted (MAM)	11 (5)	11(5)	21 (9)
Severely stunted (SAM)	4 (2)	6 (3)	7 (3)
Weight for length[e], N (%)			
Normal	169 (75)	162 (71)	170 (76)
Possible risk of overweight	44(20)	41 (18)	37 (16)
Over nutrition	12 (5)	11 (5)	10(4)
Overweight	12 (5)	8 (4)	7 (3)
Obese	0 (0)	3 (1)	3 (1)
Under nutrition	1 (1)	14 (6)	8 (4)
Wasted (MAM)	0 (0)	11 (5)	6 (3)
Severely wasted (SAM)	1 (1)	3 (1)	2 (1)
Supplementation from birth, N (%)			
No supplementation	na	221 (97)	222 (99)
Supplemented		7 (3)	3 (1)
Yes, iron	na	1 (0)	0 (0)
Yes, multivitamin	na	2 (1)	3 (1)
Yes, not specified	na	4 (2)	0 (0)

Moderate Acute Malnutrition (MAM) defined when WHO anthropometric measurement is 2 standard deviations (SD) below the mean of normal range and Severe Acure Malnutrition (SAM) defined when WHO anthropometric measurement 3 SDs below the mean of normal range
[a]missing for 5 participants
[b]missing for 10 participants, na = not applicable as this question was not asked in the first interview
[c, d, e]Missing values anthropometric measurement at birth (weight for age = 1, length for age = 3, weight for length = 7), at 6 month (weight for length = 3)

Infants' health and case management of ARI and diarrhea

At 8–10 weeks of age, 42% (5/12) of infants with reported ARI symptoms and cough in the 2 weeks prior had received cough expectorants (glycerylguaiacolate (GG)) and 25% (3/12) had received an oral bronchodilator (Table 5). Oral anti-histamines were also commonly prescribed, with a quarter of infants with cough (3/12) and one third of infants with ARI symptoms without a cough (5/17) receiving chlorpheniramine maleate (CTM). At 22–24 weeks, more than half of the infants with a cough in the 2 weeks prior had received expectorants and antihistamines (21/39 and 27/39) and 26% (10/39) and 15% (6/39) of these infants had received mucolytics and bronchodilators respectively (Table 5). With regards to an episode of diarrhea within 2 weeks of the 8–10 and 22–24 week assessments, 8% ($n = 19$) and 9% ($n = 21$) of children, respectively, had experienced diarrhea. The median frequency of diarrhea was 5 (IQR 4–7) and 4 (IQR 4–6) stools a day and the median duration of diarrhea was 2 (IQR 2–4) and 3 (IQR 2–4) days at 8–10 weeks and 22–24 weeks respectively. Use of ORS and zinc for treatment of diarrhea was low, with 5% (1/19) and 14% (3/21) of the infants experiencing diarrhea receiving ORS and 21% (4/19) and 10% (2/21) receiving zinc therapy, at 8–10 and 22–24 weeks of age respectively (Table 6). No hospitalization was reported for any episode of diarrhea.

Discussion

This is one of the first studies to describe the nutritional status, feeding practice and health status particularly ARI and diarrhea case management, in the first 6 months

Table 3 Growth velocity from birth to 22–24 weeks

	Birth	8–10 weeks	22–24 weeks	N (%)
Weight for age	Normal	Normal	Normal	194 (91)
	Normal	< − 2 SD	Normal	11 (5)
	Normal	Normal	< − 2 SD	9 (4)
	Normal	< − 2 SD	< − 2 SD	5 (2)
	Total			219
Length for age	Normal	Normal	Normal	165 (78)
	Normal	< − 2 SD	Normal	7 (3)
	Normal	Normal	< − 2 SD	15 (7)
	Normal	< − 2 SD	< − 2 SD	10 (5)
	< − 2 SD	Normal	Normal	11 (5)
	< − 2 SD	< − 2 SD	Normal	1(1)
	< − 2 SD	Normal	< − 2 SD	3 (1)
	< − 2 SD	< − 2 SD	< − 2 SD	0 (0)
	Total			212
Weight for length	Normal	Normal	Normal	171 (91)
	Normal	< − 2 SD	Normal	10 (5)
	Normal	Normal	< − 2 SD	5 (3)
	Normal	< − 2 SD	< − 2 SD	0 (0)
	< − 2 SD	Normal	Normal	1 (1)
	< − 2 SD	< − 2 SD	Normal	0 (0)
	< − 2 SD	Normal	< − 2 SD	0 (0)
	< − 2 SD	< − 2 SD	< − 2 SD	0 (0)
	Total			187

of life in Indonesia. The study was conducted alongside a rotavirus vaccine clinical trial at three separate time points after birth and has provided valuable insights into breastfeeding practices and the management of both ARI and diarrhea in two regions of Indonesia.

At the both points after birth, 5–6% of our study participants were underweight, 1–2% were severely underweight; 3–5% were wasted and 1% were severely wasted. We also found that at all three time points stunting occurred in 5–9% of study participants, with 2–3% being severely stunted. This is substantially lower than national finding in 2013 where the proportion of underweight, wasted and stunted infants in Indonesia was 19.6, 37.2 and 12.1% respectively [6]. As expected, the overall nutritional status of infants within our study was higher than the general population of infants in Indonesia since they had higher engagement with the health system through the clinical trial and improved access to early detection of nutritional problems compared with the general population. [28]. Nevertheless, it is clear that nutritional problems are still an issue in Indonesia. To address the national problems in under nutrition, the Indonesian government has engaged with the Scaling Up Nutrition (SUN) movement, a program that aims to provide country specific nutritional intervention for pregnant women and children under 5 years (i.e Vitamin A supplementation) and support breastfeeding, to improve the management of under nutrition [29]. In the 3 years since introduction of the SUN movement in 2011, the prevalence of stunted children under 5 years had decreased from 39.2 to 36.4%, with a target of 26.3% by 2025 [30].

In addition to the reported under nutrition in this study, we also identified 5% of infants who were overweight or obese. Moreover, a fifth of the total infants participating in this study were at possible risk of overweight and might need further nutritional evaluation. Improvement in the economic conditions in developing countries may increase the prevalence of overweight and obesity that co-exists with under nutrition through factors such as life styles changes (such as reducing physical activities), urbanisation and aggressive nutrition interventions for undernourished children [31]. In 2014 the Indonesian Pediatric society published a guideline for the management and prevention of childhood obesity. For children aged 0–12 months, exclusive breast-feeding is recommended up to 6 months with continuation of breastfeeding up to 12 months. Other recommendations include the introduction of a wide variety of foods, avoidance of sweetened beverages and snacks and no televisions in bedrooms [32].

In our study, 60% of women were still EBF their infant at 6 months. This was higher than the recent WHO report of 42% EBF coverage in the first 6 month of age in Indonesia in 2014 [33]. In the same year the Indonesian ministry of health reported that the EBF rate was 54% nationwide. The current national Indonesian EBF rate of 46.3% [34] is above the global average rate of EBF (37% across 75 countries), [11] although it is still below the Indonesian government's target of >75% [35]. The higher EBF rate in our study may be due to the families' engagement in the vaccine clinical trial, providing a higher exposure to health care providers and to the national program that encouraged EBF. In our study, majority of mothers reported themselves as the primary support for EBF at 6 months, and 25% of mother reported that the strongest support for EBF was from their partners. Other studies have reported that mothers who face difficulties maintaining EBF are more likely to have limited partner support [36]. To reach the targeted level of EBF in Indonesia, increasing support for mothers practicing EBF in the first 6 months, including partner education, and appropriate complementary feeding support up to 24 months, is needed. Most of the infants were reported to be breastfed for more than 10 times per day as recommended by American Academy of Pediatrics [37].

Table 4 Breastfeeding status

Feeding status	8–10 weeks $N = 228$ n (%)	24 weeks $N = 223$ n (%)
Number exclusively breastfeeding (EBF), n (%)	183 (80)	136 (60)
Introduced to formula milk, n (%)	36 (16)	33(15)
Introduced to solid food, n (%)	4 (2)	33 (15)
Introduced to both solid food and formula milk, n (%)	1(0)	22 (10)
Primary support provided for EBF[b]		
Mother herself	148 (80)	101 (70)
Mother's partner	28 (15)	36 (25)
Mother's parent/in law	3 (2)	0 (0)
Mother's friends	1 (0)	0 (0)
Other	5 (3)	8 (5)
Reason discontinuing EBF[c]	$N = 45$	$N = 87$
Inadequate breast milk supply	8 (19)	12 (16)
Not confident breast milk will be enough	5 (12)	12 (16)
Mother was sick/had to take medication	2 (5)	2 (3)
Mother had to get back to work	11 (26)	18 (25)
Other reasons[a]	10 (24)	24 (33)
Feeding frequency in a day (EBF and formula)		
Less than 6 times	4 (2)	5 (2)
6–8 times	12 (5)	11 (5)
8–10 times	34 (15)	54 (24)
More than 10 times	177 (78)	153 (69)

[a]Other reasons included baby kept crying after feeding, trial and error with formula and breast milk did not come in straightaway after birth. EBF = infants who only received breast milk in the first 6-month of life without any additional food or formula
[b]Reported by the mother as who gave her the strongest support to continue breastfeeding Captured only for those still exclusively breastfeeding
[c]some participants had more than one answer

The prescription of cough medication for ARIs in the first 6 months, including expectorants (Glyceryl Guaiacolate or Guaifenesin), antihistamines (Chlorpeniramin maleat) and mucolytics (ambroxol), was very common in our study despite it not being recommended by the Indonesian Pediatric society and the WHO. Expectorants, mucolytic agents in cough medication, antihistamines and oral bronchodilators are not recommended medication for the management of URTI in children. In addition, a systematic review reported that most cough medications in children are not effective [38, 39] and there have been a number of reports of toxicity and deaths related to cough medications in young infants, [40, 41] mostly due to Chlorpheniramin maleat (CTM) and ambroxol. In the current study, CTM is the second most commonly prescribed cough medication in infants, especially in primary health care settings. Studies reported that CTM can depress the central nervous system or cause dysrhythmias [41, 42]. Among 10 cold and cough medication-related deaths in infants <6 months of age in a US study, four had toxic levels of CTM and Ambroxol in their blood [36]. This was possibly because the dosage of cough and cold medication deemed to be safe in infants had been extrapolated from adult data with limited safety data available for use in young infants [40]. Education of mothers and health workers regarding the risk and health benefits for giving the abovementioned therapies in infants is required.

Bronchodilator use in infants under 6 months was also very common in our study for the treatment of cough. WHO guidelines recommend that bronchodilators in ARI are given by inhalation and not by oral therapy [21] and are only recommended when children present with wheeze with unclear cause or wheeze with the presence of fast breathing or chest indrawing, and not for mild cough. There is little evidence of a beneficial effect from giving oral bronchodilators for the treatment of cough alone [21]. A randomised controlled trial in India comparing the use of oral salbutamol for symptomatic relief in acute cough with placebo concluded non-superiority of oral salbutamol [43] and there was also

Table 5 Common prescriptions for acute respiratory symptoms in participants with an acute respiratory illness within the 2 weeks prior to the follow-up assessment

Medication type	Age 8–10 weeks		Age 22–24 weeks	
	ARI with cough ($N = 12$)	ARI without cough ($N = 17$)	ARI with cough ($N = 39$)	ARI without cough (N = 23)
No medication, n (%)	1 (8)	1 (6)	2 (5)	1 (4)
Cough medication (Glycerylguaiacolate), n (%)	5 (42)	0 (0)	21 (54)	4 (17)
Antihistamine (CTM), n (%)	3 (25)	5 (29)	27 (69)	10 (44)
Mucolytic (Ambroxol), n (%)	0 (0)	1 (6)	10 (26)	4 (17)
Oral Bronchodilator (Salbutamol), n (%)	3 (25)	2 (12)	6 (15)	3 (13)
Antibiotic (Amoxicillin), n (%)	3 (25)	1 (6)	2 (5)	1 (4)

Results are number (percentage)

Table 6 Common prescriptions for diarrhea in participants with an episode of diarrhea within the 2 weeks prior to the follow-up assessment

Medication type	Age 8–10 weeks (*N* = 19)	Age 22–24 weeks (*N* = 21)
No rehydration	11 (58)	13 (62)
ORS rehydration at any time	1 (5)	3 (14)
Zinc tablet	4 (21)	2 (10)
ORS rehydration at any time and zinc tablet	3 (16)	1 (5)

Results are number (percentage). ORS = Oral Rehydration Solution; A liquid given orally to prevent or correct dehydration due to diarrhea disease

little evidence, that oral salbutamol affected the mean duration of fever, cough, and noisy breathing or the time to the resolution to normal activities compared with placebo. Of most concern, 5 out of 140 Indian infants in the bronchodilator group were reported to have adverse effects including tremors [43, 44]. Salbutamol use in neonates has also been associated with supraventricular tachycardia [45]. Considering there appears to be limited or no benefit from giving oral salbutamol for the treatment of mild ARI in infants, and there are substantial safety concerns, administration of oral salbutamol is not recommended for infants and further education of health care providers in Indonesia is needed.

The use of ORS and zinc supplementation to treat diarrhea was low in our study. Currently, WHO recommends rehydration with ORS and zinc supplementation daily for 10–14 days for the treatment of acute diarrhea episodes with no or some dehydration [21]. However, most diarrhea episodes in our study were mild, with diarrhea occurring on average 4–5 times a day and lasting for 3 days during an average episode, and none required hospitalisation. Yet, the findings from our study are consistent with the low use of ORS for rehydration and zinc supplementation for treatment of diarrhea that has been identified nationally for the management of acute diarrhea, where it was reported that 33 and 17% of children under five with acute diarrhea received ORS and zinc respectively [6]. Low implementation of ORS might be due to home solutions being given over ORS (due to the ease of availability and for palatability reasons) or due to low adherence to WHO guidelines in community settings, once again raising the need for further education of healthcare workers.

There were several limitations to the current study. The general health of infants in this study would be higher than the general population as all the participants were enrolled in a clinical trial, were regularly monitored and had good engagement with the health system. However, we still found evidence of wasting, severe stunting and obesity in up to 9% of infants. In this study, we did not collect information for all episodes of ARI and diarrhea over the 6 months but rather chose to focus on case management of ARI and diarrhea in episodes that occurred within 2 weeks prior to the follow-up assessments. Given this was not our aim, we were unable to provide an estimate of the incidence of ARI and diarrhea episodes, nor report the treatment received for all episodes of ARI or diarrhea occurring within the first 6 months of life. In addition, we did not collect severity of diarrhea within this study, which may have been lower as participants were included in a rotavirus vaccine clinical trial, although both vaccine and placebo participants were included. Diarrhea severity would also have impacted on the use of ORS and zinc, but regardless use was reported to be very low with poor adherence to guidelines for diarrhea case management. There was also the potential for recall bias with ARI and diarrhea episode management, with episodes retrospectively reported by the mother. Further clarification was sought from medical reports held at the PHCs on treatment but completeness of the diagnostic and management information varied.

Conclusion

In a prospective cohort study of the nutritional status and management of acute respiratory illness and diarrhea in infants enrolled in a vaccine clinical trial in Indonesia, EBF rates at 6 months were below the Indonesian national target. Adherence to recommended WHO guidelines for case management of ARI and diarrhea in the first 6 months of life was poor, with a high use of cough medicines and oral bronchodilators. Our findings highlight the need for ongoing education of community health providers in the support of EBF and optimal case management for childhood ARI and diarrhea in Indonesia.

Abbreviations

ARI: Acute respiratory illnesses; CRF: Case report forms; CTM: Chlorpheniramine maleate; EBF: Exclusively breast feeding; GG: Glycerylguaiacolate; MAM: Moderate acute malnutrition; MDG: Millennium development goal; ORS: Oral rehydration solutions; PHCs: Primary health care clinics; SAM: Severe acute malnutrition; UNICEF: The United Nations children's emergency fund; URTI: Upper respiratory tract infections; WHO: World Health Organization

Acknowledgements

We thank all the infants and their families for their participation in this study. We also thank all the hospital and community pediatricians, doctors and midwives; the health district office staff who were involved in this study from the initiation, recruitment and follow up, Prof Stephen Michael Graham who had reviewed the manuscript and provided important insights and to all research assistants involved in the study; Rizka Dinari, Meysitha Haris, Asih Sri Utami, Niken Safitri, Dewi Setiani and Septi Kurnia Lestari.

Funding
Funding for the study was obtained from the Shepard foundation. MCRI is supported by Infrastructure Grant from the Victorian Government. First author, VO holds PhD scholarship from the Indonesia Endowment Fund for Education (LPDP), Ministry of Finance, Indonesia.

Authors' contributions
Principal investigators: MHD, VO, co-investigators: JEB, JAT, CDS, YS, CDK, EW. Designing the project: MHD, VO. Study execution and collecting material: VO, JAT, CDS, YS, EW and HN. Data analysis and interpretation: VO, MHD, KL, JEB, EW. Writing draft paper: VO, MHD, KL, JEB and EW. All authors read and approved the final manuscript.

Competing interests
All authors declare that they have no competing interests.

Author details
[1]Pediatrics Research Office, Child Health Department, Faculty of Medicine, Universitas Gadjah Mada/ DR Sardjito Hospital, Yogyakarta, Indonesia. [2]Department of Pediatrics, Faculty of Medicine, Dentistry and Health Sciences, The University of Melbourne, Melbourne, Australia. [3]Murdoch Childrens Research Institute (MCRI), The Royal Children Hospital, Melbourne, Australia. [4]Department of Pharmacology & Therapy, Faculty of Medicine, Universitas Gadjah Mada, Yogyakarta, Indonesia. [5]Department of Microbiology, Faculty of Medicine, Universitas Gadjah Mada, Yogyakarta, Indonesia. [6]Bill and Melinda Gates Foundation, Seattle, USA.

References

1. Statistics Indonesia MoHRI. The National Population and family planning board,. Indonesia demographic and health survey 2012. Jakarta: Statistics Indonesia, Ministry of Health Republic Indonesia, The National Population and Family Planning Board; 2012.
2. Department of Maternal Newborn Child and Adolescent Health (MCA/WHO). Neonatal and child health profile : Indonesia 2013. Available from: http://apps.who.int/iris/bitstream/10665/170250/1/9789240694439_eng.pdf. Accessed 20 Oct 2016.
3. Black RE, et al. Global, regional, and national causes of child mortality in 2008: a systematic analysis. Lancet. 2010;375(9730):1969–87.
4. Rudan I, Boschi-Pinto C, Biloglav Z, Mullholland K, Campbell H. Epidemiology and etiology of childhood pneumonia. Bull WHO. 2008; 86:408–16.
5. Ministry of Health Republic Indonesia. Indonesia health profile 2013. Jakarta: Ministry of Health Republic Indonesia; 2013.
6. Badan Penelitian Dan Pengembangan Kesehatan Kementerian Kesehatan RI. Riset Kesehatan Dasar : Riskesdas 2013: Kemenkes RI; 2013.
7. Hernani S. Agustina T, Sariasih T. Report on situational analysis of acute respiratory infections in children in Indonesia. Jakarta: University of Indonesia; 2009.
8. Sonego M, Pellegrin M, Becker G, Lazzerini M. Risk factors for mortality from acute lower respiratory infections (ALRI) in children under five years of age in low and middle- income countries: a systematic review and meta-analysis of observational studies. PLoS One. 2015:1–17.
9. Taylor C, Camargo C. Impact of micronutrients on respiratory infections. Nutr Rev. 2011;69(5):259–69.
10. IDAI. Jadwal imunisasi 2017 2017 [updated 18 April 2017]. Available from: http://www.idai.or.id/artikel/klinik/imunisasi/jadwal-imunisasi-2017. Accessed 28 Apr 2017.
11. WHO. Unicef. Ending preventable child deaths from pneumonia and Diarrhoea by 2025 : the integrated global action plan for pneumonia and Diarrhoea (GAPPD). France: WHO; 2013.
12. Mitra AK, Rabbani F. The importance of breastfeeding in minimizing mortality and morbidity from diarrhoeal diseases: the Bangladesh perspective. J Diarrhoeal Dis Res. 1995;13(1):1–7.
13. Walker CL, Rudan I, Liu L, Nair H, Theodoratou E, Bhutta ZA, et al. Global burden of childhood pneumonia and diarrhoea. Lancet. 2013;381(9875): 1405–16.
14. Chirico G, Marzollo R, Corrinovis S, Fonte C, Gasparoni A. Antiinfective properties of human milk. J Nutr. 2008;138:1801S–6S.
15. Hanson LA, Korotkova M. The role of breastfeeding in prevention of neonatal infection. Semin Neonatol. 2002;7(4):275–81.
16. Rowe AK, et al. Deming MS. Management of Childhood Illness at health facilities in Benin: problems and their causes. Am J Public Health. 2001; 91(10):1625–35.
17. Boonstra E, et al. Adherence to management guidelines in acute respiratory infections and diarrhoea in children under 5 years old in primary health care in Botswana. Int J Qual Health Care. 2005;17(3):221–7.
18. Forsberg BC, Petzold MG, Tomson G, Allebeck P. Diarrhoea case management in low- and middle-income countries–an unfinished agenda. Bull World Health Organ. 2007;85(1):42–8.
19. Mary E, Rimsza SN. Unexpected infant deaths associated with use of cough and cold medications. Pediatrics. 2008;5:e318–22.
20. Richard C, Dart IMP, Randall Bond G, Winston DC, Manoguerra AS, Palmer RB, Kauffman RE, Banner W, Green JL, Rumack BH. Pediatric fatalities associated with over the counter (nonprescription) cough and cold medications. Ann Emerg Med. 2009;53(April 2009):8.
21. WHO. Pocket book of hospital care for children: guidelines for the Management of Common Childhood Illnesses with limited resources. 2nd ed. Malta: WHO; 2013.
22. IDAI. Pedoman Pelayanan Medis. IDAI: Jakarta; 2011.
23. Badan Pusat Statistik. Population density of Jawa Tengah by regency/City 2013 2017 . Available from: https://klatenkab.bps.go.id/subject/153/geografi.html#subjekViewTab3. cited 4 May 2017.
24. Badan Pusat Statistik. Luas Wilayah, Banyaknya Penduduk dan Kepadatan Penduduk per Km2 menurut Kecamatan di Kabupaten Sleman, 2015 2017 . Available from: https://slemankab.bps.go.id/statictable/2016/10/12/7/banyaknya-penduduk-menurut-jenis-kelamin-dan-sex-rasio-per-kecamatan-di-kabupaten-sleman-2015.html. Accessed 4 May 2017.
25. Badan Pusat Statistik. Produk Domestik Regional Bruto Per Kapita Atas Dasar Harga Berlaku Menurut Provinsi, 2010–2015 2016. Available from: https://www.bps.go.id/linkTableDinamis/view/id/957. Accessed 25 April 2017.
26. Indonesian Ministry of National Development Planning (BAPPENAS). Penduduk Miskin dan Indeks Kemiskinan [cited 2017]. Available from: https://data.go.id/dataset/penduduk-miskin-dan-indeks-kemiskinan.
27. Badan Pusat Statistik. Jumlah Penduduk Miskin, Persentase Penduduk Miskin dan Garis Kemiskinan, 1970–2015 2017 [updated 6 March 2017]. Available from: https://bps.go.id/subject/23/kemiskinan-dan-ketimpangan.html#subjekViewTab3. Accessed 23 May 2017.
28. Ministry of Health Republic Indonesia. Basic health survey 2013. Jakarta: Ministry of Health Republic Indonesia; 2013.
29. Kementrian Kesehatan Republik Indonesia. Menuju Masyarakat Sehat yang Mandiri dan Berkeadilan. Kinerjad Dua Tahun kementrian Kesehatan Republik Indonesia. 2009–2011. Jakarta: Kementrian Kesehatan Republik Indonesia; 2011.
30. (SUN) S. Progress reported through in-country self-assessment exercise. Indonesia: Scalingupnutrition (SUN) organisation; 2015.
31. Misra A, Khurana L. Obesity and the metabolic syndrome in developing countries. J Clin Endocrinol Metab. 2008;93(11 Suppl 1):S9–30.
32. IDAI. Diagnosis, Tata Laksana dan Pencegahan Obesitas pada Anak dan Remaja. UKK Nutrisi dan Penyakit Metabolik, editor. IDAI: Jakarta; 2014.
33. Indonesia Maternal and Child Health Data 2014 . Available from: http://www.countdown2015mnch.org/country-profiles/indonesia. [Accessed 12 Sep 2016].
34. Ananta Y, Gandaputra E, Waiman E, Partiwi I, Marzuki N, Yohmi E, et al. Exclusive breastfeeding rate and factors associated with infant feeding practices in Indonesia. Paediatrica Indonesiana. 2016;56(1):24–31.
35. Ministry of Health Republic Indonesia. InfoDATIN Situasi dan Analisis ASI Ekslusif. Jakarta Selatan: Ministry of Health Republic Indonesia; 2014.
36. Poole S, Gephart S. State of the science for practice to promote breastfeeding success among young mothers. Newborn Infant Nurs Rev. 2014;14:112–8.

37. AAP. FAQs : Breastfeeding initiatives. Available from: http://pediatrics.aappublications.org/content/pediatrics/115/2/496.full.pdf. Accessed 28 April 2017.
38. Chang AB, Laundau L, Asperen P, Glasgow N, Robertson C, Marchant J, et al. Cough in children: definition and clinical evaluation. Position statement of the Thoracic Society of Australia and new Zealand. Med J Aust. 2006;184:398–403.
39. Schroeder K, Fahey T. Should we advise parents to administer over the counter cough medicines for acute cough? Systematic review of randomised controlled trials. Arch Dis Child. 2002;86:170–5.
40. Vernacchio L, Kelly J, Kaufman D, Mitchell A. Cough and cold medication use by US children 1999-2006: results from the Sloan survey. Pediatrics. 2008;122:323–9.
41. Rimza M, Newberry S. Unexpected infant deaths associated with use of cough and cold medications. Pediatrics. 2008;122:e318–22.
42. Al Khaja KA, Al Ansari TM, Damanhori AH, Sequeira RP. Evaluation of drug utilization and prescribing errors in infants: a primary care prescription-based study. Health Policy. 2007;81(2–3):350–7.
43. Gupta P, Aggarwal A, Gupta P, Sharma K. Oral Salbutamol for symptomatic relief in mild Bronchiolitis: a double blind randomised placebo controlled trial. Indian Pediatr. 2008;45:547–53.
44. Bernard D, Goepp J, Duggan A, Serwint J, Rowe P. Is oral Albuterol effective for acute cough in non-asthmatic children? Acta Paediatr. 1999;88:465–7.
45. Say B, Degirmencioglu H, Gozde Kanmaz Kutman H, Uras N, Dilmen U. Supraventricular tachycardia after nebulized salbutamol therapy in a neonate: case report. Arch Argent Pediatr. 2015;113(2):e98–100.

16

Pediatric severe asthma: a case series report and perspectives on anti-IgE treatment

Virginia Mirra, Silvia Montella and Francesca Santamaria*

Abstract

Background: The primary goal of asthma management is to achieve disease control for reducing the risk of future exacerbations and progressive loss of lung function. Asthma not responding to treatment may result in significant morbidity. In many children with uncontrolled symptoms, the diagnosis of asthma may be wrong or adherence to treatment may be poor. It is then crucial to distinguish these cases from the truly "severe therapy-resistant" asthmatics by a proper filtering process. Herein we report on four cases diagnosed as difficult asthma, detail the workup that resulted in the ultimate diagnosis, and provide the process that led to the prescription of omalizumab.

Case presentation: All children had been initially referred because of asthma not responding to long-term treatment with high-dose inhaled steroids, long-acting β_2-agonists and leukotriene receptor antagonists. Definitive diagnosis was severe asthma. Three out four patients were treated with omalizumab, which improved asthma control and patients' quality of life. We reviewed the current literature on the diagnostic approach to the disease and on the comorbidities associated with difficult asthma and presented the perspectives on omalizumab treatment in children and adolescents. Based on the evidence from the literature review, we also proposed an algorithm for the diagnosis of pediatric difficult-to-treat and severe asthma.

Conclusions: The management of asthma is becoming much more patient-specific, as more and more is learned about the biology behind the development and progression of asthma. The addition of omalizumab, the first targeted biological treatment approved for asthma, has led to renewed optimism in the management of children and adolescents with atopic severe asthma.

Keywords: Severe asthma, Omalizumab, Children, Adolescents, Asthma exacerbations

Background

Children with poor asthma control have an increased risk of severe exacerbations and progressive loss of lung function, which results in the relevant use of health resources and impaired quality of life (QoL) [1]. Therefore, the primary goal of asthma management at all ages is to achieve disease control [2–4].

According to recent international guidelines, patients with uncontrolled asthma require a prolonged maintenance treatment with high-dose inhaled corticosteroids (ICS) in association with a long-acting β_2-agonist (LABA) *plus* oral leukotriene receptor antagonist (LTRA) (Table 1) [5].

Nevertheless, in the presence of persistent lack of control, reversible factors such as adherence to treatment or inhalation technique should be first checked for, and diseases that can masquerade as asthma should be promptly excluded. Finally, additional strategies, in particular anti-immunoglobulin E (anti-IgE) treatment (omalizumab), are suggested for patients with moderate or severe allergic asthma that remains uncontrolled in Step 4 [5].

Herein, we reviewed the demographics, clinical presentation and treatment of four patients with uncontrolled severe asthma from our institution in order to explain why we decided to prescribe omalizumab. We also provided a review of the current literature that focuses on recent advances in the diagnosis of pediatric difficult asthma and the associated comorbidities, and summarizes the perspectives on anti-IgE treatment in children and adolescents.

* Correspondence: santamar@unina.it
Department of Translational Medical Sciences, Federico II University, Via Sergio Pansini 5, 80131 Naples, Italy

Table 1 Recommended options for initial controller treatment in children and adults according to GINA Guidelines [5]

	Step 1	Step 2	Step 3	Step 4	Step 5
Preferred choice	–	Low dose ICS	Low dose ICS/LABA	Medium/high dose ICS/LABA	Add anti-IgE
Alternative choices	Low dose ICS	LTRA	Medium/high dose ICS	Add tiotropium	Add tiotropium
		Low-dose theophylline	Low dose ICS + LTRA	High dose ICS + LTRA	Add low dose OCS
			Low dose ICS + theophylline	High dose ICS + theophylline	

Theophylline is not recommended for children 6–11 years, while tiotropium is not indicated in patients < 18 years
ICS inhaled corticosteroids, *LTRA* leukotriene receptor antagonist, *LABA* long-acting β_2-agonist, *anti-IgE* anti-immunoglobulin E therapy, *OCS* oral corticosteroids

Case presentations

Table 2 summarizes the clinical characteristics and the triggers/comorbidities of the cases at referral to our Institution. Unfortunately, data on psychological factors, sleep apnea, and hyperventilation syndrome were not available in any case. Clinical, lung function and airway inflammation findings at baseline and after 12 months of follow-up are reported in Table 3. In the description of our cases, we used the terminology recommended by the ERS/ATS guidelines on severe asthma [6].

Case 1

A full-term male had severe preschool wheezing and, since age 3, recurrent, severe asthma exacerbations with frequent hospital admissions. At age 11, severe asthma was diagnosed. Sensitization to multiple inhalant allergens (i.e., house dust mites, dog dander, *Graminaceae* pollen mix, and *Parietaria judaica*) and high serum IgE levels (1548 KU/l) were found. Body mass index (BMI) was within normal range. Combined treatment with increasing doses of ICS (fluticasone, up to 1000 μg/day) in association with LABA (salmeterol, 100 μg/day) plus LTRA (montelukast, 5 mg/day) has been administered over 2 years. Nevertheless, persistent symptoms and monthly hospital admissions due to asthma exacerbations despite correct inhaler technique and good adherence were reported. Parents refused to perform any test to exclude gastroesophageal reflux (GER) as comorbidity [6]. However, an *ex-juvantibus* 2-month-course with omeprazole was added to asthma treatment [7], but poor control persisted. Anterior rhinoscopy revealed rhinosinusitis that was treated with nasal steroids for six months [8], but asthma symptoms were unmodified. Treatment with omalizumab was added at age 12. Reduced hospital admissions for asthma exacerbations, no further need for systemic steroids, and improved QoL score (from 2.0 up to 6.7 out of a maximum of 7 points) were documented over the following months. Unfortunately, after one year of treatment, adherence to omalizumab decreased because of family complaints, and eventually parents withdrew their informed consent and discontinued omalizumab. Currently, by age 17, treatment includes inhaled salmeterol/fluticasone (100 μg/500 μg·day^{-1}, respectively) *plus* oral montelukast (10 mg/day). Satisfactory symptom control is reported, with no asthma exacerbations.

Table 2 Clinical characteristics of described patients with difficult asthma

	Case 1	Case 2	Case 3	Case 4
Age at asthma symptoms onset	3 years	6 years	3 years	4 years
History	Monthly asthma exacerbations/ hospital admissions	Monthly asthma exacerbations/ hospital admissions	Monthly asthma exacerbations/ hospital admissions	Monthly asthma exacerbations/ hospital admissions
	Frequent need of systemic steroids	Frequent need of systemic steroids	Several ICU admissions	Frequent need of systemic steroids
			Frequent need of systemic steroids	
Allergen sensitization	House dust mites, dog dander, *Graminaceae* pollen mix, *Parietaria judaica*	House dust mites	House dust mites, dog and cat dander, *Alternaria alternata*, *Graminaceae* pollen mix, *Artemisia vulgaris*, *Parietaria judaica*, *Olea europaea* pollen, cow milk proteins, egg, peanuts	House dust mites, dog dander, *Graminaceae* pollen mix, *Olea europaea* pollen, tomatoes, beans, shrimps, peas
Age at referral	11 years	10 years	6 years	8 years
Comorbidity	Rhinosinusitis	GER	Absent	Absent
Treatment at referral	Fluticasone (1000 μg/d) + salmeterol + montelukast	Fluticasone (1000 μg/d) + salmeterol + montelukast	Fluticasone (1000 μg/d) + salmeterol + montelukast	Fluticasone (1000 μg/d) + salmeterol + montelukast

GER Gastroesophageal reflux, *ICU* Intensive care unit

Table 3 Clinical findings at baseline and after 12 months of follow-up in patients with difficult asthma

	Case 1		Case 2		Case 3		Case 4	
	Baseline	T 12 months	Baseline	T 12 months	Baseline	T 12 months	Baseline	T 12 months
FVC (% pred)	109	127	95	97	98	95	103	113
FEV_1 (% pred)	80	78	74	85	67	94	90	85
Post BD ΔFEV_1 (%)	3	NA	7	NA	25	NA	12.1	NA
FEV_1/FVC (%)	64	87	69	73	67	82	70	66
FEF_{25-75} (% pred)	14	61	41	55	25	72	48	46
Post BD ΔFEF_{25-75} (%)	21	NA	8	NA	55	NA	69	NA
FeNO (ppb)	54	21	19	7	36	5	116	NA
QoL score	2.0	6.7	3.9	6.5	6.4	6.8	4.0	5.9
c-ACT Score	17	23	22	25	17	21	12	15
Current treatment	Fluticasone (500 μg/d) + salmeterol + montelukast		Fluticasone (100 μg/d) + salmeterol + omalizumab		Fluticasone (200 μg/d) + montelukast + omalizumab		Fluticasone (1000 μg/d) + salmeterol + montelukast	

BD bronchodilator, Δ % predicted changes from the pre-bronchodilator values, *FeNO* fractional exhaled nitric oxide, *Ppb* part per billion, *QoL* Quality of Life defined according to references [14], *c-ACT* Children Asthma Control Test evaluated according to references [79, 80], *NA* Not Available

Case 2

A full-term male, who had a recurrent severe preschool wheezing, at 6 years of age developed exercise-induced asthma. At age 10, severe asthma was diagnosed. High serum IgE levels (1300 KU/l) and skin prick tests positive to house dust mites were found. Despite a 3-year treatment with progressively increasing doses of inhaled fluticasone (up to 1000 μg/day) combined with salmeterol (100 μg/day) and oral montelukast (5 mg/day), monthly hospital admissions with systemic steroids use were reported. At age 13, a 24-h esophageal impedance/pH study demonstrated the presence of acid and non-acid GER [7]. Esomeprazole was added to asthma medications, but with an incomplete clinical benefit for respiratory symptoms. Esomeprazole was withdrawn after 3 months, and parents refused to re-test for GER. As respiratory symptoms persisted uncontrolled despite treatment, severe asthma was definitively diagnosed [6]. BMI was within the normal range and anterior rhinoscopy excluded rhinosinusitis. Inhaler technique and adherence were good; thus we considered the anti-IgE treatment option [9]. Subcutaneous omalizumab was started, with fast improvement of both symptoms and QoL score (from 3.9 up to 6.5). Seventeen months later, the dose of ICS had been gradually tapered and oral montelukast definitely discontinued. Currently, at age 14, treatment includes the combined administration of bimonthly subcutaneous omalizumab and of daily inhaled salmeterol/fluticasone (50 μg/100 μg·day^{-1}, respectively). Asthma control is satisfactory and no side effects are reported. Omalizumab has been continuously administered for 2.6 years and is still ongoing.

Case 3

A full-term male had severe preschool wheezing and, since age 3, recurrent, severe asthma exacerbations with acute respiratory failure that frequently required intensive care unit (ICU) admission. At age 6, sensitization to multiple perennial inhalant (i.e., house dust mites, dog and cat danders, *Alternaria alternata*, *Graminaceae* pollen mix, *Artemisia vulgaris*, *Parietaria judaica*, and *Olea europaea* pollen) and food allergens (i.e., egg, milk, and peanut) was diagnosed. Serum IgE levels were 2219 KU/l. Weight and height were appropriate for age and sex. The patient has been treated over 3 years with a combined scheme of high-dose inhaled fluticasone (up to 1000 μg/day) *plus* salmeterol (100 μg/day) and oral montelukast (5 mg/day), with correct inhaler technique and good adherence. Despite this, monthly hospital admissions with systemic steroids use were recorded. Rhinosinusitis and GER were excluded on the basis of appropriate testing; thus treatment with omalizumab was started when the patient was 9 years old. At age 11, adherence to treatment is satisfactory, with no side effects. More importantly, reduced hospital admissions for asthma exacerbations, no further need for systemic steroids, and improved QoL score (from 6.4 to 6.8) were reported. Finally, progressive step-down of anti-asthma treatment was started, and at present (by 11.5 years) inhaled fluticasone (200 μg/day) *plus* bimonthly subcutaneous omalizumab provide good control of symptoms. Omalizumab has been continuously administered for 2.6 years and is still ongoing.

Case 4

A full-term male had severe preschool wheezing and, since age 4, recurrent, severe asthma exacerbations with frequent hospital admissions. At age 8, multiple perennial inhalants and food sensitization (i.e., house dust mites, dog dander, *Graminaceae* pollen mix, *Olea europaea* pollen, tomatoes, beans, shrimps, and peas) and high serum IgE levels (1166 KU/l) were found. The patient has been treated over 5 years with inhaled fluticasone (up to 1000 μg/day) in association with salmeterol (100 μg/day) and oral montelukast (5 mg/day). Despite this, monthly hospital admissions with systemic steroids need were recorded. After checking the inhaler technique and adherence to treatment, comorbidities including obesity, rhinosinusitis and GER were excluded. Omalizumab was proposed, but parents refused it. By 13.6 years, despite a treatment including the association of inhaled salmeterol/fluticasone (100 μg/1000 $\mu g \cdot day^{-1}$, respectively) *plus* oral montelukast (10 mg/day), monthly exacerbations requiring systemic steroids are reported.

Discussion and conclusions

Most children and adolescents with asthma respond well to inhaled short-acting $beta_2$-agonists (SABA) on demand if symptoms are intermittent, or to low dose controller drugs *plus* as-needed SABA if the risk of exacerbations increases [1]. Nevertheless, a proportion of patients is referred to specialists because this strategy is not working and asthma is persistently uncontrolled [4]. For these children, assessment is primarily aimed at investigating the reasons for poor control. Indeed, when the child is initially referred, before the label of "severe, therapy-resistant asthma" (i.e., not responding to treatment even when factors as exposure to allergens and tobacco smoke have been considered) is assigned, three main categories need to be identified: 1) "not asthma at all", in which response to treatment is suboptimal because the diagnosis is wrong; 2) "asthma *plus*", when asthma is mild but exacerbated by one or more comorbidities; and 3) "difficult-to-treat asthma", when asthma is uncontrolled because of potentially reversible factors [10].

The reported cases highlight some aspects of the disease process that may expand the diagnosis and improve patients' care. At our institution, the severe asthma program includes a multidisciplinary approach with consultations by gastroenterologists as well as ear, nose and throat experts. Recently, sleep medicine experts joined this multidisciplinary team; thus, unfortunately, sleep-disordered breathing (SDB) could not be excluded at the time of our patients' assessment. Inhalation technique is periodically evaluated by nurses or doctors in each patient. Unfortunately, in Italy an individual prescription database is not available and thus we cannot assess patients' use of medication. In two cases, the filtering process eventually identified GER and rhinosinusitis, but poor control of asthma persisted even after comorbidities were treated. In all subjects, inhaler skills, treatment adherence, and environmental exposure to indoor/outdoor allergens as well as to second- and third-hand smoke were excluded as cause of lack of control. Eventually, three out of four patients started anti-IgE treatment; asthma control was obtained and maintenance drugs were progressively reduced. In the case that refused omalizumab therapy, pulmonary function, clinical features and controller treatment including high-dose ICS were unchanged.

Previous studies have highlighted an association between increasing asthma severity in children and reduced QoL [11–13]. Uncontrolled asthma symptoms not only affect children physically, but can impair them socially, emotionally, and educationally [13]. In line with previous observations, 3 out 4 of our cases had poor QoL, assessed by a standardized questionnaire [14]. It is well known that improving QoL in difficult asthma is not an easy task, despite a variety of treatments aimed at achieving control [12], and much more remains to be done to address the problem. Nevertheless, 2 of our 3 cases showed a remarkable improvement of QoL after one year of treatment with omalizumab.

Reduction in forced expiratory volume in the first second (FEV_1) is often used to define childhood asthma severity in treatment guidelines and clinical studies [5, 11, 15]. Nevertheless, children with severe asthma often have a normal FEV_1 that does not improve after bronchodilators, indicating that spirometry may be a poor predictor of asthma severity in childhood [6, 16, 17]. Actually, children with a normal FEV_1, both before and after β_2-agonist, may show a bronchodilator response in terms of forced expiratory flow between 25% and 75% (FEF_{25-75}) [18]. However, the utility of FEF_{25-75} in the assessment or treatment of severe asthma is currently unknown. Interestingly, all the reported cases showed normal or slightly reduced values of FEV_1 but severe impairment of FEF_{25-75}. Two cases showed a bronchodilator response in terms of FEV_1 (subjects 3 and 4), while 3 patients had a significant increase of FEF_{25-75} (cases 1, 3 and 4). Unfortunately, we could not provide the results of bronchodilator response during or after the treatment with omalizumab in any case.

Available literature on the diagnostic approach to difficult asthma in children offers a number of reviews which basically summarize the steps needed to fill the gap between a generic diagnosis of "difficult asthma" and more specific labels (i.e., "severe" asthma, "difficult-to-treat" asthma, or even different diagnoses) [3, 5, 6, 8, 10, 19–21]. So far, few original articles and case reports have been published, probably due to the peculiarity of the issue, which makes retrospective discussion of cases easier than the design of a prospective clinical study [4, 22–26]. Available knowledge mainly derives from the experience of specialized centers.

The evaluation of a child referred for uncontrolled asthma should start with a careful history focused on typical respiratory symptoms and on the definition of possible triggers. In the "severe asthma" process, it is crucial for clinicians to maintain a high degree of skepticism about the ultimate diagnosis, particularly in the presence of relevant discrepancies between history, physical features and lung function, as many conditions may be misdiagnosed as asthma. In order to simplify this process, herein we propose an algorithm for the diagnosis of difficult-to-treat and severe asthma (Fig. 1). Confirmation of the diagnosis through a detailed clinical and laboratory re-evaluation is important because in 12–50% of cases assumed to have severe asthma this might not be the correct diagnosis [10]. Several documents have indicated the main steps of the process that should be followed in children with uncontrolled asthma [3, 8, 10]. The translation of these procedures into real life practice may deeply change from one subject to another due to the variability of individual patients' history and clinical features, which will often lead the diagnostic investigations towards the most likely reason for uncontrolled asthma. For children with apparently severe asthma, the first step is to confirm the diagnosis and, before proceeding to broader investigations, to verify that the poor control is not simply determined by poor adherence to treatment, inadequate inhaler skills and/or environmental exposure to triggers. A nurse-led assessment, including a home visit, despite not being applicable in all settings, may be useful for identifying potentially modifiable factors in uncontrolled pediatric asthma [27].

A number of comorbidities have been increasingly recognized as factors that may impact asthma clinical expression and control in childhood [10, 28]. Children with uncontrolled disease should be investigated for GER, rhinosinusitis, dysfunctional breathing and/or vocal cord dysfunction, obstructive sleep apnea, obesity, psychological factors, smoke exposure, hormonal influences, and ongoing drugs [3, 6, 8, 20]. Indeed, the exact role played by comorbidities in pediatric asthma control is still debated [28]. The most impressive example is GER. Several pediatric documents recommend assessing for GER because reflux may be a contributing factor to problematic or difficult asthma [7, 29]. Nevertheless, GER treatment might not be effective for severe asthma [30, 31], as confirmed by current cases 1 and 2. There is an established evidence that chronic rhinosinusitis is associated with more severe asthma in children [32–34]. Therefore, examination of upper airways and *ad hoc* treatment if rhinosinusitis is evident are recommended in children with severe asthma [3, 8, 35]. However, intranasal steroids for rhinitis resulted in a small reduction of asthma risk in school-aged children [36], and actual placebo-controlled studies on the effect of treatment of rhinosinusitis on asthma control in children are lacking [10, 37].

Dysfunctional breathing, including hyperventilation and vocal cord dysfunction, is associated with poorer asthma control in children [8, 10, 38, 39]. Unfortunately, there is scarce literature on the effect of its treatment on the control of severe asthma in children [40]. SDB ranging from primary snoring to obstructive sleep apnea syndrome is very common in children [41], and an increased prevalence of SDB together with increasing asthma severity has been reported [42]. Interestingly, GER may also be worsened by recurrent episodes of upper airway obstruction associated with SDB, and this may further trigger bronchial obstruction. Asthma guidelines recommend the assessment of SDB through nocturnal polysomnography in poorly controlled asthmatics, particularly if they are also obese [5]. There are no studies examining whether pediatric asthma improves after SDB has been treated, for example, with nasal steroids, adenotonsillectomy, continuous positive airway pressure or weight reduction if the child is also obese [43]. The parallel increase in obesity and asthma suggests that the two conditions are linked and that they can aggravate each other [44, 45], even though the exact mechanisms that underlie this association remain unclear [46]. Indeed, other coexisting comorbidities such as SDB or GER may play a confounding role in the development of the interactions between obesity and the airways [47, 48]. Obesity is associated with increased markers of inflammation in serum and adipose tissue and yet decreased airway inflammation in obese people with asthma [49]. Several interventions, including behavioral and

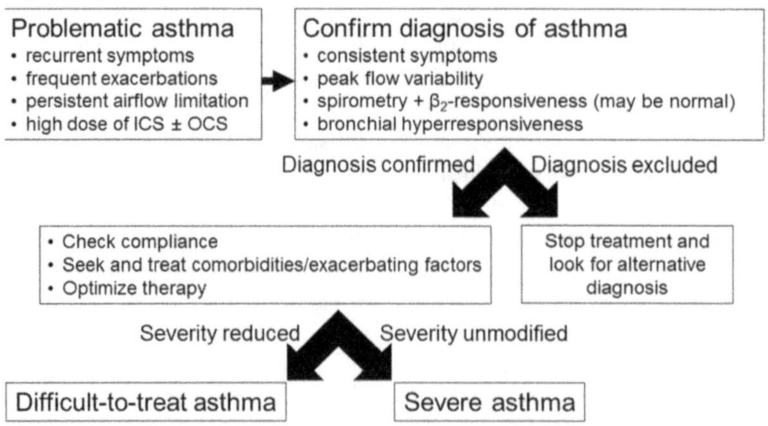

Fig. 1 A practical algorithm for the diagnosis of difficult-to-treat and severe asthma. ICS, inhaled corticosteroids; OCS, oral corticosteroids

weight reduction programs or bariatric surgery, may result in improved asthma control, quality of life and lung function in adult obese asthmatics [50]. Although reports of adolescent bariatric surgery demonstrate a significant body weight decrease, this approach is not widely available and there are no published reports on its effect on pediatric severe asthma control [51]. Finally, although it is still unclear whether food allergy is causative or shares a common pathway with difficult asthma, it might explain the loss of asthma control at least in some children and thus be considered as a comorbid condition [10, 16, 52].

In conclusion, establishing the impact of comorbidities on asthma control may be cumbersome, and an ex-juvantibus treatment is sometimes necessary to assess their role. Comorbid conditions can also worsen each other, and symptoms arising from some of them may mimic asthma [6]. Although the ability to improve pediatric severe asthma by treating comorbidities remains unconfirmed, they should be treated appropriately [9].

The vast majority of asthmatic children exhibit a mild or at most a moderate disease that can be fully controlled with low-to-medium dose ICS associated or not with other controllers [5, 6]. However, a subset of asthmatics remains difficult-to-treat [5, 6]. With the advent of biologics, these severe steroid-dependent asthmatics have alternative options for treatment, as steroid-related adverse events are common in severe asthma [53]. Omalizumab, an anti-IgE monoclonal antibody, is the only biologic therapy recommended in children with moderate-to-severe asthma by the recent guidelines [5, 6]. In Italy, this treatment is fully covered by the National Health System. Therefore, there is no influence by any funding on treatment decisions. It was approved by the US (Food and Drug Administration) in 2003 and by the European Union (European Medicines Agency) in 2005 as an add-on treatment for patients aged > 12 years with severe persistent allergic asthma and who have a positive skin test or in-vitro reactivity to a perennial aeroallergen, $FEV_1 < 80\%$ predicted, frequent daytime symptoms or nighttime awakenings, and multiple documented severe asthma exacerbations despite daily ICS *plus* a LABA [54, 55]. In 2009, it also received approval in Europe for treating patients aged 6–12 years. Figure 2 illustrates current indications for treatment with omalizumab in children and adolescents with severe asthma.

IgE antibodies, Th_2-derived cytokines and eosinophils play a major role in the development of chronic airway inflammation in asthmatic subjects [56]. Once released from plasma cells, IgE binds principally to the high-affinity IgE receptor (FcεRI) on mast cells, triggering

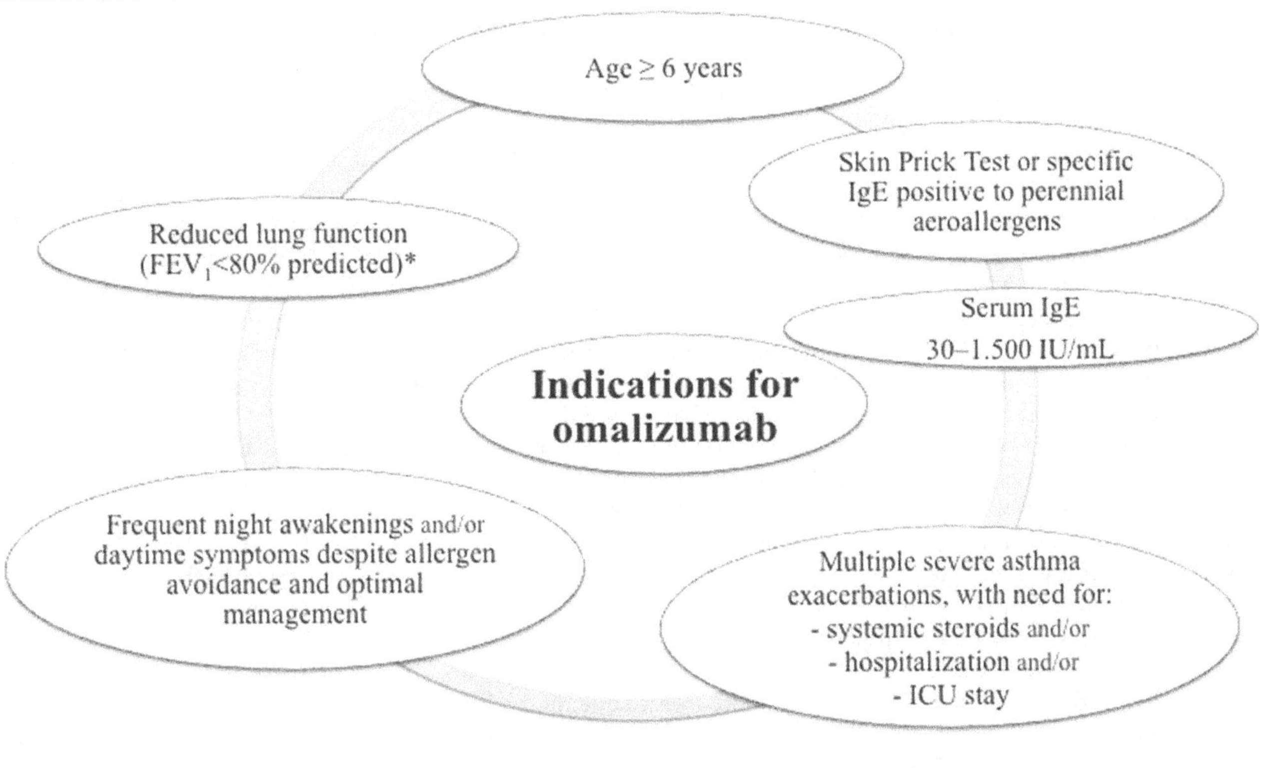

*Not applicable in children less than 12 years
Abbreviations: IgE, immunoglobulin E; FEV_1, forced expiratory volume in 1 second; ICU, intensive care unit.

Fig. 2 Indications for omalizumab in children and adolescents with severe asthma

different effector responses, including the release of mediators leading to allergic inflammatory reactions [56]. The activation of the allergic cascade by IgE, under constant allergen stimulation, leads to the establishment of chronic allergic inflammation in the airways of asthmatic patients, with IgE being a key element of the vicious circle that maintains it. Cytokines produced during the late phase and subsequent chronic inflammation stage have been directly associated with the induction of airway remodelling, indirectly implicating IgE in the process [56]. At present, omalizumab is the only commercially available recombinant humanized anti-IgE monoclonal antibody that specifically binds serum free IgE at its CH_3 domain, in the proximity of the binding site for FcεRI, thus preventing IgE from interacting with its receptor on mast cells, basophils, antigen-presenting cells and other inflammatory cells [57]. The rapid reduction of free IgE levels leads to a downregulation of the FcεRI expression on inflammatory cells and an interruption of the allergic cascade, which results in the reduction of peripheral and bronchial tissue eosinophilia and of levels of granulocyte macrophage colony stimulating factor, interleukin (IL)-2, IL-4, IL-5, and IL-13 [58]. Moreover, basophils have a relevant role in the initiation and progression of allergic inflammation, suggesting that they may represent a viable therapeutic target. Indeed, in children with severe asthma, it has been reported that omalizumab therapy is associated with a significant reduction in circulating basophil numbers, a finding that is concurrent with improved clinical outcomes [59]. This finding supports a mechanistic link between IgE levels and circulating basophil populations, and may provide new insights into one mechanism by which omalizumab improves asthma symptoms.

Several clinical controlled and real-life studies of adults with severe, inadequately controlled allergic asthma have demonstrated the efficacy and safety of omalizumab in reducing asthma-related symptoms, corticosteroid use, exacerbation rates, and healthcare resource utilization, and in improving QoL and lung function [60–63]. Fewer studies have been published in children. In two double-blind, randomized, placebo-controlled trials (RCTs) of children aged 6 to 12 years with moderate-to-severe allergic asthma, treatment with omalizumab reduced the requirement for ICS and protected against disease exacerbations, but there was little change in asthma symptom scores or spirometry [9, 64]. These findings were confirmed and extended in older children [65–67].

The results of the ICATA study, a multicenter RCT of 419 inner-city children, adolescents and young adults with persistent allergic asthma, showed that, compared to placebo, omalizumab reduces the number of days with asthma symptoms and the proportion of participants with at least one exacerbation by approximately 25% and 19%, respectively ($p < 0.001$), thus reducing the need for asthmatic symptom controllers [68]. Another multicenter RCT of inner-city children and adolescents showed that the addition of omalizumab to ongoing guidelines-based care before patients return to school reduces fall asthma exacerbations (odds ratio, 0.48), particularly in subjects with a recent exacerbation [69]. Moreover, in a real-life study of 104 children and adolescents with severe allergic refractory asthma followed over 1 year, treatment with omalizumab resulted in good asthma control in 67% of the cases ($p < 0.001$), while FEV_1 improved by 4.9% ($p = 0.02$) and exacerbation rates and healthcare utilisation decreased approximately by 30% ($p < 0.001$) [70]. The same authors also showed that, after two years of treatment, exacerbation rate and healthcare utilisation were further decreased by 83% and 100%, respectively, while level of asthma control, steroid use and lung function remained unchanged [71].

A systematic review of pediatric RCTs pooled the data of 1381 children and adolescents with moderate-to-severe allergic asthma in order to establish the efficacy of omalizumab as an add-on therapy [72]. During the stable-steroid phase, omalizumab decreased the number of patients with at least one exacerbation (risk ratio, 0.69; $p < 0.001$), the mean number of asthma exacerbations per patient (risk ratio, 0.35; $p < 0.001$), and the asthma symptom score (mean difference, 0.12; $p = 0.005$) when compared to placebo. During the steroid reduction phase, omalizumab further reduced the number of patients with at least one exacerbation (risk ratio, 0.48; $p < 0.001$) and the mean number of asthma exacerbations per patient (mean difference, 0.12; $p < 0.05$).

Given the cost of omalizumab, many authors have argued for the importance of identifying specific asthma populations who will have significant benefit from it [68, 73, 74]. In the ICATA study, baseline predictors of good response to treatment were sensitization and exposure to cockroach allergen, sensitization to house dust mite allergens, a serum IgE level of more than 100 IU per milliliter, a BMI of 25 or more, and a history of at least one unscheduled medical visit in the previous year [68].

Several studies have assessed the long-term safety of omalizumab in children and adults. A pooled analysis of 67 RCTs conducted over 2 decades on 4254 children and adults treated with omalizumab showed no association between omalizumab treatment and risk of malignancy [75]. In an RCT evaluating 225 school-aged children, omalizumab was well tolerated, there were no serious adverse events, and the frequency and types of all adverse events were similar to the placebo group [9]. These results have been further confirmed by a recent systematic review of RCTs that concluded that treatment with omalizumab does not result in increased risk of malignancy or hypersensitivity reactions [72].

While the rationale for long-term treatment with omalizumab is supported by pharmacokinetic-pharmacodynamic models [76], the duration of treatment is still under discussion. Results from published studies suggest that omalizumab should be continued for > 1 year [77, 78]. In a retrospective study of adults and children with uncontrolled severe asthma treated with omalizumab, the response to treatment was 'excellent' in 52.5% of patients, particularly in the subgroup of children aged 6 to 11 years [77]. After the discontinuation of treatment, loss of asthma control was documented in 69.2% of the patients who had received omalizumab for < 1 year, 59.1% of the subjects treated for 1–2 years, and 46.1% of the cases treated for > 2 years. Time to loss of control was shorter in younger children and longer in patients with an 'excellent' response compared with patients with a 'good' response. No early loss of control (within 6 months) was observed among patients with > 3.5 years of continuous treatment with omalizumab. Finally, 20% of patients in whom omalizumab was re-prescribed because of loss of control did not respond to the treatment anymore [77]. Despite these encouraging findings, the impact of omalizumab on the natural history of severe asthma in children deserves to be further investigated by long-term studies that will also define the criteria and timing for discontinuing the treatment.

It is well known that asthma pharmacotherapy is effective in controlling symptoms and bronchial inflammation, but cannot affect the underlying immune response, thus leading to the possibility of symptom reappearance after its discontinuation [79]. In this scenario, allergen-specific immunotherapy (AIT) has been proposed as the only therapeutic method that can modulate the underlying immune pathophysiology in allergic asthma [80].

AIT is currently indicated in children and adults with mild-moderate allergic asthma that is completely or partially controlled by pharmacotherapy and with the evidence of a clear relationship between symptoms and exposure to a specific allergen [81–84]. However, according to recent guidelines, the efficacy of AIT in asthmatic subjects is limited, and its potential benefits must be weighed against the risk of side effects and the inconvenience and costs of the prolonged therapy [5]. Moreover, severe or uncontrolled asthma (regardless of its severity) is a major independent risk factor for non-fatal or even fatal adverse reactions, thus representing a contraindication for AIT [85–87]. Finally, children with severe asthma are often sensitized to multiple allergens, thus making AIT prescription even more complicated [88].

In subjects with uncontrolled and/or severe allergic asthma, a combination of omalizumab and AIT has been proposed [88]. Surprisingly, only a few studies have addressed this issue [89–92]. However, pre-treatment with omalizumab seems to improve the efficacy and tolerability of subcutaneous AIT in children and adults with severe allergic asthma both during omalizumab treatment and after its discontinuation [89, 91, 92]. Omalizumab has also been successfully used as a supplementary treatment to AIT in order to improve asthma control in children ≥6 years with severe persistent allergic asthma [90]. Given the scarcity of studies on AIT *plus* omalizumab in children with severe allergic asthma, further research is warranted to assess risks and benefits of the combined treatment.

Children with severe asthma require a detailed and individualized approach including re-assessment for differential diagnoses, comorbidities and contributory factors, environmental triggers, lung function and inflammation, adherence and response to therapy, and QoL. Treatment of pediatric severe asthma still relies on the maximal optimal use of corticosteroids, bronchodilators and other controllers recommended for moderate-to-severe disease. However, the management of asthma is becoming much more patient-specific, as more and more is learned about the biology behind the development and progression of asthma.

In the current paper, we described the characteristics of four children with severe asthma in whom omalizumab was prescribed. A review of the relevant literature on the topic was also performed. Finally, we provided an algorithm for the diagnosis of difficult-to-treat and severe asthma in children and adolescents, based on the evidence from the literature review. As all algorithms, it is not meant to replace clinical judgment, but it should drive physicians to adopt a systematic approach towards difficult and severe asthma and provide a useful guide to the clinician.

The addition of omalizumab, the first targeted biological treatment approved for asthma, has led to renewed optimism of outcome improvements in patients with allergic severe asthma. As severe asthma is a heterogeneous condition consisting of different phenotypes, the future of asthma management will likely involve phenotypic and potentially even genotypic characterization in selected cases in order to determine appropriate therapy and thus to provide the highest possible benefit, especially if specific responder phenotypes can be identified and selected for this highly specific treatment.

Abbreviations

anti-IgE: Anti-immunoglobulin E; BMI: Body mass index; FcεRI: IgE receptor; FEF_{25-75}: Forced expiratory flow between 25% and 75%; FEV_1: Forced expiratory volume in the first second; GER: Gastroesophageal reflux; ICS: Inhaled corticosteroids; ICU: Intensive care unit; IL: Interleukin; LABA: Long-acting β_2-agonist; LTRA: Oral leukotriene receptor antagonist; QoL: Quality of life; RCTs: Randomized controlled trials; SABA: Short-acting β_2-agonists; SDB: Sleep-disordered breathing

Acknowledgements

The authors gratefully thank Dr. Marco Maglione for his contribution in the clinical assessment of the described cases. Medical writing assistance was provided by Stephen Walters on behalf of City Hills Proofreading.

Funding

No funding was secured for this study.

Authors' contributions

VM, SM and FS, authors of the current manuscript, declare that they have participated sufficiently in the work to take public responsibility for appropriate portions of the content. VM and SM carried out the initial investigations, drafted the initial manuscript, revised the manuscript, and approved the final manuscript as submitted. FS conceptualized and designed the study, and critically reviewed and approved the final manuscript as submitted. All authors read and approved the final manuscript.

Competing interests

The authors declare that they have no competing interests to disclose. Authors have no financial relationships relevant to this article to disclose.

References

1. O'Byrne PM, Pedersen S, Schatz M, Thoren A, Ekholm E, Carlsson LG, et al. The poorly explored impact of uncontrolled asthma. Chest. 2013;143:511–3.
2. National Asthma Education and Prevention Program. Expert panel report 3 (EPR-3): guidelines for the diagnosis and Management of Asthma-Summary Report 2007. J Allergy Clin Immunol. 2007;120:S94–8.
3. Hedlin G. Management of severe asthma in childhood-state of the art and novel perspectives. Pediatr Allergy Immunol. 2014;25:111–21.
4. Konradsen JR, Nordlund B, Lidegran M, Pedroletti C, Grönlund H, van Hage M, et al. Problematic severe asthma: a proposed approach to identifying children who are severely resistant to therapy. Pediatr Allergy Immunol. 2011;22:9–18.
5. Global Initiative for Asthma Report. Global strategy for asthma management and prevention (updated 2016). https://www.ginasthma.org. Accessed 07 June 2017.
6. Chung KF, Wenzel SE, Brozek JL, Bush A, Castro M, Sterk PJ, et al. International ERS/ATS guidelines on definition, evaluation and treatment of severe asthma. Eur Respir J. 2014;43:343–53.
7. Vandenplas Y, Rudolph CD, Di Lorenzo C, Hassall E, Liptak G, Mazur L, et al. Pediatric gastroesophageal reflux clinical practice guidelines: joint recommendations of the north American Society for Pediatric Gastroenterology, Hepatology, and nutrition (NASPGHAN) and the European Society for Pediatric Gastroenterology, Hepatology, and nutrition (ESPGHAN). J Pediatr Gastroenterol Nutr. 2009;49:498–507.
8. Lødrup Carlsen KC, Hedlin G, Bush A, Wennergren G, de Benedictis FM, De Jongste JC, et al. Assessment of problematic severe asthma in children. Eur Respir J. 2011;37:432–40.
9. Milgrom H, Berger W, Nayak A, Gupta N, Pollard S, McAlary M, et al. Treatment of childhood asthma with anti-immunoglobulin E antibody (omalizumab). Pediatrics. 2001;108:E36.
10. Bush A, Saglani S. Management of severe asthma in children. Lancet. 2010;376:814–5.
11. Lang A, Mowinckel P, Sachs-Olsen C, Riiser A, Lunde J, Carlsen KH, et al. Asthma severity in childhood, untangling clinical phenotypes. Pediatr Allergy Immunol. 2010;21:945–53.
12. Nordlund B, Konradsen JR, Pedroletti C, Kull I, Hedlin G. The clinical benefit of evaluating health-related quality-of-life in children with problematic severe asthma. Acta Paediatr. 2011;100:1454–60.
13. Dean BB, Calimlim BC, Sacco P, Aguilar D, Maykut R, Tinkelman D. Uncontrolled asthma: assessing quality of life and productivity of children and their caregivers using a cross-sectional internet-based survey. Health Qual Life Outcomes. 2010;8:6.
14. Juniper EF, Guyatt GH, Feeny DH, Ferrie PJ, Griffith LE, Townsend M. Measuring quality of life in children with asthma. Qual Life Res. 1996;5:35–46.
15. British Thoracic Society. Scottish Intercollegiate Guidelines Network. British guideline on the management of asthma, 2014. https://www.brit-thoracic.org.uk/guidelines-and-quality-standards/asthma-guideline. Accessed 13 Apr 2016.
16. Montella S, Baraldi E, Cazzato S, Aralla R, Berardi M, Brunetti LM, et al. Severe asthma features in children: a case-control online survey. Ital J Pediatr. 2016;42:9.
17. Fitzpatrick AM, Gaston BM, Erzurum SC, Teague WG, National Institutes of Health/National Heart, Lung, and Blood Institute Severe Asthma Research Program. Features of severe asthma in school-age children: Atopy and increased exhaled nitric oxide. J Allergy Clin Immunol. 2006;118:1218–25.
18. Simon MR, Chinchilli VM, Phillips BR, Sorkness CA, Lemanske RF Jr, Szefler SJ, et al. Forced expiratory flow between 25% and 75% of vital capacity and FEV1/forced vital capacity ratio in relation to clinical and physiological parameters in asthmatic children with normal FEV1 values. J Allergy Clin Immunol. 2010;126:527–34.
19. Hedlin G, Bush A, Lødrup Carlsen K, Wennergren G, De Benedictis FM, Melén E, et al. Problematic severe asthma in children, not one problem but many: a GA2LEN initiative. Eur Respir J. 2010;36:196–201.
20. Fitzpatrick AM, Teague WG. Severe asthma in children: insights from the National Heart, Lung, and Blood Institute's severe asthma research program. Pediatr Allergy Immunol Pulmonol. 2010;23:131–8.
21. Konradsen JR, Caffrey Osvald E, Hedlin G. Update on the current methods for the diagnosis and treatment of severe childhood asthma. Expert Rev Respir Med. 2015;9:769–77.
22. Lang AM, Konradsen J, Carlsen KH, Sachs-Olsen C, Mowinckel P, Hedlin G, et al. Identifying problematic severe asthma in the individual child—does lung function matter? Acta Paediatr. 2010;99:404–10.
23. Rao DR, Gaffin JM, Baxi SN, Sheehan WJ, Hoffman EB, Phipatanakul WJ. The utility of forced expiratory flow between 25% and 75% of vital capacity in predicting childhood asthma morbidity and severity. Asthma. 2012;49:586–92.
24. Eid N, Yandell B, Howell L, Eddy M, Sheikh S. Can peak expiratory flow predict airflow obstruction in children with asthma? Pediatrics. 2000;105:354–8.
25. Cicutto LC, Chapman KR, Chamberlain D, Downey GP. Difficult asthma: consider all of the possibilities. Can Respir J. 2000;7:415–8.
26. Wener RR, Bel EH. Severe refractory asthma: an update. Eur Respir Rev. 2013;22:227–35.
27. Bracken M, Fleming L, Hall P, et al. The importance of nurse-led home visits in the assessment of children with problematic asthma. Arch Dis Child. 2009;94:780–4.
28. De Groot EP, Kreggemeijer WJ, Brand PL. Getting the basics right resolves most cases of uncontrolled and problematic asthma. Acta Paediatr. 2015;104:916–21.
29. Grimaldi-Bensouda L, Zureik M, Aubier M, Humbert M, Levy J, Benichou J, et al. Does omalizumab make a difference to the real-life treatment of asthma exacerbations? Results from a large cohort of patients with severe uncontrolled asthma. Chest. 2013;143:398–405.
30. American Lung Association Asthma Clinical Research Centers, Mastronarde JG, Anthonisen NR, Castro M, Holbrook JT, Leone FT, et al. Efficacy of esomeprazole for treatment of poorly controlled asthma. N Engl J Med. 2009;360:1487–9.
31. Writing Committee for the American Lung Association Asthma Clinical Research Centers, Holbrook JT, Wise RA, Gold BD, Blake K, Brown ED, et al. Lansoprazole for children with poorly controlled asthma: a randomized controlled trial. JAMA 2012;307:373-381.
32. Wright AL, Holberg CJ, Martinez FD, Halonen M, Morgan W, Taussig LM. Epidemiology of physician-diagnosed allergic rhinitis in childhood. Pediatrics. 1994;94:895–901.
33. De Groot EP, Nijkamp A, Duiverman EJ, Brand PL. Allergic rhinitis is associated with poor asthma control in children with asthma. Thorax. 2012;67:582–7.
34. Rotiroti G, Roberts G, Scadding GK. Rhinitis in children: common clinical presentations and differential diagnoses. Pediatr Allergy Immunol. 2015;26:103–10.
35. Bousquet J, Khaltaev N, Cruz AA, Denburg J, Fokkens WJ, Togias A, et al. Allergic rhinitis and its impact on asthma (ARIA). 2008 update (in collaboration with the World Health Organization, GA(2)LEN and AllerGen). Allergy. 2008;63:S8–160.
36. Deliu M, Belgrave D, Simpson A, Murray CS, Kerry G, Custovic A. Impact of rhinitis on asthma severity in school-age children. Allergy. 2014;69:1515–21.
37. Brozek JL, Bousquet J, Baena-Cagnani CE, Bonini S, Canonica GW, Casale TB, et al. Allergic rhinitis and its impact on asthma (ARIA) guidelines: 2010 revision. J Allergy Clin Immunol. 2010;126:466–76.
38. Weinberger M, Abu-Hasan M. Pseudo-asthma: when cough, wheezing, and dyspnea are not asthma. Pediatrics. 2007;120:855–64.
39. De Groot EP, Duiverman EJ, Brand PL. Dysfunctional breathing in children with asthma: a rare but relevant comorbidity. Eur Respir J. 2013;41:1068–73.
40. Barker NJ, Jones M, O'Connell NE, Everard ML. Breathing exercises for dysfunctional breathing/hyperventilation syndrome in children. Cochrane Database Syst Rev. 2013;12:CD010376.
41. Section on Pediatric Pulmonology, Subcommittee on Obstructive Sleep Apnea Syndrome, American Academy of Pediatrics. Clinical practice guideline: diagnosis and management of childhood obstructive sleep apnea syndrome. Pediatrics. 2002;109:704–12.

42. Goldstein NA, Aronin C, Kantrowitz B, Hershcopf R, Fishkin S, Lee H, Weaver DE, et al. The prevalence of sleep-disordered breathing in children with asthma and its behavioral effects. Pediatr Pulmonol. 2015;50:1128–36.
43. Ross KR, Storfer-Isser A, Hart MA, Kibler AM, Rueschman M, Rosen CL, et al. Sleep-disordered breathing is associated with asthma severity in children. J Pediatr. 2012;160:736–42.
44. Santamaria F, Montella S, Greco L, Valerio G, Franzese A, Maniscalco M, et al. Obesity duration is associated to pulmonary function impairment in obese subjects. Obesity (Silver Spring). 2011;19:1623–8.
45. Sivapalan P, Diamant Z, Ulrik CS. Obesity and asthma: current knowledge and future needs. Curr Opin Pulm Med. 2015;21:80–5.
46. Rasmussen F, Hancox RJ. Mechanisms of obesity in asthma. Curr Opin Allergy Clin Immunol. 2014;14:35–43.
47. Santamaria F, Montella S, Pietrobelli A. Obesity and pulmonary disease: unanswered questions. Obes Rev. 2012;13:822–33.
48. Lang JE, Hossain J, Holbrook JT, Teague WG, Gold BD, Wise RA, et al. Gastro-oesophageal reflux and worse asthma control in obese children: a case of symptom misattribution? Thorax. 2016;71:238–46.
49. Santamaria F, Montella S, De Stefano S, Sperlì F, Barbarano F, Valerio G. Relationship between exhaled nitric oxide and body mass index in children and adolescents. J Allergy Clin Immunol. 2005;116:1163–4.
50. Van Huisstede A, Rudolphus A, Castro Cabezas M, Biter LU, van de Geijn GJ, Taube C, et al. Effect of bariatric surgery on asthma control, lung function and bronchial and systemic inflammation in morbidly obese subjects with asthma. Thorax. 2015;70:659–67.
51. Katzmarzyk PT, Bouchard C. Where is the beef? Waist circumference is more highly correlated with BMI and total body fat than with abdominal visceral fat in children. Int J Obes. 2014;38:753–4.
52. De Groot EP, Duiverman EJ, Brand PL. Comorbidities of asthma during childhood: possibly important, yet poorly studied. Eur Respir J. 2010;36:671–8.
53. Sweeney J, Patterson CC, Menzies-Gow A, Niven RM, Mansur AH, Bucknall C, et al. Comorbidity in severe asthma requiring systemic corticosteroid therapy: cross-sectional data from the optimum patient care research database and the British thoracic difficult asthma registry. Thorax. 2016; https://doi.org/10.1136/thoraxjnl-2015-207630.
54. Federal Drug Administration Advisory for Omalizumab. Available at: https://wayback.archive-it.org/7993/20170111075347/. http://www.fda.gov/Drugs/DevelopmentApprovalProcess/HowDrugsareDevelopedandApproved/ApprovalApplications/TherapeuticBiologicApplications/default.htm. Accessed 4 Feb 2018.
55. European Medicines Agency: assessment report for Xolair. Available at: http://www.ema.europa.eu/ema/index.jsp?curl=pages/medicines/human/medicines/000606/human_med_001162.jsp&mid=WC0b01ac058001d124. Accessed 7 June 2017.
56. Chung KF. Targeting the interleukin pathway in the treatment of asthma. Lancet. 2015;386:1086–96.
57. Jensen RK, Plum M, Tjerrild L, Jakob T, Spillner E, Andersen GR. Structure of the omalizumab Fab. Acta Crystallogr F Struct Biol Commun. 2015;71:419–26.
58. Holgate S, Smith N, Massanari M, Jimenez P. Effects of omalizumab on markers of inflammation in patients with allergic asthma. Allergy. 2009;64:1728–36.
59. Hill DA, Siracusa MC, Ruymann KR, Tait Wojno ED, Artis D, Spergel JM. Omalizumab therapy is associated with reduced circulating basophil populations in asthmatic children. Allergy. 2014;69:674–7.
60. Humbert M, Beasley R, Ayres J, Slavin R, Hébert J, Bousquet J, et al. Benefits of omalizumab as add-on therapy in patients with severe persistent asthma who are inadequately controlled despite best available therapy (GINA 2002 step 4 treatment): INNOVATE. Allergy. 2005;60:309–16.
61. Normansell R, Walker S, Milan SJ, Walters EH, Nair P. Omalizumab for asthma in adults and children. Cochrane Database Syst Rev. 2014;1:CD003559.
62. Lai T, Wang S, Xu Z, Zhang C, Zhao Y, Hu Y, Cao C, et al. Long-term efficacy and safety of omalizumab in patients with persistent uncontrolled allergic asthma: a systematic review and meta-analysis. Sci Rep. 2015;5:8191.
63. Abraham I, Alhossan A, Lee CS, Kutbi H, MacDonald K. "real-life" effectiveness studies of omalizumab in adult patients with severe allergic asthma: systematic review. Allergy. 2015; https://doi.org/10.1111/all.12815.
64. Lanier B, Bridges T, Kulus M, Taylor AF, Berhane I, Vidaurre CF. Omalizumab for the treatment of exacerbations in children with inadequately controlled allergic (IgE-mediated) asthma. J Allergy Clin Immunol. 2009;124:1210–6.
65. Solèr M, Matz J, Townley R, Buhl R, O'Brien J, Fox H, et al. The anti-IgE antibody omalizumab reduces exacerbations and steroid requirement in allergic asthmatics. Eur Respir J. 2001;18:254–61.
66. Holgate ST. Cytokine and anti-cytokine therapy for the treatment of asthma and allergic disease. Cytokine. 2004;28:152–7.
67. Odajima H, Ebisawa M, Nagakura T, Fujisawa T, Akasawa A, Ito K, et al. Omalizumab in Japanese children with severe allergic asthma uncontrolled with standard therapy. Allergol Int. 2015;64:364–70.
68. Busse WW, Morgan WJ, Gergen PJ, Mitchell HE, Gern JE, Liu AH, et al. Randomized trial of omalizumab (anti-IgE) for asthma in inner-city children. N Engl J Med. 2011;364:1005–15.
69. Teach SJ, Gill MA, Togias A, Sorkness CA, Arbes SJ Jr, Calatroni A, et al. Preseasonal treatment with either omalizumab or an inhaled corticosteroid boost to prevent fall asthma exacerbations. J Allergy Clin Immunol. 2015; 136:1476–85.
70. Deschildre A, Marguet C, Salleron J, Pin I, Rittié JL, Derelle J, et al. Add-on omalizumab in children with severe allergic asthma: a 1-year real life survey. Eur Respir J. 2013;42:1224–33.
71. Deschildre A, Marguet C, Langlois C, Pin I, Rittié JL, Derelle J, et al. Real-life long-term omalizumab therapy in children with severe allergic asthma. Eur Respir J. 2015;46:856–9.
72. Rodrigo GJ, Neffen H. Systematic review on the use of omalizumab for the treatment of asthmatic children and adolescents. Pediatr Allergy Immunol. 2015;26:551–6.
73. Oba Y, Salzman GA. Cost-effectiveness analysis of omalizumab in adults and adolescents with moderate-to-severe allergic asthma. J Allergy Clin Immunol. 2004;114:265–9.
74. Campbell JD, Spackman DE, Sullivan SD. The costs and consequences of omalizumab in uncontrolled asthma from a USA payer perspective. Allergy. 2010;65:1141–8.
75. Busse W, Buhl R, Fernandez Vidaurre C, Blogg M, Zhu J, Eisner MD, et al. Omalizumab and the risk of malignancy: results from a pooled analysis. J Allergy Clin Immunol. 2012;129:983–9.
76. Lowe PJ, Renard D. Omalizumab decreases IgE production in patients with allergic (IgE-mediated) asthma; PKPD analysis of a biomarker, total IgE. Br J Clin Pharmacol. 2011;72:306–10.
77. Molimard M, Mala L, Bourdeix I, Le Gros V. Observational study in severe asthmatic patients after discontinuation of omalizumab for good asthma control. Respir Med. 2014;108:571–6.
78. Busse WW, Trzaskoma B, Omachi TA, Canvin J, Rosen K, Chipps BE, et al. Evaluating Xolair persistency of response after long-term therapy (XPORT). Am J Respir Crit Care Med. 2014;189:A6576.
79. Guilbert TW, Morgan WJ, Zeiger RS, Mauger DT, Boehmer SJ, Szefler SJ, et al. Long-term inhaled corticosteroids in preschool children at high risk for asthma. N Engl J Med. 2006;354:1985–97.
80. Akdis CA. Therapies for allergic inflammation: refining strategies to induce tolerance. Nat Med. 2012;18:736–49.
81. National Heart, Lung, and Blood Institute. Expert panel report 3: Guidelines for the diagnosis and management of asthma—full report 2007. Available at: https://www.nhlbi.nih.gov/files/docs/guidelines/asthgdln.pdf. Accessed 4 Feb 2018.
82. Joint Task Force on Practice Parameters, American Academy of Allergy, Asthma and Immunology, American College of Allergy, Asthma and Immunology, Joint Council of Allergy, Asthma and Immunolgy. Allergen immunotherapy: a practice parameter second update. J Allergy Clin Immunol. 2007;120:S25–85.
83. Zuberbier T, Bachert C, Bousquet PJ, Passalacqua G, Walter Canonica G, Merk H, et al. GA(2) LEN/EAACI pocket guide for allergen-specific immunotherapy for allergic rhinitis and asthma. Allergy. 2010;65:1525–30.
84. Pajno GB, Bernardini R, Peroni D, Arasi S, Martelli A, Landi M, et al. Clinical practice recommendations for allergen-specific immunotherapy in children: the Italian consensus report. Ital J Pediatr. 2017;43:13.
85. Pitsios C, Demoly P, Bilo MB, Gerth van Wijk R, Pfaar O, Sturm GJ, et al. Clinical contraindications to allergen immunotherapy: an EAACI position paper. Allergy. 2015;70:897–909.
86. Tsabouri S, Mavroudi A, Feketea G, Guibas GV. Subcutaneous and sublingual immunotherapy in allergic asthma in children. Front Pediatr. 2017;5:82.
87. Jutel M, Agache I, Bonini S, Burks AW, Calderon M, Canonica W, et al. International consensus on allergy immunotherapy. J Allergy Clin Immunol. 2015;136:556–68.
88. Hedlin G, van Hage M. The role of immunotherapy in the management of childhood asthma. Ther Adv Respir Dis. 2012;6:137–46.
89. Lambert N, Guiddir T, Amat F, Just J. Pre-treatment by omalizumab allows allergen immunotherapy in children and young adults with severe allergic asthma. Pediatr Allergy Immunol. 2014;25:829 32.

17

Case report of severe myocarditis in an immunocompromised child with Respiratory Syncytial Virus infection

Hiroki Miura[1], Fumihiko Hattori[1], Hidetoshi Uchida[1], Tadayoshi Hata[2], Kazuko Kudo[1], Masatoki Sato[3] and Tetsushi Yoshikawa[1*]

Abstract

Background: Respiratory syncytial virus (RSV) infection is common and may be severe among patients with preexisting cardiac anomalies, but direct involvement of myocardial damage is not common in those patients. Additionally, myocardial involvement has been rarely described among immune compromised children.

Case presentation: A 4-year-old girl with acute lymphoblastic leukemia who received maintenance chemotherapy in an outpatient clinic developed systemic inflammatory response syndrome. RSV infection was confirmed by a positive rapid antigen test and serological assay. Subsequently, she was diagnosed with severe myocarditis caused by RSV infection, which was diagnosed by abnormal findings of cardiac echography and ECG and elevated biomarkers for myocardial damage. Then, she was treated in the intensive care unit for 13 days. High amounts of RSV type B RNA was detected in tracheal aspirates and serum sample.

Conclusion: This case report emphasizes that RSV infection may be associated with myocarditis in immunocompromised children receiving maintenance chemotherapy.

Keywords: RSV, Myocarditis, Leukemia, Maintenance treatment, Real-time RT-PCR

Background

Respiratory syncytial virus (RSV) is one of the most important viral causes of lower respiratory tract infection (LRTI) in infancy and childhood. It is well known that premature infants, infants with cardiac diseases, and immunocompromised patients, including leukemic children, are at high risk for more severe and complicated RSV infection. Although severe LRTI caused by RSV infection is associated with high morbidity in patients with acute lymphoblastic leukemia [1], no RSV myocarditis case has been reported in such patients. This report describes an immunocompromised child with severe myocarditis caused by RSV infection and detection of high amounts of viral genome in not only tracheal tube aspirates but also serum sample based on real-time revers transcription polymerase chain reaction (RT-PCR).

* Correspondence: tetsushi@fujita-hu.ac.jp
[1]Department of Pediatrics, Fujita Health University School of Medicine, 1-98, Dengakugakubo, Kutsukake-cho, Toyoake, Aichi 470-1192, Japan
Full list of author information is available at the end of the article

Case presentation

A 4-year-old Japanese girl with B-cell acute lymphoblastic leukemia (ALL) presented to the emergency room with febrile convulsion. The age of disease onset was 3 years and the patient received maintenance chemotherapy in our outpatient clinic. Clinical course of patient is shown in Fig. 1. The patient had a high fever (40.1 C°), tachypnea (respiratory rate 38/min), and tachycardia (pulse rate 180/min). She was diagnosed with febrile neutropenia and systemic inflammatory response syndrome (SIRS) based on her neutrophil count, which was 322/μL, as well as remarkably elevated inflammatory responses (CRP: 2.2 mg/dl; procalicitonin: 67.8 ng/mL). Chest X-ray revealed mild perihilar infiltration with normal cardiothoracic ratio (51.6%), and chest computed tomographic scanning showed bilateral consolidation and pleural effusion. Within two hours after admission, the patient's respiratory condition continued to deteriorate despite oxygen supplementation while lactate levels increased to 62.6 mg/dL. The patient was transferred to

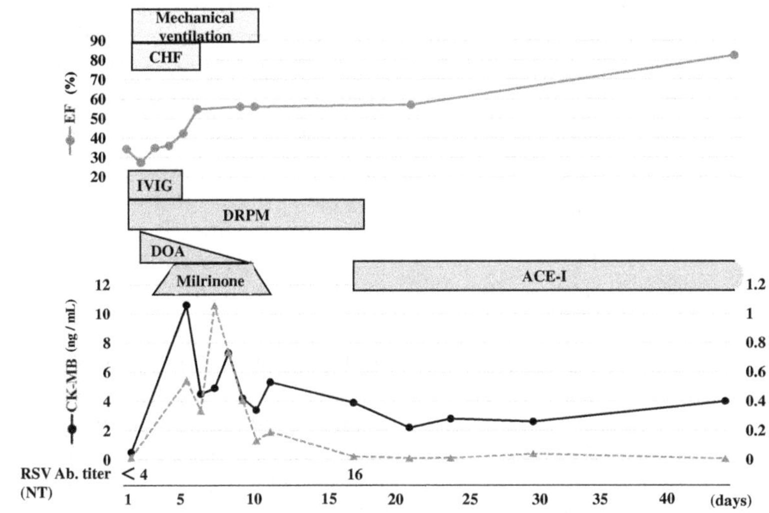

Fig. 1 Clinical course of the patient. Kinetics for the ejection fraction and biomarkers of myocardial damage. Myocardial function and myocardial damage were gradually recovered in the acute phase using intensive treatment. CHF: continuous hemofiltration; EF: ejection fraction; CPK: creatine kinase; MB: muscle and brain; ACE: angiotensin converting enzyme inhibitor

the intensive care unit for mechanical ventilation; however, her systolic blood pressure decreased gradually from 116 to 40 mmHg despite hydration and blood transfusion for volume expansion. Therefore, catecholamine administration, intravenous immunoglobulin, and continuous venovenous hemofiltration were initiated. As we suspected myocardial dysfunction, cardiac ultrasound was performed and showed depressed left ventricular function with an ejection fraction of 27%, as well as a left ventricular Tei index of 0.62 indicating global systolic and diastolic ventricular function, mitral regurgitation, and tricuspid regurgitation. An electrocardiogram showed ST-T wave change in V4-6. Furthermore, a marked increase in myocardial markers was noted, including Troponin-I 0.541 ng/mL (normal 0-0.04 ng/mL), myoglobin 91.2 ng/mL (normal 12.8-66.1 ng/mL), and CK-MB 10.6 ng/mL (0.9-5.9 ng/mL).

Two days after admission to the hospital, her systolic blood pressure improved to 120 mmHg and inotropic support was gradually reduced and stopped by day 9. In addition to the administration of milrinone for 11 days, continuous hemofiltration was carried out for 6 days to treat the heart failure. Subsequently, left ventricular function gradually improved, and myocardial markers returned to normal levels 17 days after admission to the hospital. Finally, she was discharged from the intensive care unit on day 13.

Three separate blood cultures were negative. Additionally, the patient tested negative for influenza virus, human-metapneumovirus, adenovirus, and *Group A streptococcus* using rapid antigen tests; however, RSV antigens were detected in a nasal swab at the time of hospital admission. Moreover, seroconversion of RSV antibody titers (< 4 and 16) was confirmed using a neutralizing antibody test (SRL Inc., Tokyo, Japan). In order to elucidate the pathophysiology of RSV infection, serially collected tracheal tube aspirates and serum samples were examined using real-time RT-PCR [2]. Real-time RT-PCR analysis detected high amounts of RSV type B RNA in the tracheal aspirates on day 2 (1.6×10^9 copies/ml) and day 5 (1.4×10^8 copies/ml) after the onset of the disease. Interestingly, viral RNA was also detected in the serum sample obtained on day 1 of the illness (3.2×10^4 copies/ml), but it had decreased to undetectable levels in serum samples collected on days 5 and 8.

In order to examine the pathophysiology of this severe cardiac complication caused by RSV infection, various cytokines and chemokines were measured in serially collected serum samples using the Cytometric Bead Array system (Table 1). Serum samples were serially collected before the onset of the RSV infection and on days 1, 5, 7, and 14 after illness onset. As shown in Table 1, IL-6, IL-10, IL-8, IFN-γ, MCP-1, and IP-10 were markedly elevated at the time of disease onset. The levels of these biomarkers returned to normal by 14 days after illness onset.

Discussion and conclusions

RSV infection in high risk patients, including patients with hematological malignancies, is associated with increased morbidity and mortality. Lymphopenia (lymphocyte counts of < 100/mm^3) and young age (less than 2 years of age) are predictors of RSV-related LRTI in immunocompromised children [3]. Maintenance treatment is considered to be safer than induction

Table 1 Kinetics of cytokines and chemokines level in serially collected serum samples

Day	Pre	1	5	14	17
IL-2 (pg/mL)	0.0	0.0	0.0	0.0	0.0
IL-4 (pg/mL)	0.0	0.0	0.0	0.0	0.0
IL-6 (pg/mL)	0.0	17,599.1	92.7	0.0	0.0
IL-10 (pg/mL)	0.0	150.6	1.7	0.0	0.0
TNF-α (pg/mL)	0.0	0.0	0.0	0.0	0.0
IFN-γ (pg/mL)	0.0	16.2	64.6	0.0	0.0
IL-8 (pg/mL)	0.0	5376.5	731.4	26.9	20.8
RANTES (pg/mL)	10,878.2	12,011.7	6193.2	17,193.4	20,705.5
MIG (pg/mL)	57.2	141.32	221.7	192.1	114.5
MCP-1 (pg/mL)	238.1	9009.0	667.4	231.0	314.2
IP-10 (pg/mL)	0.0	1104.5	2739.1	404.3	303.0

IL interleukin, *TNF* tumor necrosis factor, *IFN* interferon, *RANTES* regulated on activation, normal T cell expressed and secreted, *MIG* monokine induced by interferon g, *MCP* monocyte chemoattractant protein, *IP* interferon g-inducible protein

treatment because it is associated with lower levels of immunosuppression. Meanwhile, maintenance treatment carried out in outpatient clinics appears to increase the risk for community acquired RSV infection. Recently, Chu et al. [4] reported that 15/54 (28%) immunocompromised children with RSV infection who were treated in outpatient clinics were later hospitalized due to LRTI. Although RSV-related myocarditis has been demonstrated in healthy children [5–9], to the best of our knowledge, this is the first myocarditis case in association with RSV infection in an immunocompromised patient. Thus, in addition to the LRTI, RSV infection may cause myocarditis in immunocompromised children during maintenance chemotherapy in an outpatient clinic setting.

It is important to note, high amounts of RSV RNA were detected in not only the tracheal aspirates but also the serum sample obtained on day 1 of the illness. A previous study found no association between viral load, including RSV, and disease severity in bronchoalveolar lavage samples collected from hematological stem cell transplant recipients [10]. However, the detection of viral RNA in serum samples was significantly associated with patient mortality [10]. Thus, the detection of RSV RNA in serum samples may serve as a useful prognostic marker in patients with severe RSV infection. Furthermre, in the present case, biopsy of the heart tissue was not performed and thus demonstration of RSV in tissue sample was not possible. This procedure is not routinely performed in children. However, the presence of serum RSV RNA in our patient suggesting systemic viral infection may support the notion of direct invasion of RSV into myocardial tissues as suggested by previous study [6].

It has been suggested that viral invasion of the myocardium or endothelial cells and host immune responses may play important roles in the pathogenesis of viral myocarditis. Several cytokines and chemokines were clearly elevated in our patient during the acute phase of the disease, suggesting that host immune responses may contribute to the pathogenesis of RSV-related myocarditis. It has been suggested that Th1 immune responses initiated by INF-γ [11, 12] and Th1 chemokines (IP-10) [13] may play important roles in the pathogenesis of viral myocarditis. Additionally, in a murine model, MCP-1 was required for the invasion of monocytes/macrophages into the myocardium [14]. Our present findings of elevated cytokines and chemokines are consistent with the previous studies [11–14]. A large number of cases is necessary to elucidate the pathogenesis of myocarditis caused by RSV infection, indeed, this may be difficult to achieve because the incidence of this complication is extremely low. Therefore, in addition to human data, an animal model should improve our understanding of the precise pathological mechanisms of RSV-related myocarditis.

In conclusion, herein, we reported on a 4-year-old Japanese girl with ALL who suffered from severe myocarditis associated with RSV infection during maintenance treatment. RSV type B RNA was detected in both tracheal aspirates and serum samples during the acute phase of the disease. This case report emphasizes that in addition to lower respiratory tract infections, RSV infection may cause myocarditis in immunocompromised children receiving maintenance chemotherapy.

Abbreviations

ALL: Acute lymphoblastic leukemia; CK: Creatine kinase; CRP: C-Reactive Protein; ECG: Electrocardiogram; IFN: Interleukin; IL: Interleukin; IP: Interferon g-inducible protein; LRTI: Lower respiratory tract infection; MB: Muscle and brain; MCP: Monocyte chemoattractant protein; RNA: Ribonucleic acid; RSV: Respiratory syncytial virus; RT-PCR: Real-time revers transcription polymerase chain reaction

Acknowledgements

Authors thank Ms. Akiko Yoshikawa, Ms. Chieko Mori, and Ms. Yoko Osakabe of Fujita Health University School of Medicine, Toyoake, Japan who helped with collection and processing samples.

Funding

No external funding was secured for this study.

Authors' contributions

Patient's treatments and sampling were carried out by Drs. HM, FH, KK, and TY. Drs. HU and TH are pediatric cardiologist, who supported treatment of myocarditis in this patient. Biomarkers analysis was carried out by Dr. HM and TY. Real-time RT-PCR for RSV genome was performed by Dr. MS. Dr. HM drafted the initial manuscript, and Prof. TY reviewed and revised the manuscript. All authors approved the final manuscript as submitted and agree to be accountable for all aspects of the work.

Authors' information
Not applicable.

Competing interests
The authors declare that they have no competing interests.

Author details
[1]Department of Pediatrics, Fujita Health University School of Medicine, 1-98, Dengakugakubo, Kutsukake-cho, Toyoake, Aichi 470-1192, Japan. [2]Graduate School of Health Sciences, Fujita Health University, Toyoake, Aichi, Japan. [3]Department of Pediatrics, School of Medicine, Fukushima Medical University, Fukushima, Japan.

References
1. Hakim H, Dallas R, Zhou Y, Pei D, Cheng C, Flynn PM, Pui CH, Jeha S. Acute respiratory infections in children and adolescents with acute lymphoblastic leukemia. Cancer. 2016;122(5):798–805.
2. Hu A, Colella M, Tam JS, Rappaport R, Cheng SM. Simultaneous detection, subgrouping, and quantitation of respiratory syncytial virus a and B by real-time PCR. J Clin Microbiol. 2003;41(1):149–54.
3. El Saleeby CM, Somes GW, DeVincenzo JP, Gaur AH. Risk factors for severe respiratory syncytial virus disease in children with cancer: the importance of lymphopenia and young age. Pediatrics. 2008;121(2):235–43.
4. Chu HY, Chin J, Pollard J, Zerr DM, Englund JA. Clinical outcomes in outpatient respiratory syncytial virus infection in immunocompromised children. Influenza Other Respir Viruses. 2016;10(3):205–10.
5. Armstrong DS, Menahem S. Cardiac arrhythmias as a manifestation of acquired heart disease in association with paediatric respiratory syncitial virus infection. J Paediatr Child Health. 1993;29(4):309–11.
6. Bowles NE, Ni J, Kearney DL, Pauschinger M, Schultheiss HP, McCarthy R, Hare J, Bricker JT, Bowles KR, Towbin JA. Detection of viruses in myocardial tissues by polymerase chain reaction. Evidence of adenovirus as a common cause of myocarditis in children and adults. J Am Coll Cardiol. 2003;42(3):466–72.
7. Menahem S. Respiratory syncytial virus and complete heart block in a child. Cardiol Young. 2010;20(1):103–4.
8. Renko M, Leskinen M, Kontiokari T, Tapiainen T, Hedberg P, Uhari M. Cardiac troponin-I as a screening tool for myocarditis in children hospitalized for viral infection. Acta Paediatr (Oslo, Norway : 1992). 2010;99(2):283–5.
9. Menchise A. Myocarditis in the setting of RSV bronchiolitis. Fetal Pediatr Pathol. 2011;30(1):64–8.
10. Campbell AP, Chien JW, Kuypers J, Englund JA, Wald A, Guthrie KA, Corey L, Boeckh M. Respiratory virus pneumonia after hematopoietic cell transplantation (HCT): associations between viral load in bronchoalveolar lavage samples, viral RNA detection in serum samples, and clinical outcomes of HCT. J Infect Dis. 2010; 201(9):1404–13.
11. Seko Y, Takahashi N, Azuma M, Yagita H, Okumura K, Yazaki Y. Effects of in vivo administration of anti-B7-1/B7-2 monoclonal antibodies on murine acute myocarditis caused by coxsackievirus B3. Circ Res. 1998;82(5):613–8.
12. Huber SA, Feldman AM, Sartini D. Coxsackievirus B3 induces T regulatory cells, which inhibit cardiomyopathy in tumor necrosis factor-alpha transgenic mice. Circ Res. 2006;99(10):1109–16.
13. Yue Y, Gui J, Ai W, Xu W, Xiong S. Direct gene transfer with IP-10 mutant ameliorates mouse CVB3-induced myocarditis by blunting Th1 immune responses. PLoS One. 2011;6(3):e18186.
14. Yue Y, Gui J, Xu W, Xiong S. Gene therapy with CCL2 (MCP-1) mutant protects CVB3-induced myocarditis by compromising Th1 polarization. Mol Immunol. 2011;48(4):706–13.

18

Respiratory morbidity through the first decade of life in a national cohort of children born extremely preterm

Kaia Skromme[1*], Maria Vollsæter[1,2], Knut Øymar[2,3], Trond Markestad[2] and Thomas Halvorsen[1,2]

Abstract

Background: Advances in perinatal care have markedly increased the prospects of survival for infants born extremely preterm (EP). The aim of this study was to investigate hospitalisation rates and respiratory morbidity from five to 11 years of age in a prospective national cohort of EP children born in the surfactant era.

Methods: This was a national prospective cohort study of all children born in Norway during 1999 and 2000 with gestational age (GA) < 28 weeks or birth weight < 1000 grams, and of individually matched term-born controls recruited for a regional subsample. Data on hospital admissions, respiratory symptoms, and use of asthma medication was obtained by parental questionnaires at 11 years of age.

Results: Questionnaires were returned for 232/372 (62%) EP-born and 57/61 (93%) regional term-born controls. Throughout the study period, 67 (29%) EP-born and seven (13%) term-born controls were admitted to hospital (odds ratio (OR) 2.90, 95% confidence interval (CI): 1.25, 6.72). Admissions were mainly due to surgical procedures, with only 12% due to respiratory causes, and were not influenced by neonatal bronchopulmonary dysplasia (BPD) or low GA(≤ 25 weeks). Respiratory symptoms, asthma and use of asthma medication tended to be more common for EP-born, significantly so for medication use and wheeze on exercise. Neonatal BPD was a risk factor for medication use, but not for current wheeze. In multivariate regression models, home oxygen after discharge (OR 4.84, 95% CI: 1.38, 17.06) and parental asthma (OR 4.38, 95% CI: 1.69, 11.38) predicted current asthma, but neither BPD nor low GA were associated with respiratory symptoms at 11 years of age.

Conclusions: Hospitalisation rates five to 11 years after EP birth were low, but twice those of term-born controls, and unrelated to neonatal BPD and low GA. Respiratory causes were rare. Respiratory complaints were more common in children born EP, but the burden of symptoms had declined since early childhood.

Keywords: Extremely preterm, Extremely low birth weight, Asthma, Hospitalisation, Respiratory health

Background

Since the early 1990s increasing numbers of infants born extremely preterm (EP) in high-income countries have survived [1, 2]. Birth at this stage of pregnancy interrupts important developmental processes, and requires gas exchange to take place in foetal lungs, often leading to the syndrome of bronchopulmonary dysplasia (BPD) [3]. The life-long health consequences of EP birth and BPD are unknown, but there are concerns of severe future morbidities, such as chronic obstructive pulmonary disease [4], metabolic syndrome [5], cardiovascular diseases and even early death [6, 7]. Continued health surveillance is therefore important in this group, particularly for those born at less than 26 weeks gestational age (GA), as their high survival rates are fairly recent history.

Health problems may be reflected in utilisation of health care services. Children born EP more often experience repeated hospital admissions during early childhood than children born at term [8]. Most published data on later outcome pertain to groups born in the pre-surfactant era, and there is a need for population based

* Correspondence: kaia.skromme@outlook.com
[1]Department of Pediatrics, Haukeland University Hospital, N-5021 Bergen, Norway
Full list of author information is available at the end of the article

knowledge on health issues among EP-born survivors exposed to the advanced treatment facilities of the late 1990s and 2000s. Such data are of interest to a growing part of health care professionals, administrators, politicians, the EP-born individuals themselves and their families.

We have previously published data on morbidities and hospital admissions during the first five years of life in a national cohort of EP-born children [9, 10]. The aims of the present study were to investigate frequencies and causes of hospital admissions, general health issues and early predictors of health at five to 11 years of age in that same cohort, with a particular focus on respiratory outcomes.

Methods

Participants

All subjects born EP, here defined as GA 22^0 to 27^6 weeks or birth weight 500 to 999 grams, in Norway during 1999 and 2000 were included at birth and followed prospectively during their stay at the neonatal intensive care unit (NICU) [2] and at two [11], five [9, 10] and 11 years of age [12]. Of 638 eligible infants, 174 were stillborn or not resuscitated, 464 were admitted to a NICU and 372 (80%) were alive at 11 years of age.

A control group was recruited at 11 years of age for a regional subsample of participants born EP within Western Norway Regional Health Authority ($n = 61$) by inviting the next-born child of the same gender with GA > 37 weeks and birth weight (BW) > 3000 grams, identified from birth protocols at the maternity ward [12]. If that individual declined, the next-born eligible child was invited until a match was obtained.

The study was based on written parental consent and was approved by the Regional committee on Medical Research Ethics and the Norwegian Data Inspectorate.

Data collection

For the children born EP, all obstetric and paediatric departments in Norway participated in collecting data on the neonatal course and follow-up at two and five years of age, as illustrated in Fig. 1, which explains the recruitment and follow-up process of the overall study. Data on maternal health, pregnancy, delivery and NICU stay were extracted from compulsory notifications to the Medical Birth Registry of Norway. All the data were registered prospectively using forms developed for this study [2]. The children were examined by experienced paediatricians at two and five years of age, and the parents completed questionnaires on socio-demographic factors, health, development, and hospital admissions at two, five and 11 years of age. The International Study of Asthma and Allergies in Childhood (ISAAC) questionnaire was used at both five and 11 years of age to collect

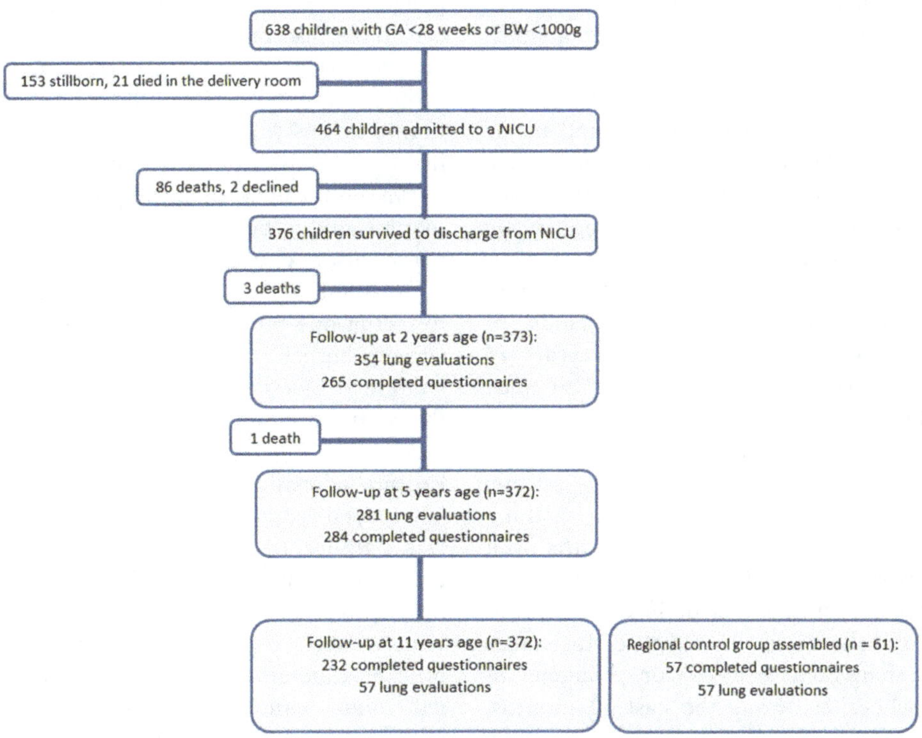

Fig. 1 Description of the Nationwide Cohort of Children Born in Norway During 1999 and 2000 at a Gestational Age <28 Weeks or with a Birth Weight <1000 Grams. *Abbreviations:* GA – Gestational Age, BW – Birth Weight, NICU – Neonatal Intensive Care Unit

data on respiratory health, as well as to compare the burden of respiratory symptoms over this timespan.

Respiratory health and hospital admissions up to five years of age have been published previously [10] and are used as background data in the current article, which reports data from five to 11 years of age. The data were collected by postal questionnaire completed by the parents when the child was 11 years old. Within the region of Western Norway the children were also examined clinically at 11 years of age, together with their matched term-controls [12].

Definitions

GA at birth was based on the national antenatal care program that includes one ultrasound examination at 17–18 weeks gestation, except for a few participants (5%) for whom GA relied on the last menstrual period because an ultrasound was not performed. Small for gestational age was defined as a BW less than the fifth percentile for GA and gender according to Norwegian growth curves [13]. Premature rupture of membranes was defined as rupture more than six days prior to labour. Prenatal steroids were recorded if given at least 24 hours before delivery or at least as two doses. BPD was defined as need of assisted ventilation or oxygen supplementation at 36 completed post-menstrual weeks [3].

At five years of age, major neurosensory disability was defined as cerebral palsy, blindness (legally classified as blind) or complete deafness. For the mothers, a minimum of three years of college education or a university degree was classified as higher education. Cerebral ultrasound findings were dichotomised to minor and major pathology, i.e. respectively periventricular haemorrhage grade 1 to 2, or a maximum of two small cysts, versus periventricular haemorrhage grade 3 to 4 or multicystic periventricular leukomalacia.

Respiratory illness as a cause for admission to hospital included airway infections and all kinds of breathing problems. Current wheeze at 11 years of age was defined by parental report during the past 12 months, while current asthma was defined as either a doctor's diagnosis of asthma combined with either respiratory symptoms or use of asthma medication in the previous 12 months, or asthma medication and symptoms in the past 12 months even if no recall of prior doctor's diagnosis. According to Lai et al. [14], severe asthma was defined as four or more episodes of wheezing, or sleep disturbances (awakened more than once a week) or problems of speaking due to wheezing during the past 12 months. Asthma medication included inhaled corticosteroids, short or long acting β_2-agonists and oral leukotriene modifiers.

Statistical methods

Data were presented as means with standard deviations or as medians with interquartile ranges. Group comparisons were performed with the Student's t-test, χ^2 test, Fisher's exact test or Mann-Whitney U-test, as appropriate. Changes in respiratory health measures were analysed using related samples McNemar's test, and point estimates with 95% confidence intervals (95% CI) were also reported to account for the children with missing responses between questionnaires.

Risk factors for admissions to hospital and for having current asthma were assessed with binary logistic regression, and results expressed as odds ratios (OR) with 95% CI. Neonatal and socio-demographic variables entered in the analyses are listed in the first column of Table 4. Multivariate risk models were constructed by entering all variables with a p-value < 0.10 in univariate regression analyses. P-values ≤ 0.05 were considered significant. As multiple hypotheses were tested in regression models utilising a dataset with limited numbers of participants, Bonferroni corrections were performed and reported in the Results section. All analyses were conducted with SPSS software version 22.0 for Windows.

Results

Questionnaires were returned for 232 (62%) of the 372 surviving children at 11 years of age. Corresponding figures at two and five years of age were 265 (71%) and 284 (76%), respectively. The ISAAC questionnaire was completed for 192 of the children at both five and 11 years of age. Table 1 accounts for differences between participants and non-participants at 11 years of age. The median GA, proportion of mothers with higher education, and proportion of infants who received surfactant and had BPD were higher among the participants, while proportions of mothers who smoked during pregnancy or had chorioamnionitis, and of boys, retinopathy of prematurity or major neurosensory disability at five years of age were lower.

On average, 1.6 term-born subjects had to be approached to recruit one consenting match for each of the 61 eligible subjects born EP within Western Norway Regional Health Authority. Questionnaires were returned for 57 (93%) of the control children.

Hospital admissions

The overall admission rate from five to 11 years of age was significantly higher for children born EP than the term-born controls (OR 2.90, 95% CI: 1.25, 6.72). The proportions of readmitted children from birth to 11 years of age are presented in Fig. 2. There were no significant differences in admission rates between those with and without BPD or between GA categories (Table 2). The 13 children with major neurosensory disability (6% of participants) accounted for 32/138 (23%) of all admissions, and 21% of the children with more

Table 1 Early Characteristics of Extremely Preterm Children Born in Norway During 1999 and 2000 at a Gestational Age < 28 Weeks or with a Birth Weight < 1000 Grams, According to Whether Response Was Given to the Parental Questionnaire at 11 Years of Age

	Parental questionnaire at 11 years of age[a]		
	Responders $n = 232$	Non-responders $n = 140$	p-value[b]
Gestational age, median (interquartile range)	27 (26–28)	26 (25–27)	**0.014**
Birth weight, median (interquartile range)	880 (766–994)	847 (715–979)	0.376
Illness severity score[c], median (interquartile range)	1 (0–2)	1 (0.5–1.5)	0.063
Length of initial stay, median (interquartile range)	92 (70–114)	89 (67–111)	0.483
Male sex	115/232 (50%)	85/140 (61%)	**0.037**
Caesarean section	159/232 (69%)	84/140 (60%)	0.094
Mother higher education	109/227 (48%)	40/120 (33%)	**0.009**
Premature rupture of membranes[d]	26/217 (12%)	13/125 (10%)	0.658
Multiple births	56/232 (24%)	27/140 (19%)	0.276
Bronchopulmonary dysplasia[e]	113/232 (49%)	52/140 (37%)	**0.030**
Patent ductus arteriosus	93/232 (40%)	50/140 (36%)	0.401
Small for gestational age[f]	46/232 (20%)	23/140 (16%)	0.414
Sepsis	52/232 (22%)	36/140 (26%)	0.468
Cerebral ultrasound findings[g]			
No pathology	152/232 (66%)	94/140 (67%)	0.814
Minor pathology	61/232 (26%)	33/140 (24%)	
Major pathology	19/232 (8%)	13/140 (9%)	
Prenatal steroids	164/232 (71%)	93/140 (66%)	0.389
Postnatal steroids	82/232 (35%)	47/140 (34%)	0.728
Mother's age, mean (standard deviation)	30 (5)	29 (6)	0.280
Chorioamnionitis	32/232 (14%)	35/140 (25%)	**0.006**
Preeclampsia	56/232 (24%)	34/140 (24%)	0.974
Retinopathy of prematurity	60/232 (26%)	52/138 (38%)	**0.017**
Smoking in pregnancy	46/191 (24%)	47/124 (38%)	**0.009**
Cerebral palsy, blind or deaf at five years of age	13/232 (6%)	20/140 (14%)	**0.004**
Home oxygen treatment	22/231 (10%)	9/124 (7%)	0.471
Surfactant	192/232 (83%)	104/140 (74%)	**0.050**
Lung disease at two years of age	62/223 (28%)	45/131 (34%)	0.195

[a]Figures are given as n (%), unless otherwise specified. Percentages were calculated from the actual response rates that varied slightly between the items
[b]Mann Whitney's U test, Student's T-test, or χ^2 test, as appropriate. Boldface denotes significant group differences
[c]A score based on lowest and highest fractional oxygen (FIO_2) requirements and the base deficit during the first 12 hours of life
[d]Defined as rupture of membranes more than six days before delivery
[e]Defined as assisted ventilation or oxygen supplementation at 36 weeks postmenstrual age
[f]Defined as less than the fifth percentile for GA and gender according to Norwegian growth curves
[g]Minor pathology defined as periventricular haemorrhage grade 1 to 2, or a maximum of two small cysts, and major pathology defined as periventricular haemorrhage grade 3 to 4 or multi-cystic periventricular leukomalacia

than one admission. The admission rate was significantly lower during 5–11 years of age than during the 0–5 year period (29%, 95% CI: 23–35% versus 75%, 95% CI: 70–80%, $P < 0.001$).

Surgery was the most common reason for admissions (Table 3), and adeno-tonsillectomies and insertion of ear ventilation tubes were significantly more common among EP-born children than controls ($p = 0.033$). Of the 67 children admitted during the study period, 45 (67%) had also been admitted before five years of age. By 11 years of age, parents of 213/372 children (57% of the total cohort) had reported a hospital admission in at least one of the three questionnaires (at two, five or 11 years of age), and 121/372 children an admission for respiratory causes (33% of the total cohort).

In multivariate regression models, a *higher* GA at birth and the presence of major neurosensory disability at five years of age were significantly associated with

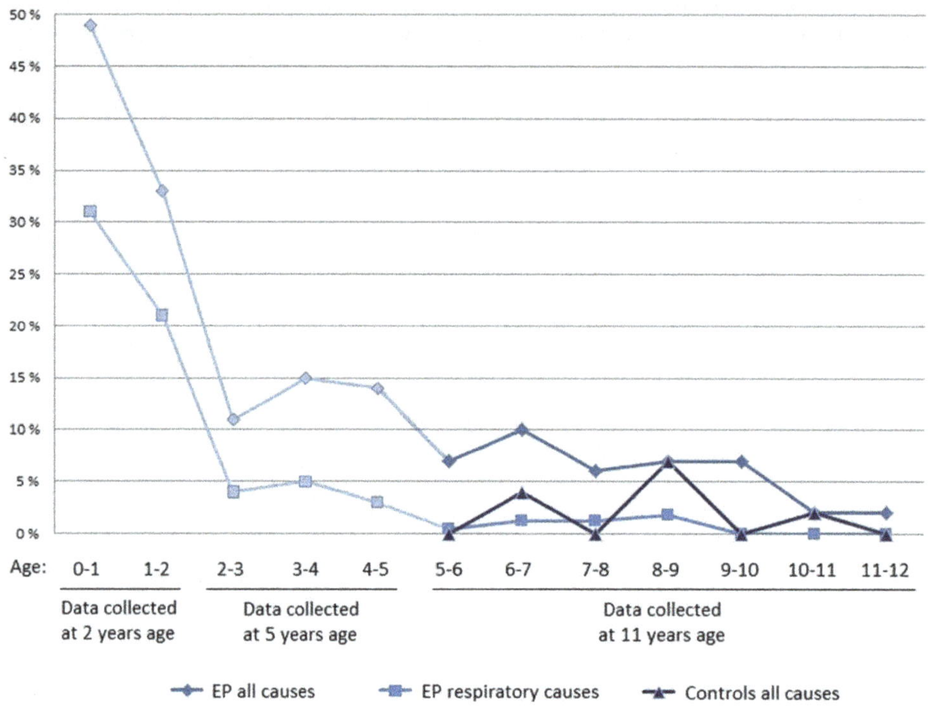

Fig. 2 Hospital Admissions from Birth to Mid-Childhood in Children Born in Norway During 1999 and 2000 at a Gestational Age < 28 Weeks or with a Birth Weight < 1000 Grams, Split by All Causes and Respiratory Causes. Also Depicted are Admissions for All Causes from Age Five to 11 Years of Age for a Regional Control Group Assembled at 11 Years of Age. *Abbreviations*: EP – Extremely Preterm

admission during the study period, while birth by caesarean section was a significant protective factor (Table 4). Adjusted for multiple hypotheses being tested, disability at five years of age and caesarean section were closest to reaching the significance limit (Bonferroni adjusted p-value 0.056 and 0.140, respectively). Removing children with major neurosensory disability at five years of age from the analysis did not alter the effect of the other variables. When added to the model, hospital admission during the third to fifth year of life was significantly associated with admission between five to 11 years of age (OR 3.48, 95% CI:1.60, 7.56), but did not alter the effect of other variables.

Respiratory health

A higher proportion of the EP-born than the term-born children had experienced wheezing and used asthma medications from five to 11 years of age, and a higher proportion of those born EP reported wheezing on exercise during the last 12 months at 11 years of age. There were no significant differences for the other ISAAC questions, but there was a general tendency towards more symptoms and treatments in the EP-born group (Table 5). However, there was a significant decline in the rates of wheezing, awakenings due to wheeze, dry cough at night, current asthma and current use of asthma medications from five to 11 years of age in the EP-born children (Table 6). The rates of parental asthma was similar for the EP- and term-born groups (17% versus 13%, $p = 0.451$), but a higher proportion of the children born EP lived in smoking households at 11 years of age (38% versus 23%, $p = 0.038$).

Significantly more EP-born children with than without neonatal BPD had experienced wheezing and used asthma medication at 5–11 years of age, and there was still a marginal difference in medication rates at 11 years of age. A significantly lower fraction of the children born at GA > 28 weeks used inhaled corticosteroids (OR 0.41. 95% CI: 0.17, 0.99), otherwise respiratory symptoms or use of asthma medications at 5–11 years of age or at 11 years of age did not differ with GA (Table 5). Of the EP-born children, 18 (8%) had by definition severe asthma at 11 years of age. Severe asthma was associated with a parental history of asthma, in that seven of 38 (18%) EP-born children with a parental history of asthma had severe asthma compared to 11 of 191 (6%) EP-born children with no such history ($p = 0.008$). In multivariate regression analyses children of older mothers were less likely to report current respiratory symptoms while a parental history of asthma was associated with both current respiratory symptoms and a diagnosis of asthma (Table 4). Likewise, BPD with home oxygen therapy after discharge remained significantly associated with current asthma (Table 4). Adjusted for multiple hypotheses being tested, the variables closest to reaching the significance level were mother's age for current respiratory symptoms (Bonferroni adjusted

Table 2 Rates and Numbers of Admissions to Hospital at Five to 11 Years of Age in Children Born in Norway During 1999 and 2000 at a Gestational Age < 28 Weeks or with a Birth Weight < 1000 Grams and a Regional Control Group Assembled at 11 Years of Age

	All participants			Neonatal bronchopulmonary dysplasia[b]			Gestational age in weeks[c]				
	Cases $n = 232$	Controls $n = 57$	*p*-values [d]	Yes $n = 165$	No $n = 207$	*p*-values [d]	≤25 $n = 99$	26–27 $n = 188$	≥28 $n = 85$	*p*-values[d] ≤ 25 vs. 26–27	*p*-values[d] 26–27 vs. ≥28
Admitted 5–11 years of age[a]											
Admitted	67 (29%)	7 (13%)	**0.010**	34 (31%)	33 (28%)	0.597	18 (36%)	31 (26%)	18 (30%)	0.193	0.576
Admitted for respiratory cause	8 (4%)	1 (2%)	1.000	6 (6%)	2 (2%)	0.158	3 (6%)	3 (3%)	2 (3%)	0.362	1.000
Admissions[e]	138	7	**0.006**	77	61	0.451	36	64	38	0.192	0.482
Admissions for respiratory cause	16 (12%)	1 (14%)	0.507	14 (41%)	2 (6%)	0.117	6	8	2	0.273	0.773
Number of admissions per child											
Once	38 (57%)	7 (100%)	0.083	17 (50%)	21 (64%)	0.355	11 (61%)	19 (61%)	8 (44%)	0.659	0.463
Twice	14 (21%)	0		7 (21%)	7 (21%)		2 (11%)	6 (19%)	6 (33%)		
Three times or more	15 (22%)	0		10 (29%)	5 (15%)		5 (28%)	6 (19%)	4 (22%)		

[a]Figures are numbers of admitted children (% of group) and admissions
[b]Defined as assisted ventilation or oxygen supplementation at 36 weeks postmenstrual age
[c]For analysis regarding gestational age, the fraction born at 26–27 weeks were selected as the reference category (those with gestational age ≥ 28 had birth weights < 1000 grams)
[d]Independent samples Mann-Whitney's U Test or χ^2 test, as appropriate. Boldface denotes significant group differences
[e]Information on admissions was given for 229 subjects

Table 3 Causes for Admission to Hospital at Five to 11 Years of Age for Extremely Preterm Children Born in Norway During 1999 and 2000 at a Gestational Age < 28 Weeks or with a Birth Weight < 1000 Grams and a Regional Control Group Assembled at 11 Years of Age

Admission causes[a]	Cases $n = 138$	Controls $n = 7$
Respiratory causes	16 (12%)	1 (14%)
Surgery	69 (50%)	6 (86%)
Hernia repairs	3	1
Adeno–tonsillectomy or ear ventilation tube insertion	31	1
Central nervous system	2	
Gastrointestinal	4	
Orthopedic procedures	13	3
Plastic surgery	4	1
Eye surgery	9	
Male genitalia	3	
Gastrointestinal	9 (7%)	0
Central nervous system	27 (20%)	0
Nutritional	3 (2%)	0
Other	2 (1%)	0
Unknown[b]	12 (9%)	0

[a]Figures are number of admissions (% of total)
[b]Parents that reported the number of admissions for their child, but failed to specify the causes

p-value 0.140) and parental asthma for both respiratory symptoms and current asthma (Bonferroni adjusted *p*-values 0.252 and 0.056, respectively).

When added to the multivariate model, lung disease diagnosed by a paediatrician at the five year follow-up was highly associated with current asthma at 11 years of age (OR 69.76, 95% CI 12.49, 389.54), but GA (OR 0.58, 95% CI: 0.36, 0.95) and BPD with home oxygen treatment (OR 13.18, 95% CI: 1.25, 138.84) also remained significant. Only 3/24 (13%) children with current asthma at 11 years of age were not considered to have lung disease at the five year follow-up.

Discussion

At 5–11 years of age, the admission rate for the EP-born children was twice that of term-born controls, but occurred mainly for children with neurosensory disabilities and for surgical reasons, such as adeno-tonsillectomy or insertion of ear ventilatory tubes. Admissions for respiratory causes were rare, and neither BPD nor GA below 26 weeks at birth was associated with increased risk. Compared to the period 2–5 years of age, hospital admissions as well as respiratory morbidity had decreased, but admission rates, respiratory symptoms, current asthma, and use of asthma medication was still more common than in the control group. Statistical associations between most tested perinatal variables and the measures of morbidity during the study period were weak, evidenced by lack of significance after Bonferroni adjustments.

The strengths of this study were primarily the nationwide and population-based recruitment base and the longitudinal follow-up design that facilitated age-related assessments from early to mid-childhood in a country with free and unlimited access to health care for children. Although follow-up was not complete, important background information was available for all EP-born children, allowing proper assessment of representativeness. Thus, the number of stillbirths, postnatal deaths and perinatal differences between participants and non-participants could be completely accounted for. Participants tended to have less disabilities and a higher GA than those lost to follow-up, but a higher fraction had BPD. The number of eligible participants ($n = 372$) reflects the occurrence rate of EP deliveries, and was comparable to most similar studies [15, 16]. The 62% follow-up rate was disappointingly low when compared to previous follow-ups of this cohort, but reflects recent tendencies of increasing attrition rates in this type of research, in Norway [17], as well as internationally [16, 18]. Estimating GA was based on ultrasound at 17–18 weeks, performed within the frames of the established national free and all-encompassing program for antenatal care. Multiple perinatal variables were assessed for potential associations with the outcomes in regression models that utilised a dataset with limited numbers of participants. Thus, in order to prevent *type I* statistical errors, Bonferroni corrected *p*-values were reported. Regrettably, we were unable to recruit term-born control subjects for the complete cohort; however, individually matched term-controls were recruited based on the "next-born-subject" principle for a regional subsample representing 20% of the national population. Thus, the control group was considered unbiased and demographically representative for the complete cohort. Nevertheless, the small size of the control group reduced statistical power in the comparative analyses, and increased the risk of making *type II* errors, particularly as most outcome events were relatively rare.

Significantly more EP than term-born control children were admitted during the study period, which is in agreement with some [19, 20], but not all [21] previous studies. Admissions for respiratory diseases were quite uncommon, which is in agreement with a previous report [22], as was our finding that neither BPD [20] nor home oxygen treatment [23] were associated with admissions during 5-11 years of age. The data fit lung function findings that have previously been reported for this cohort when they were 11 years of age, in that neonatal BPD did not predict later airway obstruction [12].

Table 4 Hospital Admissions at Five to 11 Years Age and Current Respiratory Symptoms and Current Asthma at 11 Years of Age According to Perinatal and Socio-Demographic Characteristics in Unadjusted and Adjusted Logistic Regression Models for 232 Extremely Preterm Children Born in Norway During 1999 and 2000 at a Gestational Age < 28 Weeks or with a Birth Weight < 1000 Grams

Characteristic	Admitted to hospital 5–11 years of age		Respiratory symptoms past 12 months at 11 years of age		Current asthma at 11 years of age	
	Unadjusted model OR (95% CI)	Adjusted model OR (95% CI)	Unadjusted model OR (95% CI)	Adjusted model OR (95% CI)	Unadjusted model OR (95% CI)	Adjusted model OR (95% CI)
Gestational age	1.00 (0.84, 1.19)	**1.33 (1.04, 1.71)***	0.91 (0.73, 1.13)	1.00 (0.77, 1.29)	0.82 (0.65, 1.03)	0.88 (0.65, 1.19)
Birth weight/ 50 grams	1.04 (0.96, 1.14)		1.00 (0.90, 1.12)		0.98 (0.88, 1.09)	
Mother's age / five years	0.76 (0.57, 1.01)	0.75 (0.55, 1.02)	**0.57 (0.40, 0.83)****	**0.57 (0.39, 0.84)****	0.77 (0.54, 1.10)	
Chorioamnionitis	1.81 (0.84, 3.92)		**2.40 (1.01, 5.73)***	1.97 (0.72, 5.42)	**2.51 (1.05, 5.99)***	1.76 (0.60, 5.13)
Preeklampsia	0.59 (0.29, 1.20)		1.20 (0.54, 2.66)		0.88 (0.38, 2.06)	
PROM[a]	0.91 (0.36, 2.30)		1.39 (0.48, 3.98)		0.45 (0.10, 1.99)	
Sepsis	0.76 (0.38, 1.54)		1.35 (0.61, 3.01)		1.66 (0.76, 3.66)	
Prenatal steroids	1.18 (0.63, 2.23)		0.98 (0.45, 2.11)		0.69 (0.33, 1.46)	
Caesarean section	**0.50 (0.28, 0.92)***	**0.32 (0.15, 0.71)****	0.82 (0.39, 1.72)		0.78 (0.37, 1.64)	
Multiple birth	1.86 (0.97, 3.54)	1.65 (0.78, 3.49)	0.85 (0.36, 1.97)		0.58 (0.23, 1.49)	
Male sex	1.43 (0.81, 2.54)		1.61 (0.79, 3.29)		1.02 (0.50, 2.08)	
Small for gestational age[b]	0.94 (0.46, 1.93)		0.75 (0.29, 1.92)		0.61 (0.22, 1.67)	
Surfactant	1.06 (0.50, 2.28)		1.09 (0.42, 2.82)		1.35 (0.49, 3.71)	
Postnatal steroids	1.66 (0.92, 2.99)	1.82 (0.80, 4.12)	0.86 (0.41, 1.81)		1.38 (0.67, 2.84)	
Patent ductus arteriosus	0.74 (0.41, 1.34)		1.02 (0.50, 2.09)		1.41 (0.69, 2.89)	
Retinopathy of prematurity	1.08 (0.57, 2.07)		1.47 (0.69, 3.15)		1.54 (0.72, 3.32)	
Illness severity score[c]	**1.16 (1.01, 1.33)***	1.13 (0.96, 1.31)	1.11 (0.94, 1.30)		1.16 (0.99, 1.36)	1.16 (0.96, 1.41)
Length initial stay / seven days	1.01 (0.98, 1.06)		1.03 (0.98, 1.07)		1.04 (0.99, 1.09)	1.00 (0.94, 1.07)
Bronchopulmonary dysplasia[d]						
Without home oxygen	0.96 (0.52, 1.78)	0.78 (0.37, 1.65)	1.02 (0.48, 2.18)		1.44 (0.66, 3.16)	0.92 (0.36, 2.39)
With home oxygen	2.37 (0.92, 6.10)	1.26 (0.39, 4.13)	1.65 (0.54, 5.04)		**4.04 (1.38, 11.83)***	**4.84 (1.38, 17.06)***
Cerebral ultrasound findings[e]	1.63 (0.88, 3.03)					
Minor pathology	1.28 (0.66, 2.45)	1.19 (0.57, 2.47)	1.30 (0.59, 2.88)		1.16 (0.51, 2.62)	
Major pathology	**2.54 (0.96, 6.71)**	0.76 (0.19, 2.99)	1.58 (0.48, 5.19)		1.58 (0.48, 5.19)	
Disability at five years	**9.30 (2.47, 34.99)*****	**12.33 (2.48, 61.36)****	1.63 (0.43, 6.24)		2.60 (0.76, 8.94)	
Smoking in pregnancy	1.10 (0.53, 2.27)		1.61 (0.67, 3.87)		1.12 (0.44, 2.85)	
Smoking in home	0.66 (0.36, 1.21)		0.92 (0.44, 1.92)		0.91 (0.44, 1.92)	
Single parent	1.73 (0.78, 3.83)		1.31 (0.50, 3.45)		**2.62 (1.09, 6.29)***	1.51 (0.63, 3.61)

Table 4 Hospital Admissions at Five to 11 Years Age and Current Respiratory Symptoms and Current Asthma at 11 Years of Age According to Perinatal and Socio-Demographic Characteristics in Unadjusted and Adjusted Logistic Regression Models for 232 Extremely Preterm Children Born in Norway During 1999 and 2000 at a Gestational Age < 28 Weeks or with a Birth Weight < 1000 Grams *(Continued)*

	Admitted to hospital 5–11 years of age		Respiratory symptoms past 12 months at 11 years of age		Current asthma at 11 years of age	
Characteristic	Unadjusted model OR (95% CI)	Adjusted model OR (95% CI)	Unadjusted model OR (95% CI)	Adjusted model OR (95% CI)	Unadjusted model OR (95% CI)	Adjusted model OR (95% CI)
Siblings < six years (yes/no)	0.71 (0.29, 1.72)		0.31 (0.070, 1.40)		0.61 (0.17, 2.18)	
Breast milk after discharge	1.25 (0.62, 2.53)		0.99 (0.42, 2.33)		0.65 (0.27, 1.55)	
Mother higher education	0.89 (0.50, 1.59)		1.45 (0.70, 3.02)		1.10 (0.52, 2.32)	
Parental history of asthma	0.73 (0.33, 1.65)		**3.80 (1.71, 8.45)***	**3.12 (1.33, 7.33)**	**4.00 (1.79, 8.93)***	**4.38 (1.69, 11.38)**

Abbreviations: OR odds ratio, *CI* confidence interval, *PROM* premature rupture of membranes

[a]Defined as rupture of membranes more than six days before delivery

[b]Defined as less than fifth percentile for GA and gender according to Norwegian growth curves

[c]A score based on lowest and highest fractional oxygen (FIO_2) requirements and the base deficit during the first 12 hours of life

[d]Defined as assisted ventilation or oxygen supplementation at 36 weeks postmenstrual age

[e]Minor pathology defined as periventricular haemorrhage grade 1 to 2, or a maximum of two small cysts, and major pathology defined as periventricular haemorrhage grade 3 to 4 or multi-cystic periventricular leukomalacia

$^{*}p \leq 0.05$; $^{**}p \leq 0.01$; $^{***}p \leq 0.001$. Boldface denotes significant group differences

Table 5 Respiratory Health at Five to 11 Years of Age for Extremely Preterm Children Born in Norway During 1999 and 2000 at a Gestational Age < 28 Weeks or with a Birth Weight < 1000 Grams and a Regional Control Group Assembled at 11 Years of Age

	All participants			Neonatal Bronchopulmonary dysplasia[a]			Gestational age in weeks[b]				
	Cases $n = 232$	Controls $n = 57$	OR (95% CI)	Yes: $n = 165$	No $n = 207$	OR (95% CI)	≤25 $n = 99$	26–27 $n = 188$	≥28 $n = 85$	OR (95% CI) ≤25 vs. 26–27	OR (95% CI) 26–27 vs. ≥28
Birth to 11 years of age:											
Ever diagnosed with asthma	69 (30%)	5 (9%)	**4.40 (1.69, 11.50)****	39 (35%)	30 (25%)	1.56 (0.89, 2.76)	19 (37%)	36 (30%)	14 (23%)	1.40 (0.70, 2.79)	0.72 (0.35, 1.47)
Ever used asthma medication	110 (47%)	7 (13%)	**6.31 (2.74, 14.52)*****	69 (61%)	41 (35%)	**2.98 (1.75, 5.09)*****	31 (61%)	61 (50%)	18 (30%)	1.53 (0.78, 2.97)	0.42 (0.22, 0.81)
From five to 11 years of age:											
Wheezing	60 (26%)	7 (13%)	**2.51 (1.08, 5.83)***	36 (32%)	24 (20%)	**1.83 (1.01, 3.33)***	14 (28%)	36 (30%)	10 (17%)	0.88 (0.43, 1.83)	0.47 (0.21, 1.02)
Asthma medication use	59 (27%)	3 (5%)	**6.52 (1.96, 21.65)****	35 (34%)	24 (21%)	**1.97 (1.08, 3.62)***	14 (30%)	34 (30%)	11 (19%)	1.03 (0.49, 2.17)	0.54 (0.25, 1.16)
Inhaled corticosteroids	45 (21%)	3 (6%)	**4.51 (1.35, 15.11)***	30 (29%)	15 (13%)	**2.68 (1.34, 5.33)****	9 (19%)	29 (26%)	7 (12%)	0.67 (0.29, 1.55)	**0.41 (0.17, 0.99)***
Others	49 (22%)	3 (6%)	**4.94 (1.48, 16.50)****	30 (29%)	19 (16%)	**2.09 (1.09, 4.00)***	13 (28%)	28 (24%)	8 (14%)	1.25 (0.58, 2.70)	0.51 (0.22, 1.20)
LRTI treated with antibiotics	34 (15%)	2 (4%)	**4.75 (1.11, 20.38)***	18 (16%)	16 (14%)	1.14 (0.55, 2.33)	9 (18%)	18 (15%)	8 (13%)	1.23 (0.51, 2.95)	0.88 (0.36, 2.16)
Last 12 months at 11 years of age											
Wheezing	37 (16%)	5 (9%)	1.97 (0.74, 5.27)	19 (17%)	18 (15%)	1.13 (0.56, 2.29)	10 (20%)	20 (17%)	7 (12%)	1.23 (0.53, 2.86)	0.67 (0.27, 1.68)
Number of attacks											
None	199 (86%)	52 (91%)	$P = 0.511$	97 (86%)	102 (86%)	$P = 0.929$	42 (82%)	104 (86%)	53 (88%)	$P = 0.675$	$P = 0.776$
1–3	18 (8%)	3 (5%)		10 (9%)	8 (7%)		4 (8%)	10 (8%)	4 (7%)		
4–12	7 (3%)	0 (0%)		3 (3%)	4 (3%)		3 (6%)	2 (2%)	2 (3%)		
> 12	5 (2%)	2 (4%)		2(2%)	3 (3%)		1 (2%)	3 (3%)	1 (2%)		
All the time	3 (1%)	0 (0%)		1 (1%)	2 (2%)		1 (2%)	2 (2%)	0 (0%)		
Wheeze on exercise	41 (18%)	3 (5%)	**3.86 (1.15, 12.97)***	23 (20%)	18 (15%)	1.43 (0.73, 2.83)	11 (22%)	21 (17%)	9 (15%)	1.31 (0.58, 2.96)	0.84 (0.36, 1.97)
Problem speaking due to wheezing	2 (1%)	0 (0%)	NC	0 (0%)	2 (2%)	NC	0 (0%)	1 (1%)	1 (2%)	NC	2.03 (0.13, 33.11)
Dry cough at night	37 (16%)	4 (7%)	2.48 (0.85, 7.27)	18 (16%)	19 (16%)	1.01 (0.50, 2.04)	13 (26%)	17 (14%)	7 (12%)	2.15 (0.95, 4.85)	0.81 (0.32, 2.07)
Ever awakened due to wheezing	16 (7%)	1 (2%)	4.15 (0.54, 31.95)	8 (7%)	8 (7%)	1.06 (0.38, 2.92)	5 (10%)	8 (7%)	3 (5%)	1.54 (0.48, 4.94)	0.74 (0.19, 2.91)
LRTI treated with antibiotics	5 (2%)	1 (2%)	1.24 (0.14, 10.87)	1 (1%)	4 (3%)	0.26 (0.023, 2.33)	1 (2%)	3 (3%)	1 (2%)	0.80 (0.081, 7.84)	0.66 (0.067, 6.49)
Currently at 11 years of age											
Current asthma (criteria-based)[c]	36 (16%)	4 (7%)	2.43 (0.83, 7.14)	22 (20%)	14 (12%)	1.81 (0.88, 3.75)	12 (24%)	17 (14%)	7 (12%)	1.88 (0.82, 4.30)	0.81 (0.32, 2.07)
Severe asthma (criteria-based)[d]	18 (8%)	2 (4%)	2.31 (0.52, 10.27)	7 (6%)	11 (9%)	0.65 (0.24, 1.74)	6 (12%)	8 (7%)	4 (7%)	1.88 (0.62, 5.73)	1.01 (0.29, 3.49)
Asthma medication use	34 (15%)	3 (5%)	3.09 (0.91, 10.45)	22 (20%)	12 (10%)	**2.16 (1.01, 4.60)***	10 (20%)	18 (15%)	6 (10%)	1.40 (0.59, 3.28)	0.64 (0.24, 1.70)
Inhaled corticosteroids	21 (9%)	3 (5%)	1.81 (0.52, 6.29)	15 (13%)	6 (5%)	**2.89 (1.08, 7.73)***	5 (10%)	13 (11%)	3 (5%)	0.92 (0.31, 2.74)	0.44 (0.12, 1.63)
Bronchodilators	25 (11%)	3 (5%)	2.21 (0.64, 7.58)	16 (14%)	8 (5%)	2.04 (0.86, 4.83)	9 (18%)	11 (9%)	5 (9%)	2.18 (0.84, 5.63)	0.92 (0.30, 2.77)
Singulair	7 (3%)	0 (0%)	NC	4 (4%)	3 (3%)	1.43 (0.31, 6.55)	2 (4%)	4 (3%)	1 (2%)	1.20 (0.21, 6.82)	0.50 (0.055, 4.58)

Abbreviations: OR odds ratio, *CI* confidence interval, *LRTI* Lower respiratory tract infection, *NC* non-calculable

[a]Defined as assisted ventilation or oxygen supplementation at 36 weeks postmenstrual age

[b]For analysis regarding gestational age, the fraction born at 26–27 weeks were selected as the reference category (those with gestational age ≥ 28 weeks had birth weights < 1000 grams)

[c]Defined by either (1) a doctor's diagnosis of asthma combined with either respiratory symptoms or use of asthma medication in the previous 12 months, or (2) asthma medication and symptoms in the past 12 months even if no recall of prior doctor's diagnosis

[d]Defined by four or more episodes of wheezing, or sleep disturbances (awakened more than once a week), or problems of speaking due to wheezing reported during the past 12 months (14)

*$p \leq 0.05$; **$p \leq 0.01$; ***$p \leq 0.001$. Boldface denotes significant group differences

Table 6 Respiratory Health the past 12 Months for Extremely Preterm Children Born in Norway During 1999 and 2000 at a Gestational Age < 28 Weeks or with a Birth Weight < 1000 Grams Assessed at Five and 11 Years of Age by the International Study of Asthma and Allergy in Childhood Questionnaire

	At 5 years of age $n = 284$	At 11 years of age $n = 232$	
	Rate (95% CI)	Rate (95% CI)	*p*-values[a]
Wheezing	26% (21–32%)	16% (11–21%)	**< 0.001**
Wheeze on exercise	20% (15–25%)	18% (13–23%)	0.200
Dry cough at night	23% (18–28%)	16% (11–21%)	**0.028**
Ever awakened due to wheezing	15% (11–19%)	7% (4–10%)	**0.001**
Current asthma (criteria-based)[b]	26% (21–31%)	16% (11–20%)	**< 0.001**
Severe asthma (criteria-based)[c]	13 (9–17%)	8% (4–11%)	0.064
Current use of asthma medication	26% (21–31%)	15% (10–19%)	**< 0.001**

Figures are the percentage of children with a positive response with the corresponding 95% confidence interval (95% CI)
[a]Mc Nemar's test. Boldface denotes significant rate differences
[b]Defined by either (1) a doctor's diagnosis of asthma and either respiratory symptoms or use of asthma medication in the previous 12 months, or (2) use of asthma medication and symptoms in the past 12 months even if no recall of prior doctor's diagnosis
[c]Defined by four or more episodes of wheezing, or sleep disturbances (awakened more than once a week), or problems of speaking due to wheezing reported during the past 12 months (14)

Overall, these findings suggest that effects of extremely low GAs, BPD and duration of oxygen treatment have become less important for later pulmonary health as treatment of EP-born infants has improved.

At 11 years of age, 30% of the EP-born participants had ever been diagnosed with asthma, which was low compared to published rates of 37–46% among extremely low birth weight children at age 8–14 years [19, 24]. Regarding current wheezing, wheeze on exercise and current asthma, our findings were nearly identical to those of children of similar age born at GA below 26 weeks in the EPICure study [16], while current use of asthma medication was slightly less common (15% versus 25%). Our 16% rate of current asthma was lower than rates reported for somewhat younger [25, 26] and slightly older [21] extremely low birth weight children and for very low birth weight children of similar ages [27, 28]. However, comparing the prevalence of asthma between studies [16, 21, 25–28] is complicated due to lack of common diagnostic standards. Asthma is common also in the general paediatric population, and in a cohort of 10 year old children with BWs over 2000 grams born in Oslo in 1992 and 1993, 16.1% had ever been diagnosed with asthma, and 11.1% had current asthma [29]. In the present cohort, parental asthma was a strong predictor of asthma and wheezing when assessed at 11 years of age, but not at five years of age [10]. Thus, one may speculate that the occurrence of respiratory illness induced primarily by preterm birth decreases with age, while the relative importance of causes that are commonly implicated in unselected childhood populations (e.g. genetic determinants) increases with age.

For the children with neonatal BPD in this EP-born cohort, the rates for 'asthma ever' (35%) was similar to previous reports of 19–52% [18, 19, 30], while the rate of current asthma (20%) was in the lower end of reports ranging from 19% to 37% [16, 22, 31]. Current asthma at 11 years of age was not influenced by neonatal BPD, as was also observed by others [16, 18, 31, 32]. However, more children with BPD used asthma medication, both in this and other studies [18, 33], suggesting that they nevertheless might have more respiratory symptoms.

As regards development from the period 0–5 years of age to 5–11 years of age, the admission rates had declined significantly, but were still higher in the EP than term-born children, corresponding to Norwegian registry data comparing admissions between very preterm children and term-born children at similar ages [34]. Using The International Study of Asthma and Allergies in Childhood questionnaire, we found a significant reduction in respiratory symptoms from five to 11 years of age. This was encouraging, particularly as a large population based study of Western European children that utilised the same questionnaire reported a *higher* prevalence of current wheezing at age 13–14 years of age compared to 6–7 years of age (14.3% versus 9.6%) [14].

Conclusions

In conclusion, respiratory morbidity reflected by hospital admissions and respiratory symptoms as reported by parents in validated questionnaires, were clearly less pronounced in mid-childhood than in early childhood in this nationwide cohort of EP-born children, but still more common than in a regionally recruited group of term-born children. There were few convincing associations between perinatal variables and measures of morbidity. Notably, children with low GA and a history of neonatal BPD did surprisingly well, and these variables did not influence admission rates or occurrence of current asthma in adjusted analyses.

Abbreviations

BPD: Bronchopulmonary Dysplasia; BW: Birth Weight; EP: Extremely Preterm; GA: Gestational Age; ISAAC: International Study of Asthma and Allergies in Childhood; NICU: Neonatal Intensive Care Unit; OR (95% CI): Odds Ratio (95% Confidence Interval)

Acknowledgements

We would like to thank the other members of the Norwegian Extreme Prematurity Study: Arild Rønnestad (Oslo University Hospital, Oslo), Per Ivar Kaaresen (University Hospital of North Norway, Tromsø), Theresa Farstad (Akershus University Hospital, Lørenskog), Ragnhild Støen (St. Olav's Hospital, Trondheim University Hospital, Trondheim), Siren Rettedal (Stavanger University Hospital, Stavanger), Sven Harald Andersen (Østfold Hospital, Fredrikstad), Jørgen Hurum (Innlandet Hospital, Lillehammer), Lars Tveiten (Innlandet Hospital, Elverum), Sveinung Slinde (Telemark Hospital, Skien), Janne Skranes (Ullevål University Hospital, Oslo), Jorunn Ulriksen and Kåre Danielsen (Sørlandet Hospital, Kristiansand), Jon Skranes (Sørlandet Hospital, Arendal), Sabine Brügman (Drammen Hospital, Drammen), Fabian Berqvist (Førde Central Hospital, Førde), Andreas Andreassen (Haugesund Hospital, Haugesund), Lutz Nietsch (Ålesund Hospital, Ålesund), Ingebjørg Fagerli (Nordland Hospital, Bodø), and Bjørn Myklebust (Levanger Hospital, Levanger). We are grateful for advice on statistical methods and interpretation offered by Prof. G.E. Eide, Center for Clinical Research, Haukeland University Hospital, and Department of Global Public Health and Primary Care, Lifestyle Epidemiology Research Group, University of Bergen. For technical assistance, we thank Inger Elise Engelund and Magnhild Viste, Medical Birth Registry of Norway, Locus of Registry-Based Epidemiology.

Funding

Major funding institutions: Norwegian Foundation for Health and Rehabilitation through The Unexpected Child Death Society of Norway, the Research Council of Norway, the University of Bergen and the Helse Vest Hospital Trust. Minor support: Pediatric Lung Research Fund, Haukeland University Hospital.

Availability of data and materials

According to the approvals granted for this study by The Regional Committee on Medical Research Ethics and The Norwegian Data Inspectorate, the data files are to be stored properly and in line with the Norwegian Law of Privacy Protection. The data file is not made publically available as this might compromise the respondents' privacy, particularly as some of our participating centers are small and the number of extremely preterm births very limited. Moreover, the data file is currently used by other researchers in our group to prepare future research papers. A subset of the data file with anonymized data may be made available to interested researchers upon reasonable request to Thomas Halvorsen (thomas.halvorsen@helse-bergen.no) and providing permission from The Norwegian Data Inspectorate and the other members of our research group.

Authors' contributions

KS was the responsible author of the manuscript, carried out the statistical analyses, and the interpretation of the results. MV and KØ contributed to data collection and critically reviewed and revised the manuscript. TM conceptualized and designed the study, participated in the data collection, interpretation of the results, and critically reviewed and revised the manuscript. TH participated in the data collection, interpretation of the results, and the drafting and revision of the manuscript. All authors approved the final manuscript as submitted.

Competing interests

The authors declare that they have no competing interests.

Author details

[1]Department of Pediatrics, Haukeland University Hospital, N-5021 Bergen, Norway. [2]Department of Clinical Science, Faculty of Medicine and Dentistry, University of Bergen, Bergen, Norway. [3]Department of Pediatrics, Stavanger University Hospital, Stavanger, Norway.

References

1. Stoll BJ, Hansen NI, Bell EF, Shankaran S, Laptook AR, Walsh MC, et al. Neonatal outcomes of extremely preterm infants from the NICHD neonatal research network. Pediatrics. 2010;126(3):443–56. https://doi.org/10.1542/peds.2009-2959.
2. Markestad T, Kaaresen PI, Ronnestad A, Reigstad H, Lossius K, Medbo S, et al. Early death, morbidity, and need of treatment among extremely premature infants. Pediatrics. 2005;115(5):1289–98. https://doi.org/10.1542/peds.2004-1482.
3. Jobe AH, Bancalari E. Bronchopulmonary dysplasia. Am J Respir Crit Care Med. 2001;163(7):1723–9. https://doi.org/10.1164/ajrccm.163.7.2011060.
4. Baraldi E, Filippone M. Chronic lung disease after premature birth. N Engl J Med. 2007;357(19):1946–55. https://doi.org/10.1056/NEJMra067279.
5. Hofman PL, Regan F, Jackson WE, Jefferies C, Knight DB, Robinson EM, et al. Premature birth and later insulin resistance. N Engl J Med. 2004;351(21):2179–86. https://doi.org/10.1056/NEJMoa042275.
6. Crump C, Sundquist K, Sundquist J, Winkleby MA. Gestational age at birth and mortality in young adulthood. JAMA : the journal of the American Medical Association. 2011;306(11):1233–40. https://doi.org/10.1001/jama.2011.1331.
7. Risnes KR, Vatten LJ, Baker JL, Jameson K, Sovio U, Kajantie E, et al. Birthweight and mortality in adulthood: a systematic review and meta-analysis. Int J Epidemiol. 2011;40(3):647–61. https://doi.org/10.1093/ije/dyq267.
8. Doyle LW, Ford G, Davis N. Health and hospitalistions after discharge in extremely low birth weight infants. Seminars in neonatology : SN. 2003;8(2):137–45. https://doi.org/10.1016/S1084-2756(02)00221-X.
9. Leversen KT, Sommerfelt K, Ronnestad A, Kaaresen PI, Farstad T, Skranes J, et al. Prediction of neurodevelopmental and sensory outcome at 5 years in Norwegian children born extremely preterm. Pediatrics. 2011;127(3):e630–8. https://doi.org/10.1542/peds.2010-1001.
10. Skromme K, Leversen KT, Eide GE, Markestad T, Halvorsen T. Respiratory illness contributed significantly to morbidity in children born extremely premature or with extremely low birthweights in 1999-2000. Acta Paediatr. 2015;104(11):1189–98. https://doi.org/10.1111/apa.13165.
11. Leversen KT, Sommerfelt K, Ronnestad A, Kaaresen PI, Farstad T, Skranes J, et al. Predicting neurosensory disabilities at two years of age in a national cohort of extremely premature infants. Early Hum Dev. 2010;86(9):581–6. https://doi.org/10.1016/j.earlhumdev.2010.07.009.
12. Vollsaeter M, Skromme K, Satrell E, Clemm H, Roksund O, Oymar K, et al. Children born preterm at the turn of the millennium had better lung function than children born similarly preterm in the early 1990s. PLoS One. 2015;10(12):e0144243. https://doi.org/10.1371/journal.pone.0144243.
13. Skjaerven R, Gjessing HK, Bakketeig LS. Birthweight by gestational age in Norway. Acta Obstet Gynecol Scand. 2000;79(6):440–9.
14. Lai CK, Beasley R, Crane J, Foliaki S, Shah J, Weiland S, et al. Global variation in the prevalence and severity of asthma symptoms: phase three of the international study of asthma and allergies in childhood (ISAAC). Thorax. 2009;64(6):476–83. https://doi.org/10.1136/thx.2008.106609.
15. Thunqvist P, Tufvesson E, Bjermer L, Winberg A, Fellman V, Domellof M, et al. Lung function after extremely preterm birth-a population-based cohort study (EXPRESS). Pediatr Pulmonol. 2017; https://doi.org/10.1002/ppul.23919.
16. Fawke J, Lum S, Kirkby J, Hennessy E, Marlow N, Rowell V, et al. Lung function and respiratory symptoms at 11 years in children born extremely preterm: the EPICure study. Am J Respir Crit Care Med. 2010;182(2):237–45. https://doi.org/10.1164/rccm.200912-1806OC.
17. Krokstad S, Langhammer A, Hveem K, Holmen TL, Midthjell K, Stene TR, et al. Cohort profile: the HUNT study. Norway Int J Epidemiol. 2013;42(4):968–77. https://doi.org/10.1093/ije/dys095.
18. Brostrom EB, Thunqvist P, Adenfelt G, Borling E, Katz-Salamon M. Obstructive lung disease in children with mild to severe BPD. Respir Med. 2010;104(3):362–70. https://doi.org/10.1016/j.rmed.2009.10.008.

19. Hack M, Schluchter M, Andreias L, Margevicius S, Taylor HG, Drotar D, et al. Change in prevalence of chronic conditions between childhood and adolescence among extremely low-birth-weight children. JAMA : the journal of the American Medical Association. 2011;306(4):394–401. https://doi.org/10.1001/jama.2011.1025.
20. McCormick MC, Workman-Daniels K, Brooks-Gunn J, Peckham GJ. Hospitalization of very low birth weight children at school age. J Pediatr. 1993;122(3):360–5.
21. Saigal S, Stoskopf BL, Streiner DL, Burrows E. Physical growth and current health status of infants who were of extremely low birth weight and controls at adolescence. Pediatrics. 2001;108(2):407–15.
22. Doyle LW, Cheung MM, Ford GW, Olinsky A, Davis NM, Callanan C. Birth weight <1501 g and respiratory health at age 14. Arch Dis Child. 2001;84(1):40–4.
23. Greenough A, Alexander J, Boorman J, Chetcuti PA, Cliff I, Lenney W, et al. Respiratory morbidity, healthcare utilisation and cost of care at school age related to home oxygen status. Eur J Pediatr. 2011;170(8):969–75. https://doi.org/10.1007/s00431-010-1381-6.
24. Smith LJ, van Asperen PP, McKay KO, Selvadurai H, Fitzgerald DA. Reduced exercise capacity in children born very preterm. Pediatrics. 2008;122(2): e287–93. https://doi.org/10.1542/peds.2007-3657.
25. Doyle LW. Victorian infant collaborative study G. Respiratory function at age 8-9 years in extremely low birthweight/very preterm children born in Victoria in 1991-1992. Pediatr Pulmonol. 2006;41(6):570–6. https://doi.org/10.1002/ppul.20412.
26. Hacking DF, Gibson AM, Robertson C, Doyle LW. Victorian infant collaborative study G. Respiratory function at age 8-9 after extremely low birthweight or preterm birth in Victoria in 1997. Pediatr Pulmonol. 2013; 48(5):449–55. https://doi.org/10.1002/ppul.22619.
27. Siltanen M, Savilahti E, Pohjavuori M, Kajosaari M. Respiratory symptoms and lung function in relation to atopy in children born preterm. Pediatr Pulmonol. 2004;37(1):43–9. https://doi.org/10.1002/ppul.10402.
28. Mai XM, Gaddlin PO, Nilsson L, Finnstrom O, Bjorksten B, Jenmalm MC, et al. Asthma, lung function and allergy in 12-year-old children with very low birth weight: a prospective study. Pediatr Allergy Immunol. 2003;14(3):184–92.
29. Lodrup Carlsen KC, Haland G, Devulapalli CS, Munthe-Kaas M, Pettersen M, Granum B, et al. Asthma in every fifth child in Oslo, Norway: a 10-year follow up of a birth cohort study. Allergy. 2006;61(4):454–60. https://doi.org/10.1111/j.1398-9995.2005.00938.x.
30. Kennedy JD, Edward LJ, Bates DJ, Martin AJ, Dip SN, Haslam RR, et al. Effects of birthweight and oxygen supplementation on lung function in late childhood in children of very low birth weight. Pediatr Pulmonol. 2000; 30(1):32–40.
31. Kulasekaran K, Gray PH, Masters B. Chronic lung disease of prematurity and respiratory outcome at eight years of age. J Paediatr Child Health. 2007; 43(1–2):44–8. https://doi.org/10.1111/j.1440-1754.2007.01001.x.
32. Darlow BA, Horwood LJ, Mogridge N. Very low birthweight and asthma by age seven years in a national cohort. Pediatr Pulmonol. 2000;30(4):291–6.
33. Vom Hove M, Prenzel F, Uhlig HH, Robel-Tillig E. Pulmonary outcome in former preterm, very low birth weight children with bronchopulmonary dysplasia: a case-control follow-up at school age. J Pediatr. 2013; https://doi.org/10.1016/j.jpeds.2013.07.045.
34. Klitkou ST, Iversen T, Stensvold HJ, Ronnestad A. Use of hospital-based health care services among children aged 1 through 9 years who were born very preterm - a population-based study. BMC Health Serv Res. 2017; 17(1):571. https://doi.org/10.1186/s12913-017-2498-3.

Usefulness of fetal magnetic resonance imaging for postnatal management of congenital lung cysts: prediction of probability for emergency surgery

Chiyoe Shirota[1], Takahisa Tainaka[1], Toshiki Nakane[2], Yujiro Tanaka[1], Akinari Hinoki[1], Wataru Sumida[1], Naruhiko Murase[1], Kazuo Oshima[1], Kosuke Chiba[1], Ryo Shirotsuki[1] and Hiroo Uchida[1*]

Abstract

Background: Emergency rescue lung resection is rarely performed to treat congenital lung cysts (CLCs) in neonates. Many reports have described fetal CLC treatment; however, prenatal predictors for postnatal respiratory failure have not been characterized. We hypothesized that fetal imaging findings are useful predictors of emergency surgery.

Methods: We retrospectively studied patients with CLC who underwent lung surgery during the neonatal period in our hospital between January 2001 and December 2015. The demographic data, fetal imaging findings, and intra- and postoperative courses of patients who underwent emergency surgery (Em group) were compared with those of patients who received elective surgery, i.e., non-emergency surgery (Ne group).

Results: The Em group and Ne group included 7 and 11 patients, respectively. No significant difference was noted in gestational age, time at prenatal diagnosis, birth weight, and body weight at surgery. The volumes of contralateral lung per thoracic volume were significantly smaller in the Em group than in the Ne group ($p = 0.0188$). Mediastinal compression was more common in the Em group (7/7) than in the Ne group (4/11) ($p = 0.0128$).

Conclusions: This is the report describing neonatal emergency lobectomy in patients with CLC evaluated by fetal MRI using the lung volume ratio and mediastinal shift. In patients with CLC, mediastinal shift and significant decreases in contralateral lung volumes during the fetal stages are good prenatal predictors of postnatal emergency lung resection.

Keywords: Congenital lung cysts, Fetal MRI, Emergency lobectomy, CCAM

Background

With the development of fetal ultrasonography, congenital lung cysts (CLCs) have been more frequently detected before birth. Fetal ultrasonography and magnetic resonance imaging (MRI) have been employed to determine prognosis after birth and whether interventions are required [1, 2]. CLCs are characterized by various patterns, ranging from patients without respiratory symptoms at birth to those with severe respiratory failure due to displacement of the contralateral lung [3].

Specific respiratory management and surgery for this rare disease in neonates are available only at advanced medical facilities, and elective Caesarean delivery is often required to prepare for sufficient medical intervention.

Predicting these patterns before birth could help determine treatment strategies and thus improve prognosis. Emergency rescue lung resection is rarely performed in neonates with CLCs. Many reports have described fetal treatment for CLC; however, prenatal predictors for postnatal respiratory failure have not been characterized [4–6]. We hypothesized that fetal imaging would help predict the requirement for emergency surgery.

Several reports described prenatal evaluation of CLC using ultrasonogram findings such as the lung thoracic ratio and cystic adenomatoid malformation volume ratio

* Correspondence: hiro2013@med.nagoya-u.ac.jp
[1]Department of Pediatric Surgery, Nagoya University Graduate School of Medicine, 65 Tsurumai-cho, Showa-ku, Nagoya 466-8550, Japan
Full list of author information is available at the end of the article

(CVR) [7–9]. Ultrasonography can be performed repeatedly with ease and is non-invasive; however, the accuracy of readings depends on the level of competency and technique of the practitioner. Fetal MRI is costly, and the time required to perform each scan limits its application; therefore, unlike ultrasonography, it cannot be performed repeatedly. However, fetal MRI exhibits several advantages over ultrasonography. Because the images obtained are almost three-dimensional, they are suitable for measuring volume and enable more accurate and objective evaluations. Although fetal MRI has been used for prenatal evaluation of the severity of congenital diaphragmatic hernia, its utility in evaluating the prognosis of CLC is unclear [10, 11]. The purpose of this study was to evaluate the severity and prognosis of CLC using fetal MRI, and thereby determine the appropriate treatment strategy.

Methods

Prior to this study, all protocols were approved by the ethics review board at our institution. The medical records of patients who had undergone lobectomy for CLC treatment during the neonatal period in our department between January 1, 2001 and December 31, 2015 were retrospectively reviewed. In order to avoid thoracic deformity and early infection of CLC, we performed scheduled thoracoscopic surgery at near the end of neonatal period for patients who had a stable cardiorespiratory state. We performed emergency thoracoscopic surgery for patients who had an unstable respiratory state at early neonatal period or before scheduled surgery. We performed morphometric analyses of MRI images to assess volumes (ml) of the affected lesion, affected lung, contralateral lung, thoracic cavity, and mediastinal compression. We calculated the volume of the affected lung per thoracic cavity, volume of the affected lesion per thoracic cavity, and volume of the contralateral lung per thoracic cavity. The characteristics of patients (gestational age, time at prenatal diagnosis, birth weight, age at surgery, and body weight at surgery) and peri- and postoperative courses (surgery time, blood loss, duration of intubation [days], duration of respiratory support [days], and postoperative hospital stay) were compared between the patients who underwent emergency surgery for postnatal respiratory failure—the emergency surgery (Em) group—or those who underwent elective surgery—the non-emergency surgery (Ne) group. Analyses of the MRI images were performed by radiologists who were blinded to the patients' background. The volumes were calculated using SYNAPSE VINCENT® FUJIFILM MEDICAL SOLUTION analytical software by easily combining values obtained from traced individual MRI images. A heart clearly displaced from the midline and mediastinal displacement diagnosed by a radiologist were defined as mediastinal shift. Statistical analysis was performed with the Wilcoxon test and Fisher exact test using JMP Pro 11, Statistical Discovery from SAS.

Results

All fetal MRI was performed during the third trimester. Of 21 patients who underwent surgery within 30 days after birth, three patients without prenatal diagnosis were excluded. The Em group and the Ne group included 7 and 11 patients, respectively. No significant difference was noted in gestational age, time at prenatal diagnosis, and birth weight. The age at surgery was significantly younger and the body weight at surgery was significantly smaller in the Em group than in the Ne group. (Table 1) In the emergency surgery group, prenatal diagnoses were 4 cases of congenital pulmonary airway malformation (CPAM) type I, 2 cases of CPAM type II, and 1 case of CPAM type III; and pathological diagnoses were 4 cases of CPAM type I, 2 cases of CPAM type II, and 1 case of CPAM type III. In the elective surgery group, prenatal diagnoses were 4 cases of CPAM type I, 5 cases of CPAM type II, and 2 cases of CPAM type III; and pathological diagnoses were 4 cases of CPAM type I, 5 cases of CPAM type II, and 2 cases of CPAM type III.

The fetal images of both groups showed no significant differences in the volumes of affected lesions per thoracic cavity (Em: 0.174 and Ne: 0.274; $p = 0.2090$) and affected lung per thoracic cavity (Em: 0.228 and Ne: 0.108; $p = 0.3927$). The volumes of contralateral lung per thoracic cavity were significantly smaller in the Em group (0.166) than in the Ne group (0.195) ($p = 0.0188$).

Table 1 Characteristics of patients who underwent lobectomy within 30 days of birth

	Emergency operation group $n = 7$	Non-emergency operation group $n = 11$	*p value*
Gestational age at delivery (weeks)	38 (37–40)	39 (37–40)	0.0540
Time of prenatal diagnosis (weeks)	25 (21–32)	24 (20–34)	0.8553
Body weight at birth (g)	3028 (2484–3138)	3152 (2618–3483)	0.1473
Age at operation (days)	2 (0–27)	26 (24–30)	0.0005
Body weight at operation (g)	3028 (2484–3382)	4000 (3500–6405)	0.0006

Median (range)

Mediastinal compression was more common in the Em group (7/7) than in the Ne group (4/11) ($p = 0.0128$). Concerning thoracoscopic lobectomy (Em; 4 cases, Ne; 11 cases), no significant intergroup differences were noted in surgery time (160 min and 206 min; $p = 0.4687$), although one thoracoscopic case in the Em group converted to thoracotomy due to deteriorating respiratory status. The volume of blood loss was significantly lower in the Ne group (2 ml) than in the Em group (18 ml) ($p = 0.0360$). The Em group required significantly longer intubation (19 vs 0 days; $p = 0.0014$), respiratory support (22 vs 0 days; $p = 0.0023$), and postoperative hospital stay (43 vs 10 days; $p = 0.0085$) than the Ne group (Table 2). The numbers of patients followed up for longer than 1 year after surgery were 4 and 11 in the Em group and the Ne group, respectively. No patients reported problems with daily living and growth.

In three patients who underwent fetal therapy, emergency surgery was performed at 1, 2, and 4 days of age. In the former two patients, a shunt tube was inserted at 25 and 29 weeks of gestation, and in the latter patient, cyst puncture was performed at 25 weeks of gestation. Fetal MRI was performed at 34, 34, and 39 weeks of gestation and revealed a mediastinal shift in all patients. The ratios of the contralateral lung volume to the thoracic cavity were 0.102, 0.147, and 0.207, respectively. The latter patient underwent MRI at 27 weeks of gestation, prior to fetal therapy, which indicated that the ratio of the contralateral lung volume to the thoracic cavity was 0.164, which improved to 0.207 with fetal therapy. Even though contralateral lung volume increased with fetal therapy, emergency lung resection was required.

One patient exhibited fetal hydrops on ultrasonography at 25 weeks of gestation with marked cardiac displacement, both of which improved by 33 weeks. The ratio of the contralateral lung volume to the thoracic cavity was 0.033 at 26 weeks and 0.190 at 33 weeks. Rupture of the membrane at 37 + 4 weeks resulted in vaginal delivery, with the neonate weighing 3120 g and in good respiratory condition. Although surgery had been scheduled, emergency surgery with a partial resection of the left superior and inferior lobes was performed because of respiratory difficulty on day 27 after birth.

Seven patients required emergency surgery at the age of 0, 0, 2, 2, 2, 4, and 27 days, four of whom required continuous one-lung ventilation until the surgery. The median ratio of the contralateral lung volume to the thoracic cavity was significantly lower in the Em group than in the Ne group. The respiratory status of six patients rapidly deteriorated soon after birth.

Discussion

In fetal imaging, poor resolution can prevent diagnosis of CLC. Diagnosis using ultrasonography is further complicated by artifacts caused by amniotic fluid volume, the form of the maternal body, and fetal movement—issues that are not applicable to MRI. Furthermore, the contrast of a lung cyst (LC) and the affected lung is sometimes poor and indistinct, making it difficult to accurately measure the LC and the affected lung volume. In contrast, the normal lung is easily delineated. We compensated for the influence of lung volume fluctuations by measuring the thoracic volume and calculating the thoracic ratio. Thus, evaluation of the volume of the

Table 2 Comparison of fetal magnetic resonance imaging examinations and pre-operative and post-operative status between the emergency operation and non-emergency operation groups

	Emergency operation group $n = 7$	Non-emergency Operation group $n = 11$	p value
Volume of affected lesion/thoracic cavity (ml)	0.174(0.000–0.445)	0.274 (0.152–0.389)	0.2090
Volume of affected lung/thoracic cavity (ml)	0.228(0.013–0.554)	0.108 (0.008–0.337)	0.3927
Volume of contralateral lung/thoracic cavity (ml)	0.166 (0.051–0.199)	0.195 (0.139–0.267)	0.0188
Positive for mediastinal compression (n)	7	4	0.0128
Positive for hydrops (n)	2	0	0.1373
Blood loss (ml)	18 (1–114)	2 (0–41)	0.0360
Number of intubation days after operation	19 (1–22)	0 (0–3)	0.0014
Number of respiratory support days after operation	22 (6–80)	0 (0–39)	0.0023
Postoperative hospital stay (days)	43 (21–109)	10 (7–77)	0.0085
Underwent thoracotomy (n)	3	0	
Underwent thoracoscopic surgery (n)	4	11	
Operative time for thoracoscopy (min)	160 (75–296)	206 (83–441)	0.4687
	Median (range).		

contralateral (not affected) lung and the thoracic volume provides accurate data.

The ultrasonic CVR can be repeatedly evaluated, and it is a convenient and very useful predictor. On the other hand, for congenital diaphragmatic hernia, various MRI techniques have been previously reported, of which lung volume was reported to be an effective predictor for prognosis [10]. In CLC, MRI can also be utilized to measure the congenital CVR, a useful indicator of the fetal treatment and ex-utero intrapartum treatment procedure [6, 9, 12]. CVR values over 1.6 or 2.0 have been reported to be high risk factors [6, 9, 12]. CVR can be calculated using the formula length × height × width × 0.52 / the head circumstance, using either MRI or echo images, and is a volume calculation based on the values obtained from cross sections, which differs from the three-dimensional volume measurement achieved using MRI. In our study, the ultrasonic CVR, which acts as the index of postnatal respiratory condition, was only measured in some cases. The results of our ultrasonographic examinations cannot be compared with the results of maternal MRI. Maternal MRI, which is not affected by the skill of the technician, is routinely performed in our institution when abnormalities are suspected in the fetus. To reduce the effect of the MRI performance time, the thoracic volume was used instead of the head circumstance.

Because we believed that surgery could be conducted efficiently if we waited about 30 days after birth, elective lobectomy was performed in the neonatal period (near 30 days) to avoid the risk of early cystic infection in this study period. In the neonatal period, the infant's body is small, so the operation is slightly challenging to perform; however, as the surgery does not increase the risk of complications, we believe it is feasible. In our current strategy for the treatment of congenital lung cystic disease without respiratory distress, we perform delayed lobectomy within 3–6 months to make it easier for the surgeon to perform the operation when the infant's body is a little bigger.

With advances in imaging analysis, volume measurement can be relatively easily applied, and based on the three-dimensional MRI images acquired, volume measurement could be widely used in the future. Future studies are expected to validate pulmonary volume as a predictor for the treatment and prognosis of CLC, and effective disease evaluations should be based on established reference values.

According to our results, CLC patients requiring emergency surgery for imminent respiratory failure after birth exhibited reduced fetal contralateral lung and mediastinal shift volumes. The Em group had longer postoperative hospital stays and required respiratory support for longer periods because of possible immaturity of the contralateral lung.

Patients in the Em group required one-lung ventilation or cyst puncture to maintain general condition sufficient for adequate surgery as early as possible. Such treatment is available only at limited medical facilities with an advanced system. Thus, if the requirement of emergency rescue lung surgery is prenatally determined, we cannot only select an appropriate birthing facility but also determine the type of delivery, such as elective Caesarean delivery, and timing of delivery based on the preparation of planned medical intervention.

Several studies have recommended early surgery even in asymptomatic cases based on the risk of pneumonia associated with non-treatment and reported no difference in surgery outcomes [13–19], whereas others recommended conservative management without surgery in asymptomatic cases [20] or waiting until 4–8 weeks after birth, reporting fewer complications when surgery was delayed by at least 3 months of birth [8, 21]. In the present study, we performed neonatal lobectomy in infants without respiratory distress; however, in the future, delaying lobectomy until 3–6 months of birth may not be associated with adverse outcomes.

In some cases of CLC diagnosed prenatally, we sometimes experience time-course change in cyst size detected by fetal ultrasonography. Although such possible time-course change in cyst size could affect the accuracy of our evaluation, a significant change in cyst size was not observed on a fetal ultrasonogram from the time of the third-trimester MRI scan to delivery. In our evaluation, we used MRI results performed in the third trimester even in the patients undergoing MRI examination multiple times; furthermore, instead of cyst size per se, the rate of the contralateral lung relative to the thoracic cavity was used; therefore, bias is not considered to be an issue.

Conclusions

This is the report describing neonatal emergency lobectomy in patients with congenital lung cysts detected by fetal MRI using lung volume ratio and mediastinal shift. We aim to improve the accuracy and prognostic capacity of this procedure by accumulating further clinical data. In patients with CLCs, mediastinal shift and significant decreases in contralateral lung volumes during the fetal stages are good prenatal predictors of postnatal emergency lung resection.

Abbreviations

CCAM: Congenital Cystic Adenomatoid Malformation; CLC: Congenital Lung Cyst; CVR: Cystic Adenomatoid Malformation Volume Ratio; Em Group: Emergency Surgery Group; MRI: Magnetic Resonance Imaging; Ne Group: Non-emergency Surgery Group

Acknowledgements
Not applicable.

Funding
Not applicable.

Authors' contributions
TT, AH, WS, NM, RS, and KO collected patient data. TN analyzed patient images. KC, and YT interpreted patient data regarding operation. HU and CS were main contributors in writing the manuscript. All authors read and approved the final manuscript.

Competing interests
The authors declare that they have no competing interests.

Author details
[1]Department of Pediatric Surgery, Nagoya University Graduate School of Medicine, 65 Tsurumai-cho, Showa-ku, Nagoya 466-8550, Japan. [2]Department of Radiology, Nagoya University Graduate School of Medicine, Nagoya, Japan.

References
1. Epelman M, Kreiger PA, Servaes S, Victoria T, Hellinger JC. Current imaging of prenatally diagnosed congenital lung lesions. Semin Ultrasound CT MR. 2010;31:141–57.
2. Ruano R, da Silva MM, Salustiano EM, Kilby MD, Tannuri U, Zugaib M. Percutaneous laser ablation under ultrasound guidance for fetal hyperechogenic microcystic lung lesions with hydrops: a single center cohort and a literature review. Prenat Diagn. 2012;32:1127–32.
3. Halloran LG, Silverberg SG, Salzberg AM. Congenital cystic adenomatoid malformation of the lung. A surgical emergency. Arch Surg. 1972;104:715–9.
4. Vrecenak JD, Howell LJ, Khalek N, Moldenhauer JS, Johnson MP, Coleman BG, et al. Outcomes of prenatally diagnosed lung lesions in multigestational pregnancies. Fetal Diagn Ther. 2014;36:312–9.
5. Witlox RS, Lopriore E, Oepkes D. Prenatal interventions for fetal lung lesions. Prenat Diagn. 2011;31:628–36.
6. Cass DL, Olutoye OO, Cassady CI, Moise KJ, Johnson A, Papanna R, et al. Prenatal diagnosis and outcome of fetal lung masses. J Pediatr Surg. 2011;46:292–8.
7. Usui N, Kamata S, Sawai T, Kamiyama M, Okuyama H, Kubota A, et al. Outcome predictors for infants with cystic lung disease. J Pediatr Surg. 2004;39:603–6.
8. Khalek N, Johnson MP. Management of prenatally diagnosed lung lesions. Semin Pediatr Surg. 2013;22:24–9.
9. Crombleholme TM, Coleman B, Hedrick H, Liechty K, Howell L, Flake AW, et al. Cystic adenomatoid malformation volume ratio predicts outcome in prenatally diagnosed cystic adenomatoid malformation of the lung. J Pediatr Surg. 2002;37:331–8.
10. Akinkuotu AC, Cruz SM, Abbas PI, Lee TC, Welty SE, Olutoye OO, et al. Risk-stratification of severity for infants with CDH: prenatal versus postnatal predictors of outcome. J Pediatr Surg. 2016;51:44–8.
11. Hayakawa M, Seo T, Itakua A, Hayashi S, Miyauchi M, Sato Y, et al. The MRI findings of the right-sided fetal lung can be used to predict postnatal mortality and the requirement for extracorporeal membrane oxygenation in isolated left-sided congenital diaphragmatic hernia. Pediatr Res. 2007;62:93–7.
12. Cass DL, Olutoye OO, Cassady CI, Zamora IJ, Ivey RT, Ayres NA, et al. EXIT-to-resection for fetuses with large lung masses and persistent mediastinal compression near birth. J Pediatr Surg. 2013;48:138–44.
13. Tsai AY, Liechty KW, Hedrick HL, Bebbington M, Wilson RD, Johnson MP, et al. Outcomes after postnatal resection of prenatally diagnosed asymptomatic cystic lung lesions. J Pediatr Surg. 2008;43:513–7.
14. Vu LT, Farmer DL, Nobuhara KK, Miniati D, Lee H. Thoracoscopic versus open resection for congenital cystic adenomatoid malformations of the lung. J Pediatr Surg. 2008;43:35–9.
15. Conforti A, Aloi I, Trucchi A, Morini F, Nahom A, Inserra A, et al. Asymptomatic congenital cystic adenomatoid malformation of the lung: is it time to operate? J Thorac Cardiovasc Surg. 2009;138:826–30.
16. Komori K, Kamagata S, Hirobe S, Toma M, Okumura K, Muto M, et al. Radionuclide imaging study of long-term pulmonary function after lobectomy in children with congenital cystic lung disease. J Pediatr Surg. 2009;44:2096–100.
17. Saeed A, Kazmierski M, Khan A, McShane D, Gomez A, Aslam A. Congenital lung lesions: preoperative three-dimensional reconstructed CT scan as the definitive investigation and surgical management. Eur J Pediatr Surg. 2013;23:53–6.
18. Shanmugam G, MacArthur K, Pollock JC. Congenital lung malformations–antenatal and postnatal evaluation and management. Eur J Cardiothorac Surg. 2005;27:45–52.
19. Choudhury SR, Chadha R, Mishra A, Kumar V, Singh V, Dubey NK. Lung resections in children for congenital and acquired lesions. Pediatr Surg Int. 2007;23:851–9.
20. Ng C, Stanwell J, Burge DM, Stanton MP. Conservative management of antenatally diagnosed cystic lung malformations. Arch Dis Child. 2014;99:432–7.
21. Khosa JK, Leong SL, Borzi PA. Congenital cystic adenomatoid malformation of the lung: indications and timing of surgery. Pediatr Surg Int. 2004;20:505–8.

20

Effect of childhood BMI on asthma: a systematic review and meta-analysis of case-control studies

Yosra Azizpour[1], Ali Delpisheh[2], Zahra Montazeri[3], Kourosh Sayehmiri[4*] and Behzad Darabi[5]

Abstract

Background: Asthma is a multifactorial syndrome that threatens the health of children. Body mass index (BMI) might be one of the potential factors but the evidence is controversial. The aim of this study is to perform a comprehensive meta-analysis to investigate the association between asthma and BMI.

Methods: Electronic databases including, Web of Science, Pubmed, Scopus, Science Direct, ProQuest, up to April 2017, were searched by two researchers independently. The keywords "asthma, body mass index, obesity, overweight, childhood and adolescence" were used. Random and fixed effects models were applied to obtain the overall odds ratios (ORs) and standardized mean difference (SMD). Heterogeneity between the studies was examined using I^2 and Cochrane Q statistics.

Results: After reviewing 2511 articles, 16 studies were eligible for meta-analysis according to inclusion/exclusion criteria. A meta-analysis from 11 case-control studies revealed OR of asthma and overweight as OR = 1.64; (95% Confidence Interval (CI): 1.13–2.38) and from 14 case-control studies, OR for asthma and obesity was OR = 1.92 (95% CI: 1.39–2.65), which indicated that risk of asthma in overweight and obese children and adolescence was significantly higher (1.64 and 1.92 times) than that of individuals with (*p*-value < 0.01 for underweight/normal weight in both cases). Furthermore, there was a significant relationship between asthma and BMI > 85 percentile according to SMD SMD = 0.21; (95%CI: 0.03–0.38; p-value = 0.021).

Conclusions: The results showed a significant relationship between BMI (obesity/overweight) and asthma among children and adolescents. It is important to study the confounding factors that affect the relationship between asthma and BMI in future epidemiological researches.

Keywords: Asthma, Adolescences, Body mass index, Childhood, Meta-analysis

Background

There are some hypotheses for the relationship between asthma and obesity since the number of the cases diagnosed with these two disorders over the last two decades has increased [1]. Asthma is a chronic clinical respiratory syndrome that is accompanied by the inflammation of respiratory ducts, obstruction, and airway hyper responsiveness [2]. It is caused by a combination of factors and complicated interaction between hereditary traits, air pollution, respiratory tract infection, and exposure to triggers such as cigarette smoking [3]. These factors influence the response of the disease to treatment and its severity [4]. It is estimated that 7.1 million individuals under 18 years of age were currently afflicted with asthma and 4.1 million suffered from periodic asthma or asthma attack in 2011 (United States) [5]. Over the last three decades, prevalence of obesity has doubled and quadrupled among children and adolescents [6, 7] and along with other mechanisms, obesity may cause shortness of breath as well. It is known that aggregation of soft fatty tissues around the chest increases pressure on the lungs, increases blood volume at the area, and consequently, decreases the capacity of the respiratory system. Furthermore, other mechanical

* Correspondence: sayehmiri@razi.tums.ac.ir
[4]Department of Biostatistics, Psychosocial Injuries Research Center, Ilam University of Medical Sciences, Ilam, Iran
Full list of author information is available at the end of the article

effects of obesity may cause limitations to airways and hypersensitivity [1]. So, lack of enough physical activity among asthma patients and physiological respiratory changes of obese patients may cause the two diseases to be interrelated [8].

There are four previous meta-analyses conducted by Chen [9], Flaherman [10], Egan [11] and Mebrahtu [12] in which Relative Risk (RR) or Odds Ratio (OR) for relationships between asthma and overweight among children were reported. Three of these meta-analyses are based on cohorts (Chen, Egan and Flaherman) and the other one is based on any observational studies including cohort, case-control, and cross-sectional. Chen and Egan applied subgroup analysis just for gender but they didn't conduct a cumulative meta-analysis. Flaherman considered studies that reported both high birth weight and high BMI in school aged children for cumulative meta-analysis and they reported OR and RR and applied subgroup analysis for physician diagnosis. Mebrahtu was more consistent in investigating this association by determining OR in different weight categories. We applied an intensive search and employed comprehensive analyses not only based on OR estimates, but also we considered SMD analysis, cumulative meta-analysis and adjusted ORs. Subgroup analyses for gender, age, continents, and asthma diagnosis method, year of publication and sample size were applied. In addition, case-control studies have been considered for risk ratio assessment.

Methods

This systematic review was based on Preferred Reporting Items for Systematic Reviews and Meta-Analyses (PRISMA) guidelines [13] (Additional file 1: PRISMA Checklist S1).

Criteria of research

All case-control studies on the relationship between BMI and asthma among childhood and adolescence regardless of time and place of study were considered, language was limited to English.

Search strategy

A comprehensive search was undertaken via Web of Science (1983 to 10 April of 2017), PubMed /Medline (1966 to 10 April of 2017), Scopus (1960 to 10 April of 2017), Science Direct (1823 to 10 April of 2017), ProQuest (1993 to 10 April of 2017), Google Scholar (web search engine), and Eastern Mediterranean Region databases (IMEMR) (1984 to 10 April of 2017). Medical subject headings (MeSH) keywords such as "asthma, BMI, obesity, overweight, childhood and adolescence" were used for our search in scientific journals, conferences, dissertations, theses and reports. All references to relevant articles (manually) were also investigated.

For example, the following box represents the search strategies in PubMed

1. "Asthma" [MeSH]
2. Childhood [MeSH]
3. Adolescence [MeSH]
4. #1 AND #2 AND #3
5. "Body mass Index" [MeSH]
6. #4 AND #5
7. "Obesity" [MeSH]
8. #4 AND #7
9. "Overweight" [MeSH]
10. #4 AND #9

Asthma diagnosis

The case group (asthmatic) was diagnosed either by a physician or by completion of the ISSAC (The International Study of Asthma and Allergies in Childhood) questionnaire by a parent or adolescent. The control group (non-asthmatic) consisted of those who were not diagnosed with asthma.

BMI criteria

The following criteria were considered in assessing the exposure factor (BMI): 1. Age-sex-specific BMI percentiles were obtained based on Centers for Disease Control and Prevention (CDC) growth chart (see Table 1). 2. Age-sex-specific cut-off points (underweight18.5 kg/m^2, overweight: 25 kg/m^2 and obesity 30 kg/m^2) by the International Obesity Task Force (IOTF) [14]. 3. Reference data for obesity with normal being < 85 th, obese > 85 th - <95th and very obese ≥95 th [15]. 4. The BMI percentile values with underweight being ≤P5, Malnutrition >P5- ≤ P15, normal >P15- < P85, overweight ≥P85- < P95, obese ≥P95 [16]. 5. The BMI-Z score based on CDC growth chart. 6. The overweight/obesity when the BMI- standard deviation score (SDS) units (z-score) was ≥2 [17]. (It is notable that we used BMI percentiles based on the CDC growth chart (2014) where underweight < 5th, normal ≥5th- < 85th, overweight≥85th- < 95th and obese ≥95th [18] and the categorization method of the IOTF for exposure (BMI)).

Article selection

Searching databases using keywords and extracting data from articles were done independently by two researchers (Azizpour and Sayehmiri) in order to avoid risk of bias. An abstract of each article was screened for eligibility according to inclusion/exclusion criteria and then the full text was reviewed for data extraction. In cases of disagreement between the two reviewers, a third researcher reviewed the article and a final decision was made after careful discussion. The relevant articles were selected according to inclusion/exclusion criteria.

Table 1 Case-control studies included in the research

Author	Sample	country	Exposure categorization method	Age group (year)	Asthma Diagnosis	Publication year	Time duration	Quality Score
Gennuso & et al. [48]	Case:85 Control:86	(USA)	Reference data Normal <85, Obese: ≥ 85th <95th.Very obese: ≥ 95th [15]	Case: 4-16 Control:4-16	Physician diagnosed asthma	1998	N/R	80
Vignolo & et al. [49]	Case:554 Control:625	(Italy)	BMI- (SDS) units (z-score)	Case: 2.2-16.1 Control: 2.4–16.3	Physician diagnosed asthma	2005	Case: January –December 2001 Control: April-May 2001	80
Mansell & et al. [50]	Case:134 Control:82	(USA)	Overweight >85th and non overweight <85th (CDC growth charts)	Case: 12-18 Control:12-18	Physician diagnosed asthma	2006	N/R	80
Vargas & et al. [51]	Case:213 Control:816	(USA)	Risk for overweight ≥ 85th-<95th/ overweight ≥ 95th (CDC growth charts)	Case: 3-5 Control:3-5	Physician diagnosed asthma	2007	November 2000-December 2003	90
Careneiro bertolace & et al. [52]	Case:231 Control:190	(Brazil)	Overweight :≥ 85th and Obese: ≥ 95th (CDC growth charts)	Case: 13-14 Control:13-14	Completed ISAAC questionnaire by adolescence	2008	March-December 2005	80
Henkin & et al. [40]	Case:94 Control:94	(USA) (Asian patient)	Underweight<20%, normal 20-85%, risk for overweight 85-95% & Overweight >95% (CDC growth charts	Case: 4-18 Control:4-18	Physician-diagnosed asthma	2008	N/R	100
Walders-Abramson & et al. [53]	Case:59 Control:59	(USA)	≥95th obese," 85th–95th "overweight,"15 and <85th "normal weight (CDC growth charts)	Case: 10-16 Control:10-16	Physician-diagnosed asthma	2009	December 2005-July 2007	80
Tsai & et al. [54]	Case:27 Control:27	(USA)	Age- and sex-specific cut-off points for childhood by (IOTF)	Case: 9-11 Control:9-11	Parent reported according physician-diagnosed asthma and meds use	2012	2004-2006	80
Ahmadi-afshar & et al. [55]	Case:200 Control:200	(Iran)	Overweight : BMI>85th and Obese BMI>95th (CDC growth charts)	Case: 6-15 Control:6-15	Physician-diagnosed asthma	2013	March-September 2010	80
Scepanovic & et al. [16]	Case:354 Control:354	(Montenegro)	Based on the BMI percentile values	Case: 6-15 Control: 6-15	Physician-diagnosed asthma	2013	N/R	70
Nahhas & et al. [43]	Case:632 Control:632	(Saudi Arabia)	Underweight <5th, Normal 5th-85th, Overweight 85th-94th & obese ≥ 95 (CDC growth charts)	Case: 6-8 Control: 6-8	Complete a ISAAC questionnaire by parent	2014	N/R	90
Forno & et al. [42]	Case:351 Control:327	(Puerto Rico)	BMI z scores based on CDC growth charts	Case: 6-14 Control: 6-14	Physician-diagnosed asthma	2014	March 2009 -June 2010	90

Table 1 Case-control studies included in the research *(Continued)*

Author	Sample	country	Exposure categorization method	Age group (year)	Asthma Diagnosis	Publication year	Time duration	Quality Score
Papoutsakis & et al. [41]	Case:217 Control:297	(Greece)	Age- and sex-specific cut-off points for childhood by (IOTF)	Case: 5-11 Control: 5-11	Physician-diagnosed asthma	2015	November 2007-September 2010	90
Rice & et al. [56]	Case:287 Control:96	(Peru)	Age- and sex-specific cut-off points for childhood by (IOTF)	Case: 9-19 Control: 9-19	Physician-diagnosed asthma	2015	N/R	80
Groth & et al. [57]	Case:61 Control:484	(USA)	Underweight $<5^{th}$, Normal $\geq 5^{th}$ and $< 85^{th}$, Overweight $\geq 85^{th}$ and $< 95^{th}$ obese $\geq 95^{th}$ (CDC growth charts)	Case: 12-15 Control: 12-15	Physician-diagnosed asthma	2016	2002-2004	90
Lawson& et al. [44]	Case:78 Control:451	(Canada)	Age- and sex-specific cut-off points for childhood by (IOTF)	Case: 6-14 Control: 6-14	Physician-diagnosed asthma	2017	2011	100

N/R Not reported

Inclusion criteria were case-control studies on the relationship between asthma and BMI, studies on children and adolescents (2–19 years old), and in the English language. Studies on adults, irrelevance of the subject, the relationship between BMI and asthma severity, cross-sectional and cohort studies and any relationship between breast feeding and asthma were excluded. For the quality assessment of studies we used, the Joanna Briggs Institute (JBI) Critical Appraisal Tools [19]. The quality score is determined by the range 67–100 (good), 34–66 (average), and 0–33 (bad).

Data extraction

An appropriate data extraction form was designed including author (s) name, sample size, country of study, age group (case and control), method of asthma diagnosis, year of publication, time of study, and the exposure assessment method (BMI). The following data, if available, are extracted to evaluate the association between BMI and asthma.

1. Frequency of obesity, overweight and underweight/normal in childhood and adolescence (based on CDC growth chart (2014), and IOTF) in both case and control groups (binary outcome) to obtain OR and RR.
2. Mean and standard deviation (M ± SD) of BMI based on BMI or BMI-Z score in case and control groups (continuous measure) to obtain SMD.
3. Adjusted OR to evaluate the association between BMI and asthma.
4. The above data were also collected for different gender, age, continents, and asthma diagnosis method, year of publication and sample size for the purpose of subgroup analyses.

Statistical analyses

The following three methods were employed to aggregate the extracted data and drive the summary effect of an association between asthma and BMI:

Method 1: OR and RR were calculated when classified BMI (overweight/obesity) for control and case groups were reported ($OR_i = \frac{a_i d_i}{b_i c_i}, RR = \frac{a/(a+b)}{c/(c+d)}$), then Der Simonian and Laird method (random effects model) were used to combine the OR_S or RR_S.

Cumulative meta-analysis was used for pooled estimates to show whether the year of publication or year of the new study has any essential effect on the final results.

Method 2: To derive the summary effects for studies that reported the effect size for case and control groups based on the mean and standard deviation (SD) of BMI, or BMI-Z score, we first calculated the mean difference of each study as follows:

$$SMD = \frac{\bar{X}_1 - \bar{X}_2}{S_{pooled}}$$

where

SMD: standardized mean difference.

SD: pooled standard deviation

$$S^2_{Pooled} = \frac{(n_1-1)S_1^2 + (n_2-1)S_2^2}{n_1 + n_2 - 2}$$

S_1^2: Variance of the case group

S_2^2: Variance of the control group

n_1: Number of samples in the case group

n_2: Number of samples in the control group

Afterwards, to find the overall SMD of all articles, Der Simonian and Laird method (random effects model) was used to combine the result of studies with the "metan" command (from STATA).

Method 3: Ln transformation, Ln ($_{OR}$) of each adjusted OR and associated confidence interval was calculated by using the following formula for standard error:

$$SE = \frac{\ln\left(\frac{OR_{Upper}}{OR_{Lower}}\right)}{2 \times 1.96}$$

where OR_{Upper} is upper limit of OR and OR_{Lower} is lower limit of OR [20].

Then the inverse variance method (fixed effect model) was used to obtain the overall effect size (ES), and the anti-log of the overall ES was taken to come back to the original OR, ($e^{ln\ (OR)}$).

Subgroups analyses were performed for gender, age, continent, sample size, year of publication and asthma diagnosis methods.

In addition, I^2 and Cochrane Q Statistics were used [21] to investigate the heterogeneity of the data. I^2 was considered in four levels; $I^2 = 0\%$ indicated no heterogeneity, 25% to – 50% for low, 50% to 75% for moderate, and more than 75% for high heterogeneity [22]. A random or fixed model was used according to the heterogeneity factor whereas random effects models [23, 24] were used for heterogeneous studies and fixed effects models otherwise.

Begg's test was used to check publication bias. All data analyses were performed in STATA version 10 and a p-value < 0.05 was considered as statistically significant.

Results

Literature search and data collection

In total, 2511 titles were found from which 2348 were removed after reviewing abstracts. Out of 163 potentially related articles, 30 were duplicates and 14 were removed since the ages of the participants were out of our scope. In addition, 69 cross-sectional and 23 cohort studies were also removed. Afterwards, out of 27 articles, 11 case-control studies were removed for the following reasons: Two articles were not in English (One in Romanian [25] and the other in Portuguese [26]), the population of one study was breastfeeding [27], one article studied the relationship between asthmatic with current and no current wheeze and BMI [28], four studies were on age range childhood-adult [29–32], one in which case-control groups were asthmatic with and without allergic rhinitis [33], and finally two studies focused on persistent asthma as the case group and Intermittent asthma as the control group [34, 35] (2001 to 2016). Finally, 16 case-control articles from 1998 to 2017 were entered into the study (Fig. 1).

Overall, 9 studies in the United States of America and Canada (North America), 2 in Peru and Brazil (South America), 3 in Montenegro, Greece and Italy (Europe) and 2 in Iran and Saudi Arabia (Asia) were identified with an age range of 2.2–18 years of age in case group and 2.4–18 years of age in control groups; in total 3577 individuals were in the case group and 4820 individuals were in the control group. In 13 studies, asthma was diagnosed by a physician, in 2 studies by a parent and in 1 study asthma was reported by adolescents. In 8 studies exposure was assessed according to BMI percentiles based on CDC growth charts, one study in which BMI-Z score was based on CDC growth chart, 4 studies in which BMI cut off point was based on IOTF, one study was based on reference data, one study was based on the BMI percentile values and one study was based on BMI-SDS units (z-score); also quality scores of the whole manuscript were good, see Table 1.

Overall OR for overweight individuals

Meta-analysis derived OR = 1.64 (95% CI: 1.13–2.38, *p*-value = 0.01) from 11 case-control studies reported OR of asthma and overweight; moderate heterogeneity was observed between studies (Heterogeneity chi-squared = 35.91 (df = 10) *p*-value = 0.0001 and I^2 = 72.2%) (Fig. 2a); However the reported relative risk was RR = 1.26 (95% CI: 1.07–1.48, p-value = 0.006). A cumulative meta-analysis showed that by combining the studies that were done before 2007, there was a significant association between overweight and asthma. By adding new studies from 2007 to 2012 to previous studies the cumulative effect of being overweight on asthma was not significant, while by adding studies that were done from 2013 to 2016 to previous studies, the cumulative effect of being overweight on asthma showed significant effects. (Fig. 2b). Meta-regression analysis showed that there was no significant statistical relationship between OR of asthma in overweight individuals and the year of publication. This means that the year of publication is not a reason

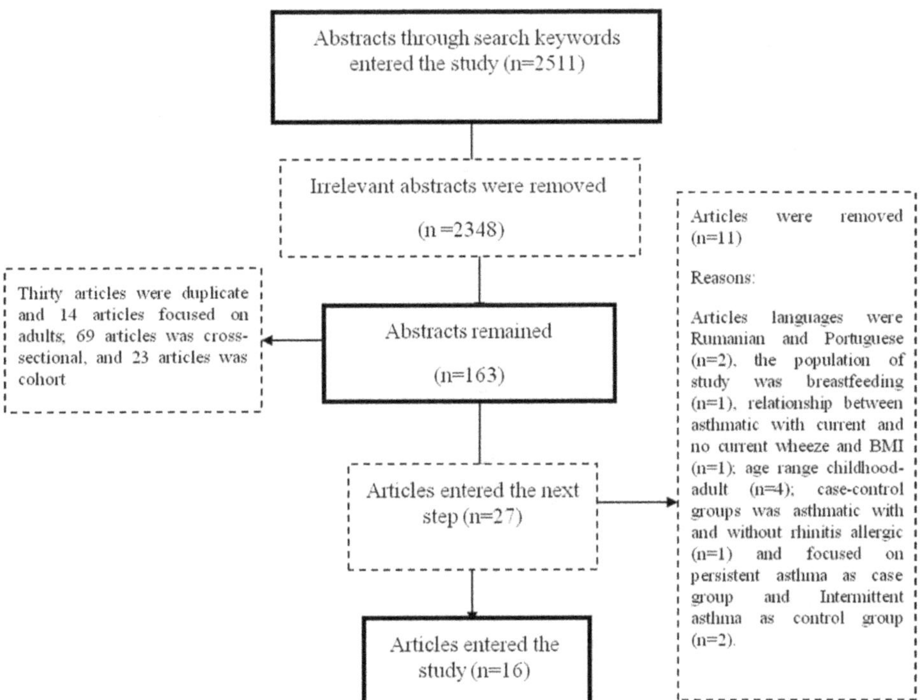

Fig. 1 Flowchart of selecting the article

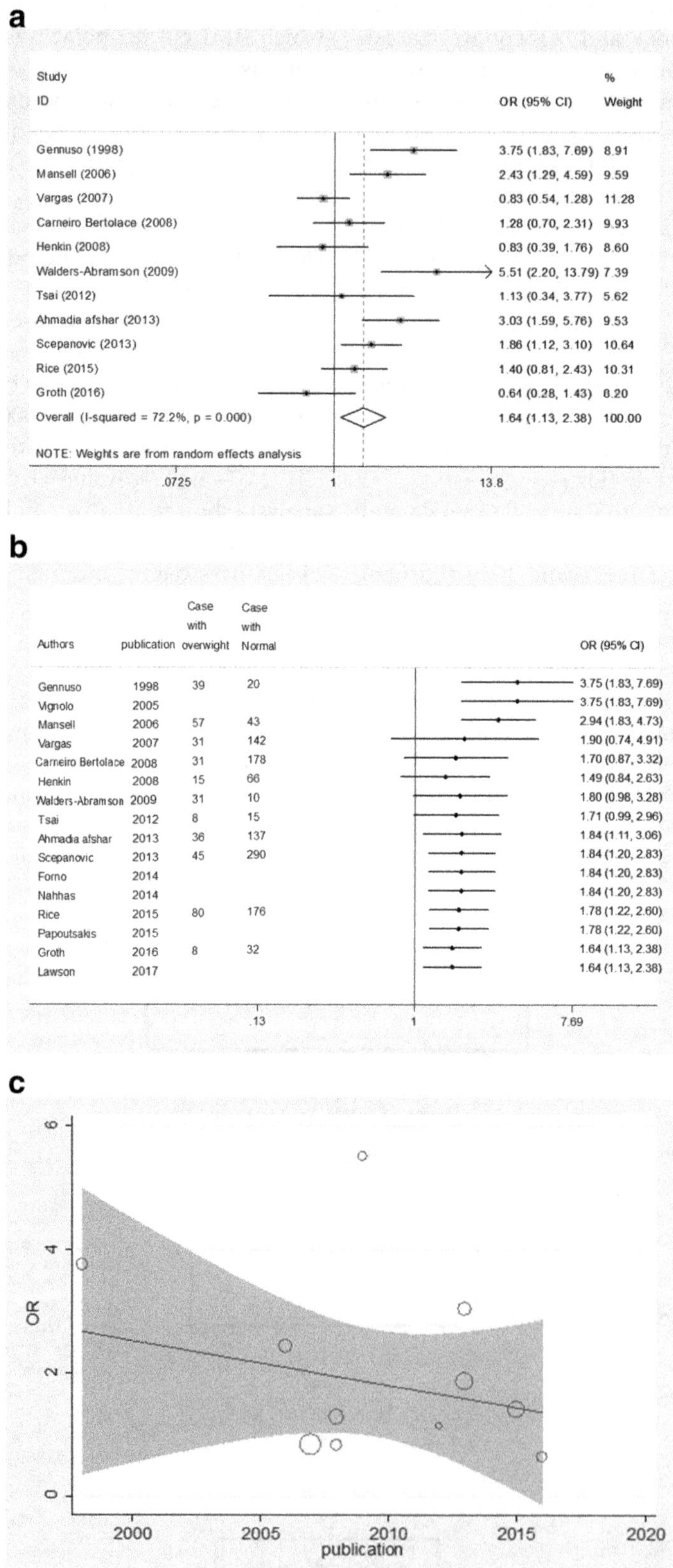

Fig. 2 Meta-analysis based on 11 case-control studies which reported asthma in overweight individuals. **a** Forest plots of estimate of overall odds ratio asthmatic **b** cumulative meta-analysis and **c** meta-regression analysis with OR of asthma in overweight individual and year of publication

for heterogeneity. (Correlation Coefficient = − 0.10, *p*-value = 0.260) (Fig. 2c).

Overall OR for obesity

In total, 14 case-control studies reported OR of asthma and obesity; meta-analysis revealed an association between them; OR = 1.92; (95% CI: 1.39–2.65, p-value = 0.0001). Furthermore, high heterogeneity was observed between studies (chi-squared = 50.49 (df = 13) *p*-value = 0.0001 and I2 = 74.3%) (Fig. 3a), as well as relative risk which was RR = 1.40; (95%CI: 1.19–1.63, *P*-value =0.0001). Cumulative meta-analysis showed that one study was done in 1998 with significant association between obesity and asthma. Adding new studies from 2005 to 2008 to previous studies showed that the cumulative effect of obesity on asthma was not significant. On the other hand, adding studies from decade of 2008 to 2017 to previous ones; a significant association was observed based on the cumulative effect of obesity on asthma (Fig. 3b). Meta-regression analysis didn't identify any significant statistical relationship between OR for asthma in obese individuals and the year of publication. This means that the reason of heterogeneity is not the year of publication (Correlation Coefficient = − 0.15, p-value = 0.08) (Fig. 3c). Overall ES of asthma based on adjusted OR.

Three studies with 740 cases and 1169 controls were reported ES = 1.30 (95% CI: 1.12–1.49; *p*-value < 0.001), that confirm a significant increased risk of asthma for individuals with BMI greater than the 85th percentile.

Overall SMD for asthma and BMI

The overall standard mean difference (SMD) based on 10 studies with 2761 cases, and 3281 controls, and the results showed a significant relationship between asthma and BMI (SMD = 0.21; 95% CI: 0.03–0.38; *p*-value = 0.021), for individuals with BMI greater than the 85th percentile.

Subgroup analyses for asthma and overweight / obesity

Analysis showed that the risk of asthma in obese and overweight children during 2009–2017 was increased in comparison with the decade of 1998–2008. Furthermore, the risk of asthma in obese and overweight girls was greater than the risk of asthma in obese and overweight boys. Asian children and adolescents had a risk of asthmatic attacks three times more likely than children in the American continent (Table 2).

Subgroup analyses based on SMD

We found that there were significant relationships between BMI (greater than the 85th percentile) and asthma in a) both genders, b) results reported in 2009–2017, c) America and the Asian continent, d) children younger than 11 years old and e) groups of children whose asthma were reported by Physicians (Table 3) according to SMD.

Bias

In order to evaluate the publication bias of studies, Begg's test and the Funnel plot were employed. For articles related to overweight children, the *p*-value = 0.312 (Fig. 4a); for articles related to obesity the *p*-value =0.090 (Fig. 4b) and this identified that publication bias was not significant which shows that the majority of the query articles had the same opportunities to be published.

Discussion

We determined that the risk of asthma in individuals who were overweight and obese was 1.64 times and 1.92 times more likely than individuals who were underweight/normal weight respectively. The ES obtained from a combination of adjusted the OR in BMI > 85 percentile was 1.30 (significant difference). Moreover, according to SMD, the relationship between asthma and BMI was significant. Beuther et al. noted that, based on the studies of animals, inflammation of airways due to allergic/non-allergic factors increased through the use of leptin from internal and external sources [36]. The relationship between obesity and asthma could be explained by a number of hypotheses, for example, obesity through hormonal influences or mechanisms of genetic factors which may have direct effects on immune system response or phenotype of asthma. Furthermore, an increased risk of asthma may be explained by a combination of genetic predisposition factors with birth weight, movement of the body that uses energy, and nutrition, as potentially linked to obesity [37]. So asthma is an outcome of a complicated combination of environmental and genetic factors for which we do not have thorough knowledge [38, 39]. However, the key point is that along with the increased risk of asthma with obesity, there are internal and external factors that count as confounders which might influence the relationship between asthma and BMI. The results from our meta-analyses showed a significant relationship between overweight/obesity and asthma, but the important result is that by removing the confounding factors, the effect size was reduced from 1.64 and 1.92 (in the overweight/obese) to 1.30. In this review, five studies reported adjusted OR according to different sets of confounding factors. The confounding factors in Henkin's research were atopic dermatitis, allergic rhinitis, and other allergies [40]; in Papoutsakis' research OR was adjusted for age, gender, education, atopic background of parents, calorie intake, breastfeeding, and physical activity score [41]; Forno et al. considered family income, the asthma record of

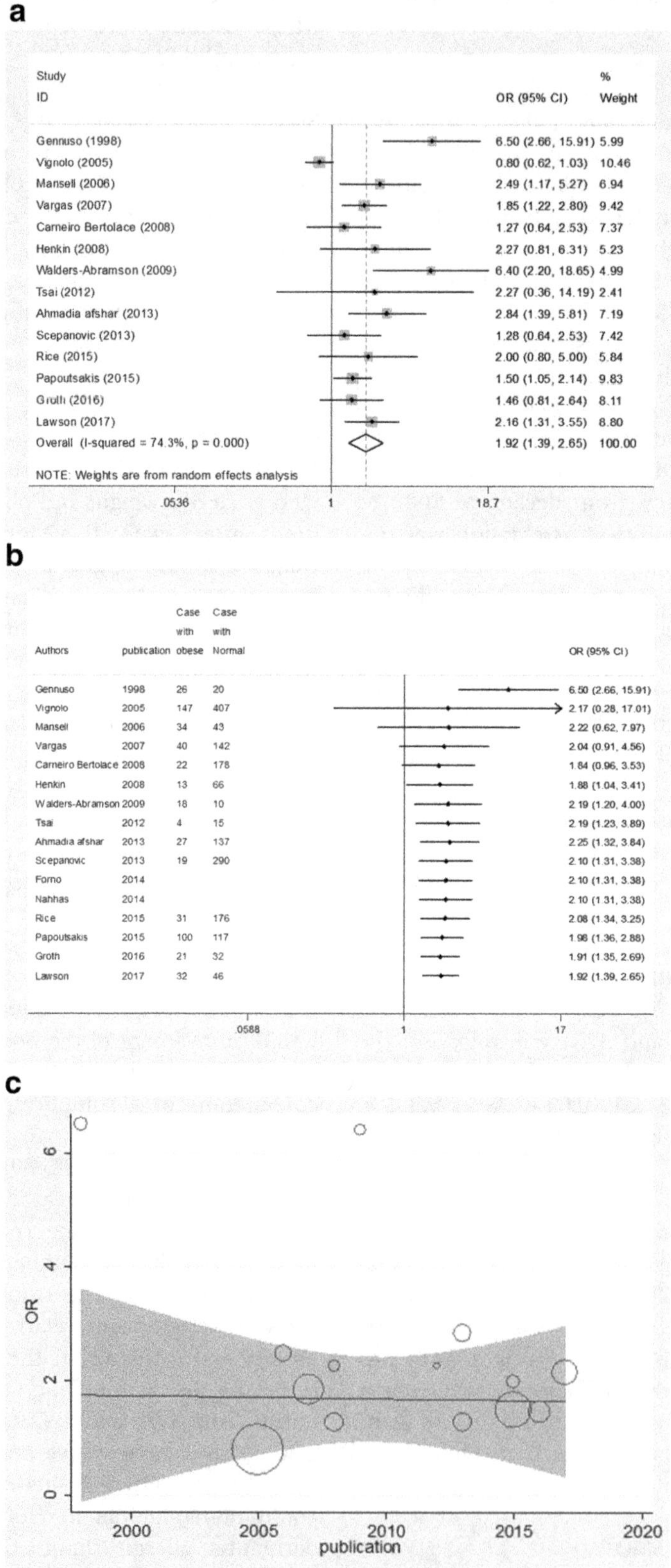

Fig. 3 Meta-analysis based on 14 case-control studies which reported asthma in obesity individuals. **a** Forest plots of estimate of overall odds ratio asthmatic **b** cumulative meta-analysis and **c** meta-regression analysis with OR of asthma in obese individual and year of publication

Table 2 The risk of asthma in obese and overweight children based on OR

Variables	Overweight			Obesity	
	Group	Study	OR (95% CI)	Study	OR (95% CI)
Year of publication	1998–2008	5	1.49 (0.84–2.63)	6	1.88 (1.04–3.41)
	2009–2017	6	1.80 (1.07–3.03)	8	1.90 (1.43–2.53)
Age	< 11 year	2	0.86 (0.58–1.29)	2	1.65 (1.26–2.15)
	> 12 year	3	1.30 (0.64–2.64)	3	1.61 (1.09–2.37)
	Mix	6	2.19 (1.35–3.55)	8	2.27 (1.26–4.06)
Gender	Male	2	1.46 (0.64–3.34)	2	1.14 (0.62–2.09)
	Female	2	1.51 (0.88–2.58)	2	1.65 (0.95–2.89)
Continents	America	9	1.50 (0.97–2.33)	10	2.21 (1.65–2.98)
	Europe	1	1.86 (1.12–3.10)	3	1.12 (0.70–1.79)
	Asia	1	3.03 (1.59–5.76)	1	2.84 (1.39–5.81)
Sample	< 500	8	2.00 (1.31–3.04)	8	2.71 (1.80–4.07)
	> 500	3	1.04 (0.56–1.93)	6	1.41 (0.98–2.03)
Report of Asthma	Physician	10	1.69 (1.11–2.56)	13	2.00 (1.42–2.82)
	Parent	1	1.28 (0.70–2.31)	1	1.27 (0.64–2.53)

parents, age, gender, and race to adjust the OR [42]; Also Nahhas considered the parents' age, birth weight, education, smoker parents, physical activity, exposure to animals, watching TV, allergens, and gender as confounding factors [43]. Lawson et al. considered age, gender, mother's education, having a asthmatic record in the family, early respiratory illness, smoker mother, smoking during pregnancy, dog at home in last 12 months, cleaning or playing in pens or corrals regularly and farm dwelling as factors to adjust the OR [44].

Analyses based on OR in the subgroups showed that overweight and obesity increased the risk of asthma in both genders (girls more than boys); however, the relationship was not significant, probably due to a small number of studies and sample size, so we need more studies dealing with a larger sample size to obtain more accurate results. Moreover, a significant association was identified between BMI and the risk of asthma in both genders (girls more than boys) based on SMD. The SMD is a calculated quantitative index based on the difference between the means in the case and control groups (continuous variable) which follows a normal distribution. This index has more precision than OR since OR is calculated on the basis of frequency of variables. In addition, the two articles that found significant SMD are different from the articles which found insignificant OR in terms of the exposure factor. Chen et al. reported that obese and overweight boys were at higher risk of asthma compared to girls [9] but the results of Egan et al. found a significant relationship between overweight and asthma in boys and obesity and asthma in girls [11].

Table 3 The risk of asthma in obese and overweight children based on SMD

Variables	Group	Study	SMD (95% CI) Overweight and Obesity
Year of publication	1998–2008	3	0.07 (−0.19–0.32)
	2009–2017	7	0.26 (0.08–0.45)
Age	< 11 year	3	0.40 (0.11–0.68)
	> 12 year	3	0.14 (−0.06–0.35)
	Mix	4	0.12 (−0.09–0.33)
Gender	Male	3	0.35 (0.25–0.44)
	Female	3	0.58 (0.19–0.98)
Continents	America	5	0.15 (0.03–0.26)
	Europe	3	0.06 (−0.15–0.26)
	Asia	2	0.52 (0.35–0.68)
Sample	< 500	4	0.27 (0.04–0.49)
	> 500	6	0.17 (−0.07–0.41)
Report of Asthma	Physician	8	0.17 (0.02–0.31)
	Parent	2	0.31 (−0.23–0.86)

Obesity is firmly connected to breathing disorders and influences the function of the lungs. In fact, the high percentage of excessive body fat compresses the lungs and limits the free air movement because of its mechanical effect on the airways via central body fat [45]. Gender, atopy, family history of asthma (non-modifiable), and obesity (one of the few modifiable) are risk factors for asthma [46]. Even though exercise has minimal impact on lung function in asthmatic children, it should still be recommended by health care providers [47]. The difference in risks by continent may indicate the effect of the environment or race on the hazard of asthma. In general, healthcare providers overseeing obese kids and wishing to control their asthma should consider

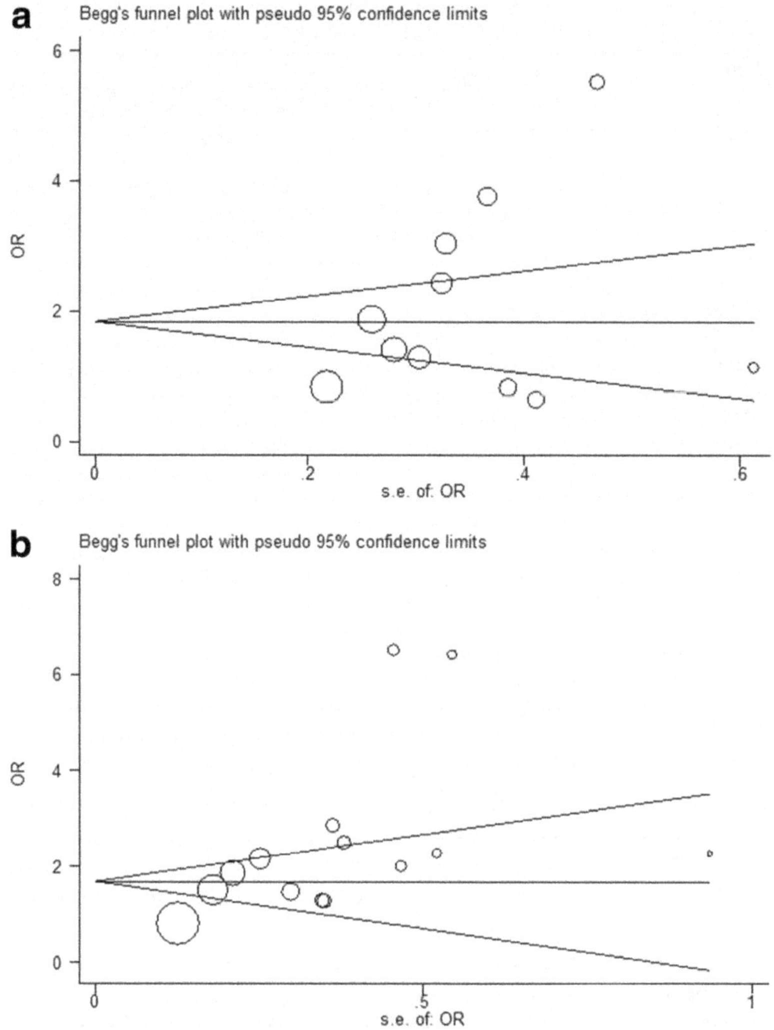

Fig. 4 Begg's funnel plot (pseudo 95% confidence limits) showings the effect of publication bias. **a** Overweight group and **b** Obese group

interventions such as weight loss, physical activity, and normalization of nutrient levels. Monitoring of complications related to obesity with designed prospective and clinical trial studies should also be taken into account.

Limitations

One of the main limitations of this research was the variety of methods used in reporting the results e.g., some studies reported M ± SD (mean ± standard deviation) and others reported OR. In addition, definitions of obesity and overweight were not consistent over different studies. The number of studies was also another limitation. Furthermore, meta-analysis for case-control studies cannot identify the causal-temporal relationships between BMI and asthma.

Conclusion

Based on our findings, we noted that BMI is a significant factor when it comes to asthma. We found that obesity and being overweight increase the risk of asthma. A thorough investigation to recognize the confounding factors on the relationship between asthma and BMI is also important for future epidemiological research.

Abbreviations

BMI: Body mass index; CDC: Centers for Disease Control and Prevention; CI: Confidence interval; ES: Effect size; IOTF: International Obesity Task Force; ISSAC: The International Study of Asthma and Allergies in Childhood; JBI: Joanna Briggs Institute; MeSH: Medical subject headings; OR: Odds ratio; ORs: Odds ratios; PRISMA: Preferred Reporting Items for Systematic Reviews and Meta-analyses; RR: Relative risk; SD: Standard deviation; SDS: Standard deviation score; SMD: Standardized mean difference

Acknowledgments

Student Research Committee of Ilam University of Medical Science has supported this study.

Funding
The study was conducted based on research plan No.:22/52/2888 approved by Student Research Committee of Ilam University of Medical Science.

Authors' contributions
YA, KS conceived the idea and preformed the literature search. YA, AD, KS contributed to the literature search, data extraction and study selection. KS preformed all the statistical analyses. YA, KS interpreted the results. YA wrote the manuscript. ZM and BD contributed in designing the study, and were involved in drafting and revising the manuscript it. All authors approved the final version of the manuscript.

Competing interests
The authors declare that they have no competing interests.

Author details
[1]Department of Clinical Epidemiology, Student Research Committee, Ilam University of Medical Sciences, Ilam, Iran. [2]Department of Clinical Epidemiology, Psychosocial Injuries Research Center, Ilam University of Medical Sciences, Ilam, Iran. [3]School of Epidemiology, Public Health and Preventive Medicine, Faculty of Medicine, University of Ottawa, Ottawa, Canada. [4]Department of Biostatistics, Psychosocial Injuries Research Center, Ilam University of Medical Sciences, Ilam, Iran. [5]Department of Pediatrics, Faculty of Medicine, Ilam University of Medical Sciences, Ilam, Iran.

References
1. Sutherland E. Obesity and asthma. Immunol Allergy Clin N Am. 2008;28: 589–602. https://doi.org/10.1016/j.iac.2008.03.003.
2. World Health Organization (WHO). "Asthma Fact sheet number 307"2011, [online]. Available at: https://web.archive.org/web/20110629035454/http:// www.who.int/mediacentre/factsheets/fs307/en/.
3. Esposito S, Principi N. Asthma in children: are chlamydia or mycoplasma involved? Paediatr Drugs. 2001;3:159–68.
4. Choudhry S, Seibold MA, Borrell LN, Tang H, Serebrisky D, Chapela R, et al. Dissecting complex diseases in complex populations: asthma in latino americans. Proc Am Thorac Soc. 2007;4:226–33. https://doi.org/10.1513/pats. 200701-029AW.
5. American Lung Association."Trend in asthma Morbidity and mortality" 2012, [online]. Available at: www.lung.org/assets/documents/research/asthma-trend-report.pdf.
6. National Center for Health Statistics. Health, United States, 2011: With Special Features on Socioeconomic Status and Health. Hyattsville, MD; U.S. Department of Health and Human Services; 2012.
7. Ogden CL, Carroll MD, Kit BK, Flegal KM. Prevalence of childhood and adult obesity in the United States, 2011-2012. JAMA. 2014;311:806–14. https://doi. org/10.1001/jama.2014.732.
8. Attaran D, Tohidi M, Asna-Ashari AM, Ismaii H, Khadivi E, Gharaei SH. Evaluation of the correlation between body mass index and the severity of asthma in recently diagnosed patients. Iran J Otorhinolaryngol. 2011;3:93–8.
9. Chen YC, Dong GH, Lin KC, Lee YL. Gender difference of childhood overweight and obesity in predicting the risk of incident asthma: a systematic review and meta-analysis. Obes Rev. 2013;14:222–31. https://doi. org/10.1111/j.1467-789X.2012.01055.x.
10. Flaherman V, Rutherford GW. A meta-analysis of the effect of high weight on asthma. Arch Dis Child. 2006;91(4):334–9. https://doi.org/10.1136/adc. 2005.080390.
11. Egan KB, Ettinger AS, Bracken MB. Childhood body mass index and subsequent physician-diagnosed asthma:a systematic review and meta-analysis of prospective cohort studies. BMC Pediatr. 2013;13:121. https://doi. org/10.1186/1471-2431-13-121
12. Mebrahtu TF, Feltbower RG, Greenwood DC, Parslow RC. Childhood body mass index and wheezing disorders: a systematic review and meta-analysis. Pediatr Allergy Immunol. 2015;26:62–72. https://doi.org/10.1111/pai.12321.
13. Moher D, Liberati A, Tetzlaff J, Altman DG, PRISMA G. Preferred reporting items for systematic reviews and meta-analyses: the PRISMA statement. PLoS Med. 2009;6:e1000097. https://doi.org/10.1371/journal.pmed.1000097.
14. Cole TJ, Bellizzi MC, Flegal KM, Dietz WH. Establishing a standard definition for child overweight andobesity worldwide: International survey. BMJ. 2000; 320:1240–3. https://doi.org/10.1136/bmj.320.7244.1240.
15. Must A, Dallal GE, Dietz WH. Reference data for obesity :85th and 95th percentiels for body mass index(wt/ht2) and triceps skinfold thickness. Am J Clin Nutr. 1991;53:839–46.
16. Scepanovic A, Perovic A, Bozic-Krstic V. Nutritional status (BMI) in children suffering from asthma. Arch Biol Sci. 2013;65:1157–62.
17. Rolland-Cachera MF, Bellisle F, Deheeger M. Nutritional status and food intake in adolescents living in western Europe. Eur J Clin Nutr. 2000;54:S41–6.
18. Centers for Disease Control and prevention (CDC). 'Healthy Weight - it's not a diet, it's a lifestyle: What is a BMI percentile?', 2014, [online]. Available at: http://www.cdc.gov/healthyweight/assessing/bmi/childrens_bmi/about_ childrens_bmi.html
19. The Joanna Briggs Institute Critical Appraisal tools . URL: http://joannabriggs. org/research/critical-appraisal-tools.html.
20. Sayehmiri K. Applied by statistics and method of research. Ilam: University of medical sciences; 2016.
21. Higgins JP, Thompson SG, Deeks JJ, Altman DG. Measuring inconsistency in meta-analyses. BMJ. 2003;327:557–60. https://doi.org/10.1136/bmj.327.7414.557.
22. Ades AE, Lu G, Higgins JP. The interpretation of random-effects meta-analysis in decision models. Med Decis Mak. 2005;25:646–54. https://doi.org/ 10.1177/0272989X05282643.
23. Rothstein HR, Sutton AJ, Borenstein M. Publication bias in meta-analysis: prevention, assessment and adjustments. New York: John Wiley & Sons; 2006.
24. Hartung J, Knapp G, Sinha B. Statistical metaanalysis with applications. New York: John Wiley & Sons; 2008.
25. Valean C, Tatar S, Nanulescu M, Leucuta A, Ichim G. Relationship between asthma and obesity in school age students. Pneumologia 2009;58:55–8.
26. Mendes AA, Strassburger MJ, Franz LB, Busnello MB, Battisti ID, Strassburger SZ. Estado nutricional antropométrico e qualidade de vida em escolares com asma. Sci Med. 2016;26(4):ID24492.
27. Mai XM, Becker AB, Sellers EA, Liem JJ, Kozyrskyj AL. The relationship of breast-feeding, overweight, and asthma in preadolescents. J Allergy Clin Immunol. 2007;120:552–6. https://doi.org/10.1016/j.jaci.2007.05.004.
28. Mai XM, Nilsson L, Axelson O, Bråbäck L, Sandin A, Kjellman NI, et al. High body mass index, asthma and allergy in Swedish schoolchildren participating in the international study of asthma and allergies in childhood: phase II. Acta Pediatr. 2003;92:1144–8.
29. Brenner JS, Kelly CS, Wenger AD, Brich SM, Morrow AL. Asthma and obesity in adolescents: is there an association? J Asthma. 2001;38:509–15.
30. Poongadan MN, Gupta N, Kumar R. Lifestyle factors and asthma in India — a case-control study. Pneumonol Alergol Pol. 2016;84(2):104–8. https://doi. org/10.5603/PiAP.2016.0008.
31. Silverberg JI, Silverberg NB, Lee-Wong M. Association between atopic dermatitis and obesity in adulthood. Br J Dermatol. 2012;166(3):498–504. https://doi.org/10.1111/j.1365-2133.2011.10694.x.
32. Gordon B, Hassid A, Bar-Shai A, Derazne E, Tzur D, Hershkovich O, et al. Association between asthma and body mass index and socioeconomic status: a cross-sectional study on 849 659 adolescents. Respirology. 2016; 21(1):95–101. https://doi.org/10.1111/resp.12645.
33. Musaad SM, Patterson T, Ericksen M, Lindsey M, Dietrich K, Succop P, et al. Comparison of Anthropometric Measures of Obesity in Childhood Allergic Asthma: Central Obesity is Most Relevant. J Allergy Clin Immunol. 2009;123: 1321–7. https://doi.org/10.1016/j.jaci.2009.03.023.
34. Silveira DH, Zhang L, Prietsch SO, Vecchi AA, Susin LR. Association between dietary habits and asthma severity in children. Indian Pediatr. 2015;52:25–30.
35. Silveira DH, Zhang L, Prietsch SO, Vecchi AA, Susin LR. Nutritional status, adiposity and asthma severity and control in children. J Paediatr Child Health. 2015;51:1001–6. https://doi.org/10.1111/jpc.12882.
36. Beuther DA, Weiss ST, Sutherland ER. Obesity and asthma. Am J Respir Crit Care Med. 2006;174:112–9. https://doi.org/10.1164/rccm.200602-231PP.
37. Noal RB, Menezes AM, Macedo SE, Dumith SC. Childhood body mass index and risk of asthma in adolescence: a systematic review. Obes Rev. 2011;12: 93–104. https://doi.org/10.1111/j.1467-789X.2010.00741.x.

38. Martinez FD. Genes, environments, development and asthma: a reappraisal. Eur Respir J. 2007;29:179–84. https://doi.org/10.1183/09031936.00087906.
39. Miller RL, Ho SM. Environmental epigenetics and asthma :current conceptsnd call for studies. Am J Respir Crit Care Med. 2008;177:567–73. https://doi.org/10.1164/rccm.200710-1511PP.
40. Henkin S, Brugge D, Bermudez OI, Gao X. A case-control study of body mass index and asthma in Asian children. Ann Allergy Asthma Immunol. 2008;100:447–51. https://doi.org/10.1016/S1081-1206(10)60469-3.
41. Papoutsakis C, Chondronikola M, Antonogeorgos G, Papadakou E, Matziou V, Drakouli M, et al. Associations between central obesity and asthma in children and adolescents: a case-control study. J Asthma. 2015;52:128–34. https://doi.org/10.3109/02770903.2014.954291.
42. Forno E, Acosta-Perez E, Brehm JM, Han YY, Alvarez M, Colon-Semidey A, et al. Obesity and adiposity indicators, asthma, and atopy in Puerto Rican children. J Allergy Clin Immunol. 2014;133:1308–14. https://doi.org/10.1016/j.jaci.2013.09.041.
43. Nahhas M, Bhopal R, Anandan C, Elton R, Sheikh A. Investigating the association between obesity and asthma in 6- to 8-year-old Saudi children: a matched case–control study. NPJ Prim Care Respir Med. 2014;24:14004. https://doi.org/10.1038/npjpcrm.2014.4.
44. Lawson JA, Chu LM, Rennie DC, Hagel L, Karunanayake CP, Pahwa P, et al. Prevalence, risk factors, and clinical outcomes of atopic and nonatopic asthma among rural children. Ann Allergy Asthma Immunol. 2017;118(3): 304–10. https://doi.org/10.1016/j.anai.2016.11.024.
45. Kopelman P, Caterson I, Dietz W. Clinical obesity in adults and children. London: Wiley-Blackwell; 2006.
46. Willeboordse M, Van de Kant KD, De Laat MN, Van Schayck OC, Mulkens S, Dompeling E. Multifactorial intervention for children with asthma and overweight (Mikado): study design of a randomised controlled trial. BMC Public Health 2013;13:494. https://doi.org/10.1186/1471-2458-13-494.
47. Wanrooij VH, Willeboordse M, Dompeling E, Van de Kant KD. Exercise training in children with asthma: a systematic review. Br J Sports Med. 48: 2014, 1024–31. https://doi.org/10.1136/bjsports-2012-091347.
48. Gennuso J, Epstein LH, Paluch RA, Cerny F. The relationship between asthma and obesity in urban minority children and adolescents. Arch Pediatr Adolesc Med. 1998;152:1197–200.
49. Vignolo M, Silvestri M, Parodi A, Pistorio A, Battistini E, Rossi GA, et al. Relationship between body mass index and asthma characteristics in a Group of Italian Children and Adolescents. J Asthma. 2005;42(3):185–9.
50. Mansell AL, Walders N, Wamboldt MZ, Carter R, Steele DW, Devin JA, et al. Effect of body mass index on response to methacholine bronchial provocation in healthy and asthmatic adolescents. Pediatr Pulmonolo. 2006; 41:434–40. https://doi.org/10.1002/ppul.20368.
51. Vargas PA, Perry TT, Robles E, Jo CH, Simpson PM, Magee JM, et al. Relationship of body mass index with asthma indicators in head start children. Ann Allergy Asthma Immunol. 2007;99(1):22–8.
52. Bertolace Mdo P, Toledo E, Jorge PP, Liberatore Junior Rdel R. Association between obesity and asthma among teenagers. Sao Paulo Med J. 2008;126:285–7.
53. Walders-Abramson N, Wamboldt FS, Curran-Everett D, Zhang L. Encouraging physical activity in pediatric asthma: a case-control study of the wonders of walking (WOW) program. Pediatr Pulmonolo. 2009;44:909–16. https://doi.org/10.1002/ppul.21077.
54. Tsai SY, Ward T, Lentz MJ, Kieckhefer GM. Daytime physical activity levels in school-age children with and without asthma. Nurs Res. 2012;61:252–9. https://doi.org/10.1097/NNR.0b013e318255679c.
55. Ahmadiafshar A, Tabbekhha S, Mousavinasab N, Khoshnevis P. Relation between asthma and body mass index in 6-15 years old children. Acta Med Iran. 2013;51:615–9.
56. Rice JL, Romero KM, Galvez Davila RM, Meza CT, Bilderback A, Williams DL, et al. Association between adherence to the Mediterranean diet and asthma in Peruvian children. Lung. 2015;193:893–9. https://doi.org/10.1007/s00408-015-9792-9.
57. Groth S, Rhee H, Kitzman H. Relationships among obesity, physical activity and sedentary behavior in young adolescents with and without lifetime asthma. J Asthma. 2016;53(1):19–24. https://doi.org/10.3109/02770903.2015.1063646.

21

Epidemiology and clinical characteristics of acute respiratory tract infections among hospitalized infants and young children in Chengdu, West China, 2009–2014

Jiayi Chen[1,2], Pengwei Hu[1,3], Tao Zhou[1], Tianli Zheng[1], Lingxu Zhou[1,4], Chunping Jiang[1] and Xiaofang Pei[1*]

Abstract

Background: Acute respiratory infection (ARI) is the leading cause of morbidity and mortality in pediatric patients worldwide and imposes an intense pressure on health care facilities. Data on the epidemiology profiles of ARIs are scarce in the western and rural areas of China. The purpose of the current study is to provide data on the presence of potential pathogens of ARIs in hospitalized children in Chengdu, west China.

Methods: Respiratory specimens were obtained from hospitalized patients (under 6 years old) with ARIs in a local hospital in Chengdu. Eight respiratory viruses were identified by PCR and 6 respiratory bacteria by biochemical reactions and Analytical Profile Index (API). Pathogens profiles, clinical characteristics and seasonality were analyzed.

Results: Fifty-one percent of patients were identified with at least one respiratory pathogen. Human rhinovirus (HRV) (23%), Respiratory syncytial virus (RSV) (22.7%) was the most commonly identified viruses, with *Klebsiella pneumoniae* (11.5%) the most commonly identified bacterium in the study. The presences of more than one pathogen were found, and multiple viral, bacterial, viral/bacterial combinations were identified in 14.9, 3.3 and 13.9% of patients respectively. Respiratory viruses were identified throughout the year with a seasonal peak in December–February. Pathogens profiles and clinical associations were different between infants (< 1 year of age) and older children (> 1 year of age). Infants with ARIs were more likely to have one or more viruses than older children. Infants identified with multiple pathogens had significantly higher proportions of tachypnea than infants that were not.

Conclusions: This study demonstrated that viral agents were frequently found in hospitalized children with ARI in Chengdu during the study period. This study gives us better information on the pathogen profiles, clinical associations, co-infection combinations and seasonal features of ARIs in hospitalized children, which is important for diagnoses and treatment of ARIs, as well as implementation of vaccines in this area. Moreover, future efforts in reducing the impact of ARIs will depend on programs in which available vaccines, especially vaccines on RSV, HRV and *S. pneumoniae* could be employed in this region and new vaccines could be developed against common pathogens.

Keywords: Acute respiratory infections, Epidemiology, Clinical characteristics, Pediatrics, West China

* Correspondence: xxpeiscu@163.com
[1]Department of Public Health Laboratory Sciences, West China School of Public Health (No.4 West China Teaching Hospital), Sichuan University, 16#, Section 3, Renmin Road South, Chengdu 610041, Sichuan, People's Republic of China
Full list of author information is available at the end of the article

Background

Acute respiratory infections (ARIs) remain one of the most common major public health threats [1]. There were approximate 11.9 million episodes of severe acute lower respiratory infections (ALRI) resulted in hospital admissions in young children worldwide [2], and ARIs-related pneumonia was one of the leading cause of death that due to infectious disease in China (> 30,000 deaths annually) as well as globally (935,000 in 2013) [3, 4]. There were, as have been suggested, associations of several viral agents with ARIs, such as: respiratory syncytial virus (RSV), human rhinovirus (HRV), human metapneumovirus (HMPV), influenza virus (IFV), parainfluenza virus (PIV), adenovirus (ADV) and human bocavirus (BoV), accounting for about 35–87% of children with ARI [5]. Viral co-infections occurred in 4–33% of children hospitalized with ARIs, and may indicate an increasing risk for clinical outcome [6, 7]. Further, bacterial infections such as: *Streptococcus pneumoniae, Haemophilus influenzae, Staphylococcus aureus, Pseudomonas aeruginosa* and *Klebsiella pneumoniae,* et al., were commonly observed in the later stage of diseases due to immune-compromised viral infections [8].

Similarities among ARI symptoms hampers the diagnostic and therapeutic efficacy among infected children, and inappropriate medication options may lead to the potential of viral escape mutants or bacterial resistance [8]. The composition of ARIs is geographically diverse and is largely associated with the epidemic status of each ARIs and climate conditions [9, 10]. The prevalence of ARIs varies from 14.6 to 94.3% among hospitalized children with respiratory infections in some metropolitan cities such as Beijing, Shanghai and Shenzhen in China [11–14]. However, in the underdeveloped interior areas of China, epidemiology profiles of ARIs are seldom reported. Chengdu is a mega-city in the southwest of China and has a population of more than 15 million people. Flu vaccination rates were pretty low in this area, which were 2.18, 1.69, 1.82 and 1.63% respectively from 2010 to 2013 [15]. The purpose of the current study is to investigate the profiles of respiratory pathogens and epidemiology characteristics of ARIs in hospitalized children in Chengdu. The results were expected to help improve diagnosis and optimization of therapeutic regimens of ARIs in this area.

Methods

Study design and patient population

The cross-sectional study was conducted monthly at a sentinel tertiary women's and children's hospitals in Chengdu, West China, from September 2009 to February 2014. A total of 1992 hospitalized children younger than 6 years old that presented symptoms of ARIs were recruited. Inclusion criteria for cases were (i) acute infection, for example fever, WBC anomaly, shivering; (ii) respiratory symptoms such as cough, rhinorrhea, pharyngalgia, expectoration, nose/throat congestion, shortness of breath, abnormal breathing sounds or dyspnea. The study protocol was approved by the Medical Ethics Committee of Sichuan University and written informed consents were obtained from the parents or the caregiver before collecting samples.

Samples including nasopharyngeal aspirates, sputum, throat swabs, blood and bronchoalevlar lavage fluid were collected by qualified medical personnel. The demographic information and medical records of the participated patients were also collected. All samples were delivered to the Microbiology Laboratory of Department of Public Health Laboratory Sciences, Sichuan University immediately after collection samples via cold chain transportation and stored at − 80 °C.

Pathogen analysis

Nasopharyngeal aspirates, sputum, throat swabs and bronchoalevlar lavage fluid were used for respiratory virus analyses. Viral RNA and DNA were extracted by Viral Nucleic Acid Extraction Kit (Geneaid, Taiwan District) according to the manufacturer's instructions. cDNA were synthesized with reverse transcription kit (BIO-RAD, California, US). Primers and multiplex PCR conditions for IFV [16], RSV [16], PIV [17], ADV [18], HMPV [13], human coronavirus (HCoV) [19], HBoV [20] and HRV [17] have been described previously. Primers were synthesized by Life Technology Corp. (Shanghai, China) and PCRs were performed using PCR Mastermix (Tiangen Company, China) and the S1000™ Thermal Cycler (BIO-RAD, California, US). Respiratory viruses were initially identified by the size of PCR products following agarose gel electrophoresis, with confirmation by DNA sequencing (Life Technology Corp., Shanghai, China).

Nasopharyngeal aspirates, sputum, blood and bronchoalevlar lavage fluid were used for bacterial analyses. For isolation of bacteria, specimens were cultured on sheep blood agar, chocolate agar and MacConkey's agar plates. Isolated bacteria were primarily evaluated by colonial morphology, Gram staining, and were finally identified by biochemical reactions and API system. *S. pneumoniae* were differentiated by Optochin sensitivity and *Group A streptococcus* were identified by bacitracin sensitivity. *P. aeruginosa* and *K. pneumoniae* were identified by API 20E. *H. influenzae, S. aureus* were differentiated by API HN, API Staph respectively.

Statistical analysis

The collected data were analyzed through SPSS version 19.0. Descriptive statistics were done in the form of means, frequencies and ranges of the variables. Continuous variables were expressed as means with their standard deviations. Categorical variables such as age groups and their associations with proportions of certain pathogens were analyzed using the chi-square test or the Fisher's exact test. Significant differences, associations and interrelationships of the variables were assessed at a level of $P < 0.05$.

Results

Profile of enrolled patients

The median age of the patients was 9 months (ranged from 1 days to 6 years old), with 54% of patients under 1 year of age. Of 1992 enrolled children, 1185 were boys and 807 were girls (gender ratio of 1.47: 1). Cough was found in 1354 (68.0%) of the children, followed by fever (51.9%, 1033) and expectoration (29.0%, 578). The median number of days between symptom onset and hospitalization was 10 days. 52.5% (1045/1992) of the patients were diagnosed with pneumonia by chest X-ray. Among all the cases, 9 children died during the study period, including 8 boys and 1 girl.

Results of pathogen analysis

Respiratory viruses were analyzed in 1764 samples. HRV testing was added in 2012 and HRV was analyzed in 795 samples. One or more respiratory viruses were identified in 51.0% of the patients (Table 1). HRV (23.0%, 183/795) and RSV (22.7%, 401/1764) were the most commonly identified viruses in hospitalized children, followed by PIV (13.4%, 236/1764), HBoV (8.4%, 149/1764) and ADV (6.2%, 110/1764). Other viruses such as IFV (4.4%), HMPV (2.2%) and HCoV (0.6%) were identified in small proportions. Multiple viral combinations in samples were found, including 223 dual, 37 triple and 3 quadruple combinations. Common combinations are listed in Table 2.

Six respiratory bacteria were analyzed among 1816 samples. One or more respiratory bacteria were identified in 26.2% (475/1816) of the patients. The most commonly detected bacteria were *K. pneumoniae* (11.5%, 209/1816), *S. pneumoniae* (9.5%, 173/1816) and *S. aureus* (4.0%, 73/1816), followed by *H. influenzae* (2.5%), *P. aeruginosa* (1.9%), and *Group A streptococcus* (0.4%). Multiple bacterial combinations in samples were found, including 52 dual and 8 triple bacterial combinations. *K. pneumoniae*/*S. pneumoniae* co-infection was the most frequent combination. Eight viruses and 6 bacteria were tested in 1728 samples, among which 883 (51.1%) were identified with at least one respiratory pathogen. 240 (27.2%, 240/883) were viral/bacterial combination among positive cases.

Among 9 death cases, 6 patients were identified with at least 1 respiratory pathogen, including 2 boys with single virus (IFV, HRV respectively), 2 boys with dual virus (PIV/HRV, PIV/HBoV respectively), 1 boy with triple virus (RSV/PIV/HRV) and 1 girl with both virus and bacteria (PIV/*S.pneumoniae*). None of the pathogens was identified in the rest of 3 boys.

Respiratory pathogens and clinical characteristics

A univariate analysis was conducted to find associations between demographic and clinical characteristics with infection (Table 3). Infants tended to have a higher proportion of virus infection than older children ($P < 0.001$), with those from 6 to 12 months of age having the highest proportion (67.4%) ($P < 0.001$). Infants identified with viruses had higher proportion of fever ($P < 0.001$), cough ($P < 0.001$), runny nose ($P = 0.007$), expectoration ($P < 0.001$) and diarrhea ($P = 0.031$) than infants that were not. Older children with viral infections had a higher proportion of tachypnea

Table 1 Pathogen profiles and distributions of viral agents among age groups

	< 6 months, $n = 799$		6 months-1 year, $n = 193$		1-3 years, $n = 351$		> 3 years, $n = 421$		All ages, $n = 1764$	
	No.%	Mixed	No.%	Mixed	No.%	Mixed	No.%	Mixed	No.%	Mixed
Positive	414 (51.8)[a]		130 (67.4)		194 (55.3)		162 (38.5)		900 (51.0)[a]	
Single	297 (33.0)[b]		92 (10.2)		127 (14.1)		121 (13.4)		637 (70.8)[b]	
Mixed	117 (13.0)[c]		38 (4.2)		68 (7.6)		40 (4.4)		263 (29.2)[b]	
IFV	29 (3.2)[b]	21 (72.4)[c]	11 (1.2)	8 (72.7)	18 (23.1)	15 (83.3)	20 (25.6)	8 (40.0)	78 (4.4)[a]	52 (66.7)
RSV	212 (23.6)	69 (32.5)	61 (6.8)	27 (44.3)	82 (9.1)	29 (35.4)	46 (5.1)	24 (52.2)	401 (22.7)	149 (37.2)
PIV	91 (10.1)	47 (51.6)	42 (4.7)	23 (48.9)	61 (6.8)	30 (49.2)	42 (4.4)	16 (38.1)	236 (13.4)	116 (49.2)
ADV	29 (3.2)	22 (75.9)	25 (2.8)	10 (40.0)	33 (3.7)	20 (60.6)	23 (2.6)	9 (39.1)	110 (6.2)	61 (55.5)
HPMV	20 (2.2)	10 (50.0)	4 (0.4)	3 (75.0)	8 (0.9)	7 (87.5)	6 (0.7)	1 (16.7)	38 (2.2)	21 (55.3)
CoV	7 (0.8)	6 (85.7)	1 (0.1)	0 (0.0)	1 (0.1)	1 (100.0)	2 (0.2)	1 (50.0)	11 (0.6)	8 (72.7)
HBoV	62 (6.9)	26 (41.9)	19 (2.1)	10 (52.6)	44 (4.9)	23 (52.3)	24 (2.7)	13 (54.2)	149 (8.4)	72 (48.3)
HRV	95 (20.4)[d]	47 (49.4)	17 (3.7)	7 (41.2)	27 (5.8)	22 (81.5)	44 (9.5)	14 (31.8)	183 (23.0)[e]	90 (49.2)

[a]Case number and percentage by age group
[b]Case number and percentage among all positive cases
[c]Co-infection cases of each virus detected and percentages of number of positive cases
[d]Positive cases in the group that were analyzed for HRV was 465
[e]HRV was analyzed in 795 samples (HRV testing was added in 2012)

Table 2 Common combinations of analyzed pathogens

	No.
Virus Combinations	
RSV + PIV	40
RSV + ADV	25
RSV + HRV	23
PIV + HBoV	18
HBoV+HRV	14
RSV + PIV + HRV	9
Virus/Bacteria Combinations	
RSV + *S. pneumoniae*	22
RSV + *K. pneumoniae*	16
IFV + *S. pneumoniae*	12
HRV+ *S. pneumoniae*	11
HRV+ *K. pneumoniae*	10

($P = 0.007$) than younger children (less than 1 year of age). In the virus-positive group, infants with viral co-infections had a significantly higher proportion of tachypnea ($P = 0.033$) than that with single viral infections.

Demographic and clinical features for each analyzed respiratory virus were also examined. PIV and ADV were usually recognized in children aged from 6 to 12 months, whereas HBoV was mostly found in 1 to 3 years group, while HRV was found in all age groups (Table 1). PIV was associated with fever, cough and expectoration while HRV with cough, expectoration and diarrhea (Data not shown).

Among children tested for respiratory bacteria, older children had higher proportion of bacterial infections than infants ($P = 0.010$). *K. pneumoniae* was usually detected in infants and *S. pneumoniae, H. influenzae* were more common in older children. Infants with bacterial infections had higher proportion of cough ($P < 0.001$) and expectoration ($P = 0.048$).

Among 1728 children (with complete viral and bacterial workups), infants identified with any pathogen (Table 4) had higher proportions of fever ($P < 0.001$), cough ($P < 0.001$), runny nose ($P = 0.011$), expectoration ($P < 0.001$) and diarrhea ($P = 0.009$) than infants that were not. Pathogen-positive older children had a higher proportion of chest pain ($P = 0.037$). In the pathogen positive group, infants with viral/bacterial co-infection had significantly higher proportions of cough ($P = 0.007$) and tachypnea ($P = 0.025$).

Considering diagnoses and etiology, pneumonia was taken into consideration. Older children had significantly higher proportion of pneumonia ($P < 0.001$) than infants, with the highest rate observed in children 1 to 3 years of age. Infants identified with bacterial had a higher proportion of pneumonia than older children, and *S. aureus* ($P = 0.004$) and *S. pneumonia* ($P = 0.009$) were associated with pneumonia.

Seasonal distributions

Seasonal distributions of respiratory pathogens were estimated by admission dates for the included children. The seasonal detection rates ranged from 7.4 to 79.7% with a mean rate of 49.5%. Overall, viral infections were more likely to occur in winter months (December to February) with a decline in summer months (June to August) (Fig. 1). The same distribution was observed for ADV (Fig. 2). PIV and HRV were detected all year, with their detection peaks often in autumn. HBoV infections showed a peak in the summer season of 2010 and 2012. No regular seasonal variations with IFV and HPMV were observed during the study period.

Discussion

To the best of our knowledge, this study is the first study to investigate the role of 8 respiratory viruses and 6 respiratory bacteria in ARIs among hospitalized children in Chengdu district, west China over a 5-year period. Therefore, these findings may be useful nationally and internationally equally.

The results confirmed a frequent viral etiology among 51% of children aged < 6 years presenting ARIs. A review of studies on positive proportions of respiratory viruses among

Table 3 Clinical characteristics in infants with viral or bacterial workups

Clinical characteristics	Any Virus $n = 544$	No Virus $n = 448$	*P* Value	Any Bacteria $n = 241$	No Bacteria $n = 773$	*P* Value
Fever (> 37.5 °C)	208 (38.2)	108 (24.1)	0.000**	85 (35.3)	239 (30.9)	0.235
Cough	366 (67.3)	177 (39.5)	0.000**	171 (71.0)	379 (49.0)	0.000**
Runny nose	71 (13.1)	34 (7.6)	0.007**	28 (11.6)	76 (9.8)	0.465
Expectoration	146 (26.8)	66 (14.7)	0.000**	63 (26.1)	154 (19.9)	0.048*
Tachypnea	95 (17.5)	66 (14.7)	0.261	35 (14.5)	126 (16.3)	0.546
Dyspnea	93 (17.1)	94 (21.0)	0.122	47 (19.5)	145 (18.8)	0.851
Diarrhea	70 (12.9)	38 (8.5)	0.031*	27 (11.2)	85 (11.0)	1.000
Pneumonia	279 (51.3)	211 (47.1)	0.189	143 (59.3)	361 (46.7)	0.001**

* $P < 0.05$, ** $P < 0.01$

Table 4 Clinical characteristics in infants with complete viral and bacterial workups

Clinical characteristics	Any Pathogen $n = 332$	No Pathogen $n = 653$	*P* Value	Virus Alone $n = 412$	Bacteria Alone $n = 113$	Virus/Baccteria Co-infection $n = 128$	*P* Value
Fever (> 37.5 °C)	69 (20.8)	243 (37.2)	0.000**	158 (38.3)	37 (32.7)	48 (37.5)	0.559
Cough	105 (31.6)	433 (66.3)	0.000**	262 (63.6)	71 (62.8)	100 (78.1)	0.007**
Runny nose	23 (6.9)	80 (12.3)	0.011*	52 (12.6)	10 (8.8)	18 (14.1)	0.455
Expectoration	44 (13.3)	166 (25.4)	0.000**	103 (25.0)	22 (19.5)	41 (32.0)	0.077
Tachypnea	57 (17.2)	104 (15.9)	0.649	69 (16.7)	9 (8.0)	26 (20.3)	0.025*
Dyspnea	69 (20.8)	117 (17.9)	0.301	70 (17.0)	25 (22.1)	22 (17.2)	0.445
Diarrhea	24 (7.2)	83 (12.7)	0.009**	56 (13.6)	13 (11.5)	14 (10.9)	0.680
Pneumonia	341 (52.2)	146 (44.0)	0.014*	198 (48.1)	64 (56.6)	79 (61.7)	0.002**

* $P < 0.05$, ** $P < 0.01$

patients with ARIs in different parts of China, such as Beijing [14] Shanghai [11], Shenzhen [12], Wuhan [21], Lanzhou [22], indicated high variability. Different incidences may be attributed to different age groups, samples collected, inclusion criteria, diagnostic methods, target pathogens and seasonality.

IFV, RSV, HPMV and HRV were the most commonly detected viruses in most regions. HRV and RSV were equally predominant in our study period. RSV is a major respiratory virus that causes respiratory illness including bronchiolitis, pneumonia, and wheezing [23]. RSV may bring about annual epidemics worldwide because of virus variability [24]. It is reported that RSV epidemic was associated with the alternate circulation of multiple genotypes and with the change of G protein [25]. HRV are usually associated with upper respiratory tract infections and are responsible for one half of all "common colds" [26]. The implementation of molecular methods has revealed HRV as an etiologic agent in lower respiratory tract infections (LRTI), associated with recurrent wheezing and asthma in infancy [26, 27].

Clinical presentations of respiratory infections may be overlapping and could not discriminate between respiratory viruses. However, infants identified with respiratory virus tended to have more severe symptoms, particularly those in the 7–12 months of age group. Age and exposure were two crucial factors for infection [8]. Immune status of infants is different from adults, and the amount of maternal antibodies attenuate distinctly, which would make infants susceptible to respiratory viral infections. The onset of disease is an interplay of immune pathology and viral pathology and prevention measures need to be taken into account [28].

It has been suggested that multiplex PCR techniques demonstrate a high detection rate of viral co-infections [29]. In this target population, mixed respiratory virus had

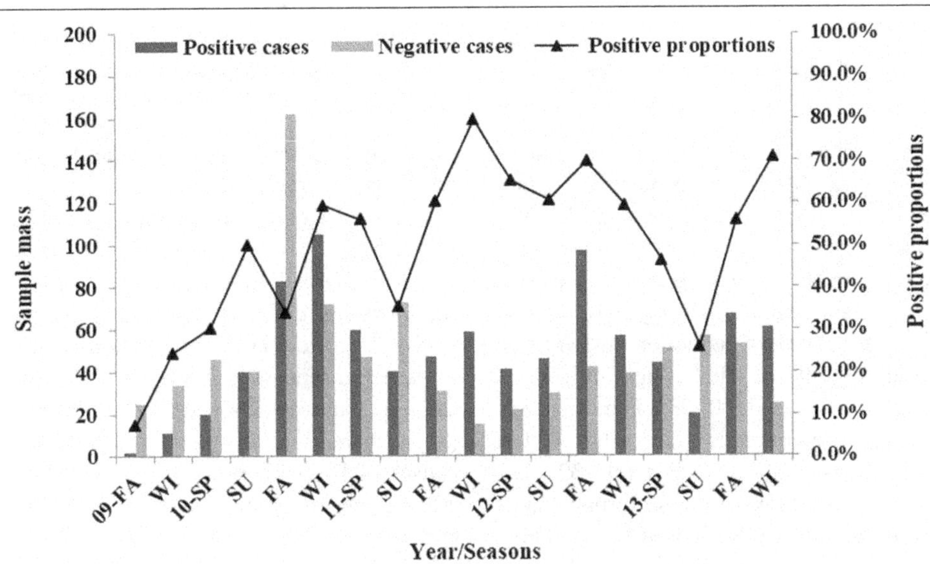

Fig. 1 Seasonal distribution of ARIs in hospitalized children, Nov 2009 - Feb 2014. Spring (SP); Summer (SU); Fall (FA); Winter (WI)

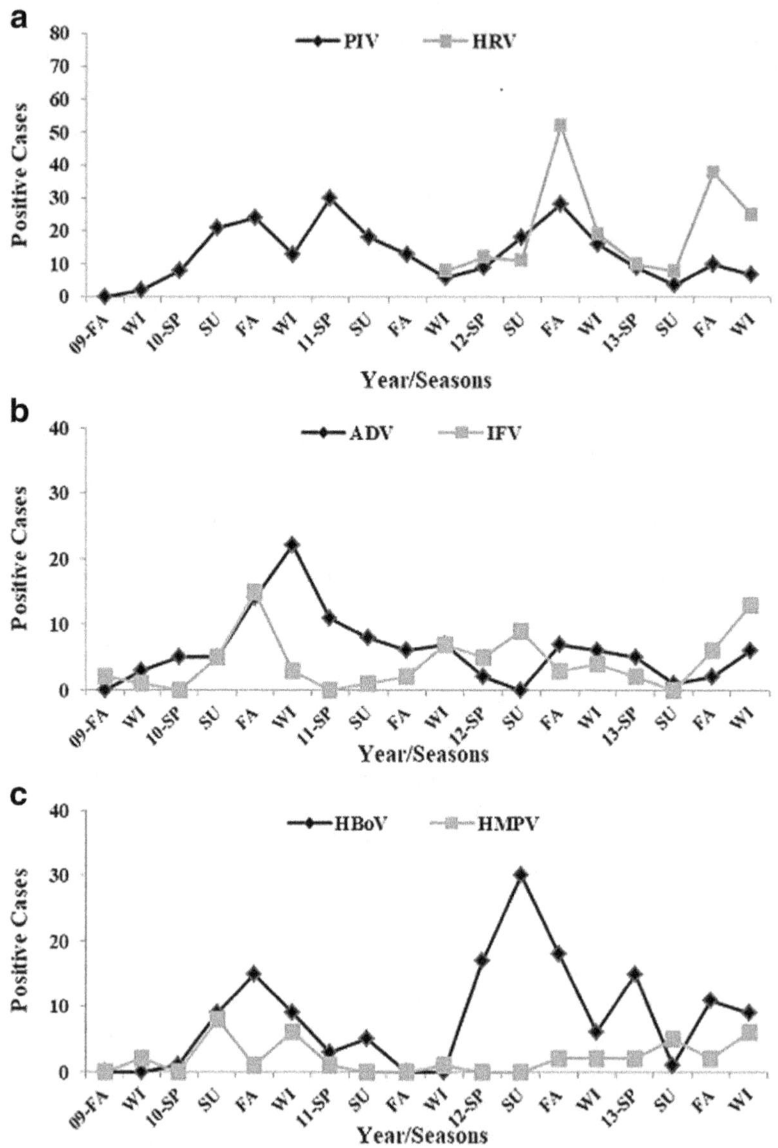

Fig. 2 Seasonal distributions of respiratory viruses in hospitalized children, Nov 2009- Feb 2014. Spring (SP); Summer (SU); Fall (FA); Winter (WI)

a proportion of 14.9%, with RSV/PIV the most frequent combination. Previous research showed proportions of viral co-infection ranged from 4.0 to 24.7%, with RSV, IFV, HPMV the common viruses present in co-infections. Different incidence of co-infection may be due to high single infection rates of certain viruses, overlapping epidemic seasons, target pathogens as well as methodology. Evidence for increased clinical severity of viral single infections versus co-infections is controversial [30–33]. The impact of co-infection on clinical presentations may rely on the specific agent involved, as well as viral load [32, 33]. Experimental studies of simultaneous respiratory infections are scarce. However, one study showed by mathematical modeling, found that one virus can block replication of another due to competition for resources, which may have implications for the treatment regimens of simultaneous viral infections [34].

Despite vaccination, pneumonia still remains a serious public health issue in the world [35]. In this study, children > 1 year seemed to suffer more from bacterial infections than younger children. The WHO reports that pneumonia is the forgotten killer of children and one of the main disease burdens worldwide [36]. Pneumonia is the most serious result of ARIs and is often due to bacterial infection [37]. *S. pneumoniae, H. influenzae type b* are the leading causes of bacterial pneumonia in children worldwide [38, 39]. Under-nutrition, lack of breast-feeding, crowding, exposure to indoor air pollution, low birth weight and diarrhea have been identified as risk factors for pneumonia [40, 41]. Etiologic studies could provide information on the prevalence of bacterial infections, which may help achieve a reduction in child mortality.

The incidence of respiratory viral/bacterial co-infection in young children ranged from 1 to 44% [42]. In the current study, we observed a respiratory viral/bacterial co-infection proportion of 13.9% (240/1728). *S.pneumoniae, S. aureus, H. influenzae* and *Pseudomonas* species were common bacterial co-pathogens. Influenza pandemics over the last 100 years have strengthened the association of bacterial super-infection and influenza infection [42, 43]. There are mounting data indicating that virus infection can predispose to bacterial colonization and overgrowth, which adversely affect the pathogenesis of respiratory infections [44, 45]. Disruption of the epithelial barrier, up regulation of adhesion proteins, production of viral factors and alterations in immune responses are several known mechanisms [44, 45]. Increased morbidity with bacterial co-infections was found in children, leading to increased duration of mechanical ventilation, longer hospital stays and admission to pediatric intensive care units [42, 46]. However, the statistical association was weak and sporadic in some studies, and additional longitudinal cohort studies may be needed to reveal the contribution of bacterial to viral ARIs.

There was a paucity of study that was conducted for etiologies of ARIs among hospitalized children in this area. Including 14 different respiratory pathogens (both viruses and bacteria), recruiting almost 2000 hospitalized children, over 5-year period, this current study revealed pathogens profiles, co-infection pattern, clinical features, and seasonality among hospitalized children with ARIs in Chengdu, west China. There are however some limitations in this study. Outpatients were not recruited and the study lacked an asymptomatic control group. Positive rates may be somewhat lower as other potential viral pathogens were not included (e.g. enteroviruses, HCoV NL63 and HKU1). In addition, virus genotyping and strain identification (such as HRV A/B/C) would be helpful for understanding viral epidemics and associated disease severity.

Conclusions

In conclusion, this 5-year consecutive surveillance research confirmed that respiratory viruses, especially RSV and HRV, were the leading potential cause of ARIs in hospitalized children in Chengdu, west China. Co-infections were associated with severity of illness in infants, who tended to have increased risks of ARIs. This study gives us better information on the pathogen profiles, clinical association, co-infection combinations, and seasonal features of ARIs in hospitalized children in this area. Moreover, future efforts in reducing the impact of ARIs will depend on a commitment to fund and implement programs to utilize available vaccines, especially vaccines on RSV, HRV and *S. pneumoniae* in in this region, and to develop new vaccines against common pathogens.

Abbreviations

ADV: Human adenovirus; ARI: Acute respiratory infection; HBoV: Human bocavirus; HCoV: Human coronavirus; HMPV: Human metapneumovirus; HRV: Human rhinovirus; IFV: Influenza virus; LRTI: Lower respiratory tract infection; PCR: Polymerase chain reaction; PIV: Parainfluenza virus; RSV: Respiratory syncytial virus

Acknowledgements

We gratefully thank to all patients who participated in this study, and to Research Center for Public Health and Preventive Medicine, West China School of Public Health, Sichuan University for providing experimental resources.

Funding

This study was supported by National Mega Projects of Science and Technology in 13th Five-Year Plan of China: Technical Platform for Communicable Disease Surveillance Project (2017ZX10103010-002).

Authors' contributions

PXF and CJY designed the research; CJY, HPW, ZT, ZTL, ZLX, JCP performed the research and acquired data; CJY, HPW, ZT, ZTL analyzed the data; CJY, HPW, ZT, ZTL, JCP and PXF wrote the paper; JCP and PXF revised the manuscript; PXF approved the final version to be published. All authors read and approved the final manuscript.

Competing interests

The authors declare that they have no competing interests.

Author details

[1]Department of Public Health Laboratory Sciences, West China School of Public Health (No.4 West China Teaching Hospital), Sichuan University, 16#, Section 3, Renmin Road South, Chengdu 610041, Sichuan, People's Republic of China. [2]Research Center for Occupational Respiratory Diseases, West China School of Public Health (No.4 West China Teaching Hospital), Sichuan University, 16#, Section 3, Renmin Road South, Chengdu 610041, Sichuan, China. [3]Shenzhen Nanshan Center for Disease Control and Prevention, 95#, Nanshang Road, Shenzhen 518054, Guangdong, China. [4]Chongqing Yuzhong District Center for Disease Control and Prevention, 254#, Heping Road, Yuzhong District, Chongqing 400010, China.

References

1. Shi T, McLean K, Campbell H, Nair H. Aetiological role of common respiratory viruses in acute lower respiratory infections in children under five years: A systematic review and meta-analysis. J Glob Health. 2015;5:010408.
2. Nair H, Simões EAF, Rudan I, Gessner BD, Azziz-Baumgartner E, et al. Global and regional burden of hospital admissions for severe acute lower respiratory infections in young children in 2010: a systematic analysis. Lancet. 2013;381:1380–90.
3. Rudan I, Chan KY, Zhang JSF, Theodoratou E, Feng XL, et al. Causes of death in children younger than 5 years in China in 2008. Lancet. 2010;375:1083–9.
4. Liu L, Oza S, Hogan D, Perin J, Rudan I, et al. Global, regional, and national causes of child mortality in 2000–13, with projections to inform post-2015 priorities: an updated systematic analysis. Lancet. 2015;385:430–40.
5. Doan Q, Enarson P, Kissoon N, Klassen TP, Johnson DW. Rapid viral diagnosis for acute febrile respiratory illness in children in the Emergency Department. Cochrane Database Syst Rev. 2014;15(9):CD006452.

6. Sung RY, Chan PK, Tsen T, Li AM, Lam WY, et al. Identification of viral and atypical bacterial pathogens in children hospitalized with acute respiratory infections in Hong Kong by multiplex PCR assays. J Med Virol. 2009;81:153–9.
7. Ruuskanen O, Lahti E, Jennings LC, Murdoch DR. Viral pneumonia. Lancet. 2011;377:1264–75.
8. Tregoning JS, Schwarze J. Respiratory viral infections in infants: causes, clinical symptoms, virology, and immunology. Clin Microbiol Rev. 2010;23: 74–98.
9. Zhang Y, Yuan L, Zhang Y, Zhang X, Zheng M, et al. Burden of respiratory syncytial virus infections in China: Systematic review and meta-analysis. J Glob Health. 2015;5:020417.
10. Nair H, Brooks WA, Katz M, Roca A, Berkley JA, et al. Global burden of respiratory infections due to seasonal influenza in young children: a systematic review and meta-analysis. Lancet. 2011;378:1917–30.
11. Dong W, Chen Q, Hu Y, He D, Liu J, et al. Epidemiological and clinical characteristics of respiratory viral infections in children in Shanghai. China Arch Virol. 2016;161:1907–13.
12. Wang H, Zheng Y, Deng J, Wang W, Liu P, et al. Prevalence of respiratory viruses among children hospitalized from respiratory infections in Shenzhen. China Virol J. 2016;13:39.
13. Cai X, Wang Q, Lin G, Cai Z, Lin C-X, et al. Respiratory Virus Infections Among Children in South China. J Med Virol. 2014;86:1249–55.
14. Zhang C, Zhu N, Xie Z, Lu R, He B, et al. Viral etiology and clinical profiles of children with severe acute respiratory infections in China. PLoS One. 2013;8: e72606.
15. Jiao W. Analysis on Influenza Vaccination Status in Chengdu, 2010–2013. J Prev Med Inf. 2015;31:688–90.
16. Coiras M, Pérez-Breña P, García M, Casas I. Simultaneous detection of influenza A, B, and C viruses, respiratory syncytial virus, and adenoviruses in clinical samples by multiplex reverse transcription nested-PCR assay. J Med Virol. 2003;69:132–44.
17. Coiras MT, Aguilar JC, García ML, Casas I, Pérez-Breña P. Simultaneous detection of fourteen respiratory viruses in clinical specimens by two multiplex reverse transcription nested-PCR assays. J Med Virol. 2004;72:484–95.
18. Allard A, Girones R, Juto P, Wadell G. Polymerase chain reaction for detection of adenoviruses in stools samples. J Clin Microbiol. 1991;29:2683.
19. Woo PCY, Lau SKP, Chu C-M, Chan K-H, Tsoi H-W, et al. Characterization and complete genome sequence of a novel coronavirus, coronavirus HKU1, from patients with pneumonia. J Virol. 2005;79:884–95.
20. Kapoor A, Simmonds P, Slikas E, Li L, Bodhidatta L, et al. Human Bocaviruses Are Highly Diverse, Dispersed Recombination Prone, and Prevalent in Enteric Infections. J Infect Dis. 2010;201:1633–43.
21. Liu J, Ai H, Xiong Y, Li F, Wen Z, et al. Prevalence and correlation of infectious agents in hospitalized children with acute respiratory tract infections in Central China. PLoS One. 2015;10:e0119170.
22. Jin Y, Zhang RF, Xie ZP, Yan KL, Gao HC, et al. Newly identified respiratory viruses associated with acute lower respiratory tract infections in children in Lanzou, China, from 2006 to 2009. Clin Microbiol Infect. 2012;18:74–80.
23. Nair H, Nokes DJ, Gessner BD, Dherani M, Madhi SA, et al. Global burden of acute lower respiratory infections due to respiratory syncytial virus in young children: a systematic review and meta-analysis. Lancet. 2010;375:1545–55.
24. Agoti CN, Mwihuri AG, Sande CJ, Onyango CO, Medley GF, et al. Genetic relatedness of infecting and reinfecting respiratory syncytial virus strains identified in a birth cohort from rural Kenya. J Infect Dis. 2012;206:1532–41.
25. Hu P, Zheng T, Chen J, Zhou T, Chen Y, et al. Alternate circulation and genetic variation of human respiratory syncytial virus genotypes in Chengdu, West China, 2009–2014. J Med Virol. 2017;89:32–40.
26. Jacobs SE, Lamson DM, St George K, Walsh TJ. Human rhinoviruses. Clin Microbiol Rev. 2013;26:135–62.
27. Message SD, Laza-Stanca V, Mallia P, Parker HL, Zhu J, et al. Rhinovirus-induced lower respiratory illness is increased in asthma and related to virus load and Th1/2 cytokine and IL-10 production. Proc Natl Acad Sci U S A. 2008;105:13562–7.
28. Gern JE, Brooks GD, Meyer P, Chang A, Shen K, et al. Bidirectional interactions between viral respiratory illnesses and cytokine responses in the first year of life. J Allergy Clin Immunol. 2006;117:72–8.
29. Cilla G, Onate E, Perez-Yarza EG, Montes M, Vicente D, et al. Viruses in community-acquired pneumonia in children aged less than 3 years old: High rate of viral coinfection. J Med Virol. 2008;80:1843–9.
30. Asner SA, Science ME, Tran D, Smieja M, Merglen A, et al. Clinical disease severity of respiratory viral co-infection versus single viral infection: a systematic review and meta-analysis. PLoS One. 2014;9:e99392.
31. Franz A, Adams O, Willems R, Bonzel L, Neuhausen N, et al. Correlation of viral load of respiratory pathogens and co-infections with disease severity in children hospitalized for lower respiratory tract infection. J Clin Virol. 2010; 48:239–45.
32. Martin ET, Kuypers J, Wald A, Englund JA. Multiple versus single virus respiratory infections: viral load and clinical disease severity in hospitalized children. Influenza Other Respir Viruses. 2012;6:71–7.
33. Goka EA, Vallely PJ, Mutton KJ, Klapper PE. Single, dual and multiple respiratory virus infections and risk of hospitalization and mortality. Epidemiol Infect. 2015;143:37–47.
34. Pinky L, Dobrovolny HM. Coinfections of the Respiratory Tract: Viral Competition for Resources. PLoS One. 2016;11:e0155589.
35. Nohynek H, Madhi S, Grijalva CG. Childhood bacterial respiratory diseases: past, present, and future. Pediatr Infect Dis J. 2009;28:S127–32.
36. UNICEF. Pneumonia The Forgotten Killer of Children. New York and Geneva: UNICEF/WHO; 2006.
37. Ma HM, Lee KP, Woo J. Predictors of viral pneumonia: The need for viral testing in all patients hospitalized for nursing home-acquired pneumonia. Geriatr Gerontol Int. 2013;13:949–57.
38. Watt JP, Wolfson LJ, o'Brien KL, Henkle E. knoll MD, et al. Burden of disease caused by Haemophilus influenzae type b in children younger than 5 years: global estimates. Lancet. 2009;374:903–11.
39. O'Brien KL, Wolfson LJ, Watt JP, Henkle E, Deloria-Knoll M, et al. Burden of disease caused by Streptococcus pneumoniae in children younger than 5 years: global estimates. Lancet. 2009;374:893–902.
40. Walker CLF, Rudan I, Liu L, Nair H, Theodoratou E, et al. Global burden of childhood pneumonia and diarrhoea. Lancet. 2013;381:1405–16.
41. Poll Tvd OSM. Pathogenesis, treatment, and prevention of pneumococcal pneumonia. Lancet. 2009;374:1543–56.
42. Thorburn K, Riordan A. Pulmonary bacterial coinfection in infants and children with viral respiratory infection. Expert Rev Anti-Infect Ther. 2012;10:909–16.
43. McCullers JA. The co-pathogenesis of influenza viruses with bacteria in the lung. Nat Rev Microbiol. 2014;12:252–62.
44. Bosch AA, Biesbroek G, Trzcinski K, Sanders EA, Bogaert D. Viral and bacterial interactions in the upper respiratory tract. PLoS Pathog. 2013;9:e1003057.
45. Hendaus MA, Jomha FA, Alhammadi AH. Virus-induced secondary bacterial infection: a concise review. Ther Clin Risk Manag. 2015;11:1265–71.
46. Nguyen T, Kyle UG, Jaimon N, Tcharmtchi MH, Coss-Bu JA, et al. Coinfection with *Staphylococcus aureus* increases risk of severe coagulopathy in critically ill children with influenza A (H1N1) virus infection. Crit Care Med. 2012;40: 3246–50.

22

YKL-40 levels are associated with disease severity and prognosis of viral pneumonia, but not available in bacterial pneumonia in children

Xingge Yang and Guangyao Sheng*

Abstract

Background: Viral pneumonia is the main type of community-acquired pneumonia (CAP) in children. YKL-40, a chitinase-like protein, is regarded as a biomarker of the degree of inflammation.

Methods: Children who were diagnosed with CAP, including viral pneumonia, bacterial pneumonia, and dual infection, were included in the cohort study. The pathogenic diagnosis depended on PCR and immunoassay test. YKL-40 levels were examined twice by enzyme-linked immunoassay (ELISA).

Results: Serum YKL-40 levels were higher in patients with pneumonia than in healthy controls. The admission levels of YKL-40 in serum and Bronchoalveolar lavage (BALFs) indicated a positive correlation with the serum levels of C-reactive protein and other inflammatory cytokines (IL-6 and TNF-α). The disease severity have no correlation with the admission serum levels of YKL-40. Meanwhile, reductions in YKL-40 levels from initial admission levels to day 5 post-admission were correlated with disease severity. The multiple logistic analysis indicated the decreased extent of serum YKL-40 level as an independent prognostic predictor of severe cases in patients with viral pneumonia.

Conclusions: Reductions in serum YKL-40 levels on day 5 after receiving therapy is a possible prognostic biomarker for children with viral pneumonia.

Keywords: YKL-40, Children pneumonia, Biomarker

Background

Worldwide, 450 million patients are diagnosed with pneumonia, and approximately 4 million people die from this illness each year [1–3]. It is estimated that 156 million cases in children occur annually, and of these, 151 million occur in developing countries such as China [1]. Viral pneumonia is the most common community-acquired pneumonia (CAP) and a cause of lung infection in children. Approximately, 100 million cases occur every year in children, which accounts for the majority of patients with viral pneumonia [2]. The prognosis depends on various risk factors, including age, immune status, co-infection with bacterial pathogens and the type of pathogenic virus [4, 5]. The first evaluation as recommended by WHO paper cited by the authors should rely on clinical signs and symptoms, the requirement of supplemental oxygen administration and or ventilatory support, still lacking a rapid and safe method to ensure a diagnosis, exception made for bronchoalveolar lavage or lung biopsy [6].

But the study about the biomarker for evaluation of disease severity and prognosis is still infrequent, which lead to that pediatrician failed to precisely estimate the prognosis. Thus more intensive therapy including admission to the intensive care unit (ICU) more positively and preventive use of antibiotic drugs are not performed. Therefore, it is crucial for clinicians to investigate the

* Correspondence: shengguangyaoo@163.com
Pediatrics, the First Affiliated Hospital of Zhengzhou University, No. 1 East Jianshe Road, Zhengzhou 450052, Henan, China

biomarkers applicable for the prediction and assessment of prognosis.

YKL-40 is a chitinase-like protein and regarded as a pro-inflammatory cytokine mainly secreted by macrophages, which are involved in the inflammatory response and tissue injury [7, 8]. Hsiang-Ling Wang et al. have revealed that the prognostic value in a cohort of adult CAP and the plasma level of YKL-40 is positively correlated with the severity of CAP depicted by pneumonia severity index (PSI) and CURB-65 score [9]. YKL-40 has been recognized as a prognostic biomarker for ILD (interstitial lung disease) [10, 11]. Its role as a predictor of outcome in hypersensitivity pneumonia (HP) has also been proved in a recent HP cohort study [12]. But its role in predicting the prognosis of children with pneumonia, especially those with viral pneumonia, is not known.

The aim of present aim is to prove the clinical utility value of YKL-40 in BALF in children with pneumonia. Our study suggest that a clinician could evaluate their patient's prognosis with two consecutive measurements of their YKL-40 serum levels, immediately after admission and day 5 after therapy initiation.

Materials and method

Study subjects and design

Children who were diagnosed with CAP, including viral pneumonia, bacterial pneumonia, and dual infection, were consecutively enrolled and their demographic and clinical data were retrospectively analyzed. The age of all children enrolled in the retrospectively study is ranging from 0.8 to 9.6. The mean age was 2.3 years old. The serum levels of YKL-40 in admission and at 5th day after therapy were measured. The clinical outcomes (including the incidence of entrance of ICU, mechanical ventilation and sepsis) and diseased severity was recorded. The correlation between admission levels of YKL-40 or decreased percentage after therapy and clinical prognosis in children with viral infection, bacterial infection and co-infection were analyzed and described respectively. The children who had a history of asthma, or immunodeficiency disease were excluded. The diagnosis of pneumonia was based on clinical characteristics, biochemical examination, cough, fever, and radiography. The diagnostic criteria of pneumonia included the presence of inflammatory exudation (alveolar or interstitial) by the chest X-ray with the simultaneous clinical manifestation of pulmonary infection, including fever, cough and difficult breathing. All patients diagnosed with pneumonia received the standard therapy according to the relevant guidelines for the CAP management in children and adult patients [13, 14].

All children or healthy volunteers enrolled in this study were in-patients at our institution from 2014 to 2017. The healthy volunteers included the out-patient children with no evidence of inflammation-related disease requiring a medical examination and collection of serum or blood samples. The retrospective observation study was approved by Medical ethic committee of the First Affiliated Hospital of Zhengzhou University. Informed consent was obtained from all study subjects.

Pathogenic diagnosis

The sputum specimen was collected from children patients with pneumonia once the diagnosis was verified by chest X-ray. Gram stain, sputum culture were performed for the detection of specific bacterial strains including the *Pneumococcus* and *Haemophilus influenzae* as has been previously described [15]. The diagnosis of viral infection depended on the detection of the viral antigen by quantitative real-time PCR or multiplex RT-PCR following the standard protocols [16]. RNA was extracted from sputum specimens using Trizol (Invitrogen, USA). cDNA was synthesized by reverse transcription. The cyclic temperature settings were 95 °C, 30 s; 60 °C, 30 s; 65 °C, 30 s; amplified by 40 cycles with the last at 65 °C for 7 min. Human cytomegalovirus (CMV), adenovirus (AV) and parainfluenza virus(PIV) was assayed by fluorescent real-time PCR (BIO-RAD iCycler). For CMV detection, the forward and reverse primers were CMV-F: 5′-AACTGTACGTGCTG TGTGTACTAACTC-3′ and CMV-R: 5′-CTCGATAAT GCGTTGTGCACCCCATAA-3′, respectively. For AV detection, the primers were AV-F: 5′-TGCGTAGTA GCCCTGGTGAA -3′; AV-R:5′-CATGTAGCGTGGTC GATGGTTC-3′; HPIVs-R: AGGTGACCGTGGGT CCACATG;HPIVs-F:ACTGTAGTAGGTTGTAGCTAG. The cyclic temperature settings were 95 °C, 30 s; 60 °C, 30 s; 70 °C, 30 s; amplified, 40 cycles.

Definition of endpoint events and evaluation of diseased severity

The endpoint event for prognostic evaluation is the the incidence of sepsis secondary to pneumonia, use of mechanical ventilation and admission in Intensive Care Unit. The disease severity of the pneumonia was determined by the WHO recommended child pneumonia classification standard and based on clinical signs as previously mentioned, including the non-severe pneumonia, severe pneumonia and very severe pneumonia [17, 18]. To overcome the limitation of disease assessment by relying solely on the admission levels of YKL-40, we detected the levels of YLK-40 in the serum twice, immediately and on day 5 after admission. We calculated the reduction degree represented by the decreased percentage of YKL-40 levels on day 5 after receiving therapy and then ranked the reduction degree as follows: low group, ≤20%; median group, > 20% but ≤50%; and high group > 50%).

YKL-40 and other inflammatory cytokine assays

BALF was collected via fiber optic bronchoscope as previously described [19]. The patient's serum was collected twice, in admission (once the diagnosis was made immediately and prior to commencement of therapy) and on day 5 after admission. YKL-40 and other inflammatory cytokines, including C-reactive protein, interleukin (IL)-6, IL-10, and TNF-α, were examined in serum and BALF samples by enzyme-linked immunoassay (ELISA). The serum levels of YKL-40 were repeatedly measured respectively in admission and at 5th day after admission. The levels of BALF was measured only on admission.

Mechanical ventilation

For children with severe pneumonia, the mechanical ventilation was applied according to synchronized intermittent mandatory ventilation (SIMV) combination with positive end expiratory pressure (PEEP). The tidal volume was kept in 10-12 ml/kg in these children. The weaning from mechanical ventilation was according to the improvement of blood oxygen saturation (FiO2 > 350) and normalization of respiratory rate (< 30 times /min) in autonomous respiration.

Statistical analysis

Data were analyzed using SPSS software (SPSS, IL, USA) and were presented as the mean ± SD. The comparison between two groups was conducted by the Student t-test or Wilcoxon's rank test for continuous variables and the Chi-squared or Fisher's exact test for categorical variables. ANOVA was used for the multiple-group comparison. To overcome the limitation of disease assessment by relying solely on the admission levels of YKL-40, we detected the levels of YLK-40 in the serum twice, immediately and on day 5 after admission. We calculated the reduction degree represented by the decreased percentage of YKL-40 levels on day 5 after receiving therapy and then ranked the reduction degree as follows: low group, ≤20%; median group, > 20% but ≤50%; and high group > 50%) for the Spearman's correlation analysis between the reduction degree of serum levels of YKL-40 and diseased severity. Spearman's correlation coefficient was obtained for correlation analysis. Univariate and multiple logistic regression analyses were used to analyze the prognostic factors. A *p*-value of < 0.05 was considered as statistically significant.

Results

Characteristics of study subjects

Total of 321 subjects were enrolled in this study, including 50 healthy volunteers. The demographic characteristics and laboratory data of the study subjects are shown in Table 1. Regarding the age of the study subjects, no significant differences were found among the groups, including the sole viral, bacterial, and dual infection groups. The disease severity was divided into three classes according to the World Health Organization classification of pneumonia. At baseline, none of the subjects were receiving treatment with corticosteroids; they were all enrolled at the time of diagnosis before receiving therapy. The infection by *Pneumococcus* was detected in the 145 children and the infection by *Haemophilus influenzae* was detected in 67 children with pneumonia by sputum examination including direct smearing and sputum culture. The AV, CMV and HPIVs infection was found in 35, 45, 63 children respectively, which indicated that the HPIVs is the major viral pathogen in children viral pneumonia in our institution.

Admission YKL-40 levels in serum and BALFs of children with CAP

Compared with the healthy controls, serum levels of YKL-40 in children with pneumonia was significantly higher (Fig. 1a). To verify the type of pneumonia was distinguished by YKL-40 levels in the serum or BALF, we compared the levels of YKL-40 in serum and BALF samples in the viral pneumonia and bacterial pneumonia groups (Fig. 1b). We observed no significant difference between the admission levels of YKL-40 in the serum of patients with viral pneumonia, bacterial pneumonia, or co-infection. But the levels of YKL-40 in the BALF specimens of patients with bacterial pneumonia were however significantly higher than those with sole viral pneumonia ($P = 0.012$), and the levels of YKL-40 in the BALF specimens were statistically higher than in the serum specimens from the same individuals ($P = 0.007$). However, in the sole viral pneumonia group, increased levels of YKL-40 in the BALF specimens as compared with the serum specimens was not observed.

The correlation between admission levels of YKL-40 and other inflammatory biomarkers

The levels of IL-6, TNF-α, and C-reactive protein were positively correlated with the serum levels of YKL-40, but the IL-10 levels were negatively correlated with YKL-40 levels in all 3 pneumonia subgroups (Fig. 2a). These results provide evidence that the YKL-40 is a pro-inflammatory cytokine accelerating tissue injury and might have an adverse effect on tissue repair and inflammation resolution. The levels of YKL-40 in the BALF specimens were also slightly positively correlated with the serum levels of C-reactive protein but not with the levels of IL-6 and TNF-α in all study subjects (Fig. 2b).

The correlation between admission serum levels of YKL-40 and the disease severity of viral pneumonia

The correlation between the admission serum levels of YKL-40 and severity of pneumonia was analyzed using

Table 1 Baseline demographic and clinical characteristics of study participants

Characteristics	Healthy controls ($N=50$)	Viral Pneumonia ($N=104$)	Bacterial Pneumonia ($N=110$)	Co-infection ($N=66$)	P value[b]
Age (years)	2.3(0.8–9.6)	1.8(0.2–8.9)	2.2(1.2–12.1)	2.4(0.5–9.7)	0.38
Gender (male, %)	34(68)	66(63)	52(47)	39(59)	0.31
Serum YLK-40 (ng/ml)	6.30 ± 2.27	18.48 ± 4.63	19.38 ± 3.34	19.32 ± 2.87	< 0.001
TNF-α (pg/ml)	NA	12.4 ± 7.85	13.6 ± 9.28	14.5 ± 10.23	0.24
IL-6 (pg/ml)	NA	32.3 ± 11.25	35.6 ± 8.17	39.5 ± 12.1	0.26
hsCRP (mg/dl)	NA	161.38 ± 34.78	158.25 ± 26.90	170.93 ± 29.36	0.34
IL-10 (pg/ml)	NA	83.96 ± 14.89	95.36 ± 8.98	84.36 ± 16.98	0.07
BALFs YLK-40 (ng/ml,n)	NA	26.45 ± 3.65(18)	34.87 ± 5.42(34)	33.63 ± 2.50(21)	0.02
Severity					
Not Severe (%)	NA	55.7	47.3	51.5	0.08
Severe (%)	NA	24.6	32.7	11.2	0.12
Very Severe (%)	NA	19.7	30.0	27.3	0.13
PO_2 (mmHg)	NA	98.1 ± 1.0	97.2 ± 2.5	97.0 ± 3.6	0.41
SO_2 (mmHg)	NA	95.5 ± 1.8	94.5 ± 1.3	94.9 ± 0.9	0.55
WBC (10^9/L)	NA	9.8 ± 4.3	13.9 ± 3.5	14.2 ± 4.4	0.008
PCT (ng/ml)	NA	0.65 ± 0.26	1.33 ± 0.49	1.59 ± 0.87	0.02
Glucocorticoid use[a], n(%) a	NA	20(19.2)	14(12.8)	12(18.2)	0.43

Abbreviations: *BALF* Bronchoalveolar Lavage Fluids, *CRP* high sensitive C-reactive protein, *WBC* white blood cell, *PCT* procalcitonin

[a] Values at the period of hospitalization before colleting the serum sample at the second time

[b] P value < 0.05 was considered significant

the Spearman's correlation coefficient; no significant correlation was observed (Fig. 3a, b and c). We further performed the Spearman's correlation analysis in the different subgroups, and no obvious correlation was shown between the serum levels and disease severity, regardless of the type of pneumonia.

The reduction degree of YKL-40 serum levels after standard therapy serves as an independent risk factor of viral pneumonia in children

Previous results have demonstrated that the admission levels of YKL-40 do not correlate with the disease severity. To determine a correlation with the severity of pneumonia, a univariate correlation analysis was performed. We found a negative correlation between the reduction degree of YLK-40 levels for the severity of disease and the median length of hospital stay (Fig. 4a and b) in the viral pneumonia group, but not in the bacterial pneumonia or co-infection groups (data not shown). In other words, the higher the percentage reduction in YKL-40 levels indicated the shorter hospital stay in the children with viral pneumonia. The logistic regression analysis identified the independent prognosis factors that were associated with the mechanical

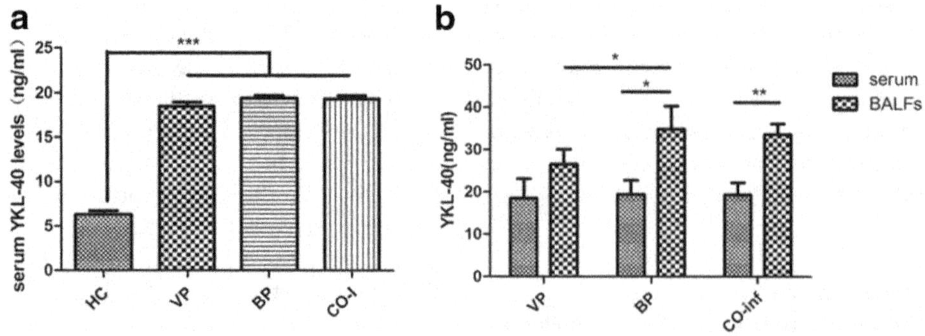

Fig. 1 The admission serum and BALFs levels of YKL-40 in healthy control and child pneumonia. **a**. The serum levels of YKL-40 in healthy volunteers and different kinds of infectious pneumonia of children. VP, viral pneumonia. BP, bacterial pneumonia. CO-I, co-infection. **b**. The difference between the serum and BALFs levels as well as the BALFs levels among the VP, BP and co-infection. All data presented by mean ± SD. *** $P < 0.001$ ** $P < 0.01$ * $P < 0.05$

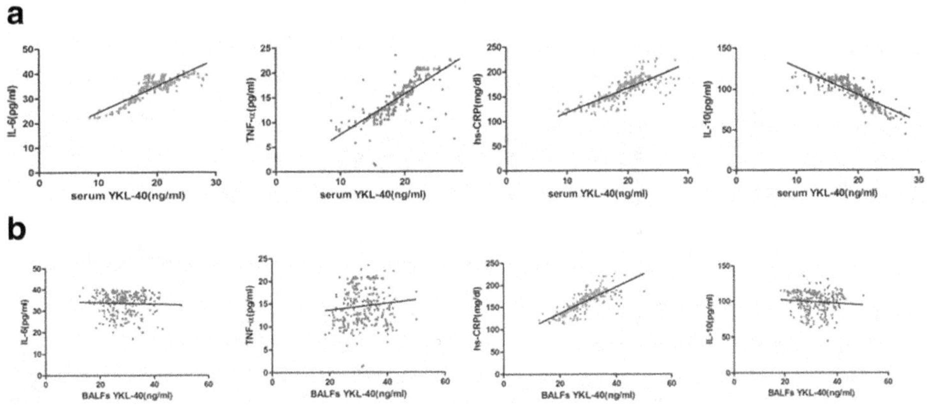

Fig. 2 The linear correlation analysis between YKL-40 levels and classic inflammatory cytokine. **a**. The correlation between serum levels of YKL-40 and proinflammatory cytokine in circulating, including respectively pro-inflammatory IL-6 ($r^2 = 0.73$, $P < 0.0001$), TNF-α ($r^2 = 0.58$, $P < 0001$), hs-CRP ($r^2 = 0.61$, $P < 0.0001$) and anti-inflammation IL-10 ($r^2 = 0.67$, $P < 0.0001$). **b**. The correlation between BALFs levels of YKL-40 and proinflammatory cytokine in circulating, respectively in IL-6 ($r^2 = 0.0019$, $P = 0.46$), TNF-α ($r^2 = 0.011$, $P = 0.0785$), hs-CRP ($r^2 = 0.084$, $P < 0.0001$) and IL-10 ($r^2 = 0.0079$, $P = 0.14$). The slight correlation only emerged in between the circulating hs-CRP levels and BALFs levels. The data represented by mean ± SD, and $P < 0{,}05$ defined as significantly statistic difference

ventilation and ICU admission rates. The factors evaluated in the multivariate logistics regression model included age, history of previous pneumonia, procalcitonin levels, degree reduction of YKL-40 levels, and infectious type (Table 2). The independent risk factors for mechanical ventilation were identified as the age, infectious type, history of previous pneumonia, and reduction degree of YKL-40 levels. The independent risk factors for ICU admission were identified as the age, infectious type, and degree reduction of YKL-40 levels. For sepsis onset, the reduction degree of YKL-40 levels was the only independent risk factor.

Discussion

The present study revealed the usefulness of YKL-40 in the prognostic assessment of child pneumonia at first, especially in viral pneumonia. Although we could not demonstrate a positive correlation between serum level of YKL-40 and disease severity, the degree of reduction of YKL-40 levels on day 5 after admission could be considered as a prognostic biomarker and might guide the clinical decisions in children with pneumonia (e.g., need more intensive therapy and care, including mechanical ventilation or admission to ICU).

YKL-40, a recently discovered protein, is involved in airway inflammation, a potential biomarker of asthma, and a member of the chitinase and chitinase-like protein family. It is secreted in the airway mucosa by the inflammatory cells that reside in the bronchial mucosal and airway epithelial cells [20–22]. Chitinase might contribute to the inflammation and bronchial remolding in T helper 2 (Th2)-airway inflammation, an immune response mediated condition. It has been reported that YKL-40 levels were increased in children with asthma and were correlated with the markers of disease severity [21]. The prognosis of hypersensitivity pneumonitis is also correlated with the serum levels of YKL-40 [12]. The admission level of YKL-40 in the serum could

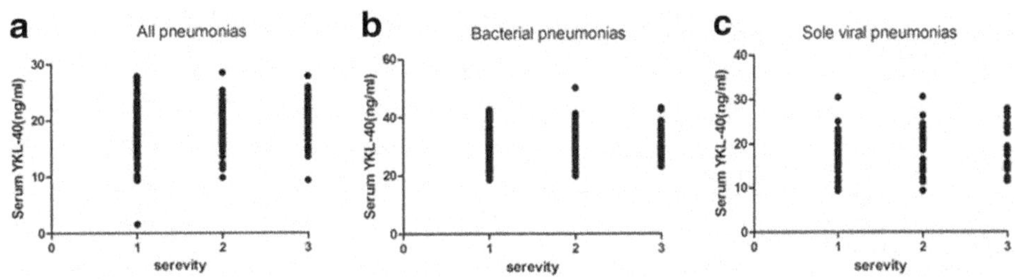

Fig. 3 The spearman correlation analysis between diseased severity and serum levels of YKL-40. **a**. The spearman correlation between severity and serum levels in all child pneumonia patients. No significant correlation was observed (spearman $r = 0.066$, $P = 0.28$). **b**. The correlation between severity and serum levels in children patients with bacterial infection (spearman $r = 0.16$, $P = 0.09$). **c**. The correlation between severity and serum levels in sole viral pneumonia patients (spearman $r = -0.19$, $P = 0.12$). No significant correlation between admission levels and severity in all children with viral or bacterial pneumonia. X axis represents the severity of childhood pneumonia. Non-severe pneumonia = 1, severe pneumonia = 2, very severe pneumonia = 3

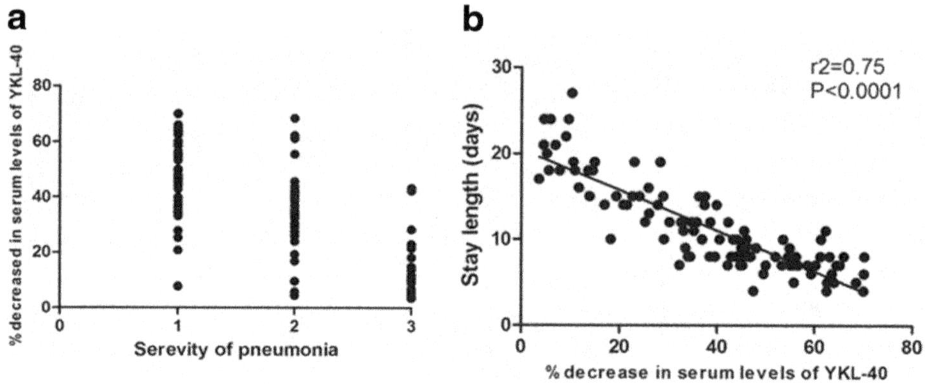

Fig. 4 The correlation between decreased percentage of serum levels of YKL-40 after 5th days and diseased severity. **a**. The correlation analysis between severity class and decreased percentage (spearman $r = -0.68$, $P < 0.0001$). The negative correlation was verified by the spearman correlation analysis. X axis represents the severity of childhood pneumonia. Non-severe pneumonia = 1, severe pneumonia = 2, very severe pneumonia = 3. **b**. The correlation analysis between severity class and median length of hospital stay ($r^2 = 0.75$, $P < 0.0001$). The hospitalization stays period was negatively correlated with decreased extent after admission. $P < 0.05$ defined as significant statistic difference

predict disease progression and estimate mortality risk in patients with hypersensitivity pneumonitis. Meanwhile, in a cohorts of adults with CAP, the serum level was correlated with the pneumonia severity index, CURB-65 scores, length of hospital stay, and APACHE-II scores, which suggested that the levels of YKL-40 might have the potential to guide the treatment of CAP in adults [8].

We found that the higher admission level of YKL-40 in children with pneumonia than healthy volunteers. And the increased YKL-40 levels in BALFs compared to the serum levels was observed in the children with bacterial infection. In children with sole viral infection, the significant difference between the serum levels and BALFs levels of YKL-40, which might be attributed to the infiltrates being confined to within the pulmonary

Table 2 Logistics regression analysis for the factors associated with the prognosis of pneumonia

	OR	95% CI	*P* value
Rate of sepsis: Yes (45, 16.1%), No (235, 83.9%)			
Age (continuous variable)	1.21	0.85,1.54	0.652
Previous pneumonia(binary variable)	0.92	0.85,1.24	0.096
Decreased extent of YKL-40 (classified variable)	2.84	2.16,3.65	0.008
Infectious type (unordered variable)	1.23	0.97,1.48	0.078
Procalcitonin (continuous variable)	1.12	1.03,1.22	0.044
Mechanical ventilation rate: Yes (31, 11.1%), No (249, 88.9%)			
Age (continuous variable)	1.235	1.156,1.366	0.023
Previous pneumonia (binary variable)	2.02	1.68,2.26	0.034
Decreased extent of YKL-40 (classified variable)	1.69	1.26,2.08	0.012
Infectious type (unordered variable)	1.63	1.21,2.27	0.028
Procalcitonin (continuous variable)	1.021	0.916,1.148	0.189
Intensive Care Unit admission rate: Yes (36, 12.9%), No (244, 87.1%)			
Age (continuous variable)	1.23	1.12,1.51	0.041
Previous pneumonia (binary variable)	1.21	0.93,1.87	0.267
Decreased extent of YKL-40 (classified variable)	3.21	2.68,4.79	0.016
Infectious type (unordered variable)	1.35	1.21,1.45	0.030
Procalcitonin (continuous variable)	1.09	0.91,1.17	0.526

Data are presented as hazard ratios, representing the relative risk of adverse therapeutic events and poor prognosis. The independent risk factors of mechanical ventilation including the age, infectious type, infections history in the previous and decreased extent of YKL-40. The age, infectious type, decreased extent of YKL-40 not associated with the increased rate of mechanical ventilation but also considered as the independent risk factors of ICU admission

interstitial lesion in most cases of viral pneumonia. But it did not predict the disease severity of pneumonia in children, which differs for the finding in adults. A previous study found that immune dysfunction was associated with increased disease severity in infants [23, 24]. This suppression of the adaptive immune response also has an adverse influence on the prognosis in septic children [25]. Therefore, the fact that there is no correlation between admission levels of YKL-40 and diseased severity might be attributed to the YKL-40 levels, which are decreased in the immunocompromised status of the severe cases in children, relative to the mild and slight cases [26]. In addition, the results are different from the finding in adults with CAP as mentioned in the introduction section. Therefore the admission levels of circulating YKL-40 have little correlation with the severity of pneumonia, which might be due to the immune suppression status for severe infectious pneumonia in children.

We noticed that the YKL-40 levels of BALF specimens were higher than the peripheral circulation in bacterial pneumonia, which support the fact suggestion that YKL-40 is secreted by the locally infiltrated inflammatory cells. To verify the correlation between the serum levels of classical pro-inflammatory cytokines and the BALF levels of YLK-40, we performed a linear correlation analysis. The levels of YKL-40 in the BALF specimens is positively correlated with the serum levels of CRP, which suggested that the level of YKL-40 in BALF specimens represented only the activity of inflammation at the lesion location rather than the systemic inflammation due to the endotoxin release or inflammation cascade. However, the difficulty in obtaining BALF samples limits its utilization for the repeated detection of admission levels of YKL-40 for monitoring diseased status. In a previous study associated with cystic fibrosis, Fantino et al. revealed that only the airway local levels of YKL-40 reflected the activity in lung tissue for the infant and young children with early cystic fibrosis [27]. The results above demonstrated that YKL-40, secreted by neutrophils, often serves as a confined inflammatory cytokine and is enriched in local inflammatory tissue rather than being released into the peripheral circulation. Therefore, it also could partly explain why the admission levels of YKL-40 were not correlated with the disease severity of pneumonia.

Eventually, to illustrate the predictive value in the evaluation of reduction degree serum levels of YKL-40 in children viral pneumonia, we applied the multivariable logistic regression analysis to explore the independent risk factors that might be correlated with prognosis. We found the reduction degree of YKL-40 is negative correlated with the admission of ICU, incidence of mechanical ventilation and sepsis. The results demonstrated that the reduction degree of YKL-40 levels, serving as a pro-inflammatory cytokine, was associated with the prognosis of child pneumonia, including the median length of stay, sepsis rate, mechanical ventilation rate, and ICU admission rate.

Study limitation

In the study, there were still several study limitations that should be taken into account in further and in-depth investigation. At first, we could not collect the BALF specimen because of the difficulty in the taking samples although the fact that the secretion of YKL-40 were produced by local inflammatory cells resident in respiratory tract. Secondly, the predictive value of degree of reduction in serum levels YKL-40 after 5 days compared than the admission levels was only available in the children with sole viral pneumonia, which might limit the more comprehensive application of this biomarker in clinical practice.

Conclusions

In conclusion, the degree of reduction of YKL-40 in the serum has a potential value in the prognostic assessment and prediction of disease severity. The YKL-40 levels in BALF specimens might reflect inflammatory activity at the lesion location and disease severity. Our study indicated that dynamically monitoring the levels of this inflammatory cytokine has potential value in the assessment of infectious diseases in children. More prospective clinical trials are needed to verify our finding.

Abbreviations

BALF: Bronchoalveolar lavage; CAP: Community-acquired pneumonia; ELISA: Enzyme-linked immunoassay; HP: Hypersensitivity pneumonia; ICU: Intensive care unit; IL: Interleukin; ILD: Interstitial lung disease; PSI: Pneumonia severity index; Th2: T helper 2

Acknowledgements

Not applicable

Funding

Not applicable

Authors' contributions

In this work, both authors conceived the study and designed the experiments; contributed to the data collection, performed the data analysis and interpreted the results; YXG wrote the manuscript; SGY contributed to the critical revision of article; both of them read and approved the final manuscript.

Competing interests

The authors declare that they have no competing interests.

References

1. Ruuskanen O, Lahti E, Jennings LC, Murdoch DR. Viral pneumonia. Lancet. 2011;377:1264–75.
2. Walker CLF, Rudan I, Liu L, Nair H, Theodoratou E, Bhutta ZA, et al. Global burden of childhood pneumonia and diarrhoea. Lancet. 2013;381:1405–16.
3. Bhutta ZA, Das JK. Global burden of childhood diarrhea and pneumonia: what can and should be done? Pediatrics. 2013;131:634–6.
4. Floyd J, Wu L, Hay Burgess D, Izadnegahdar R, Mukanga D, Ghani AC. Evaluating the impact of pulse oximetry on childhood pneumonia mortality in resource-poor settings. Nature. 2015;528:S53–9.
5. Chiu CY, Chen CJ, Wong KS, Tsai MH, Chiu CH, Huang YC. Impact of bacterial and viral coinfection on mycoplasmal pneumonia in childhood community-acquired pneumonia. J Microbiol Immunol Infect. 2015;48:51–6.
6. Boyd K. Back to the basics: community-acquired pneumonia in children. Pediatr Ann. 2017;46:e257–61.
7. Libreros S, Iragavarapu-Charyulu V. YKL-40/CHI3L1 drives inflammation on the road of tumor progression. J Leukoc Biol. 2015;98:931–6.
8. Kastrup J. Can YKL-40 be a new inflammatory biomarker in cardiovascular disease? Immunobiology. 2012;217:483–91.
9. Wang HL, Hsiao PC, Tsai HT, Yeh CB, Yang SF. Usefulness of plasma YKL-40 in management of community-acquired pneumonia severity in patients. Int J Mol Sci. 2013;14:22817–25.
10. Furuhashi K, Suda T, Nakamura Y, Inui N, Hashimoto D, Miwa S, et al. Increased expression of YKL-40, a chitinase-like protein, in serum and lung of patients with idiopathic pulmonary fibrosis. Respir Med. 2010; 104:1204–10.
11. Johansen JS, Milman N, Hansen M, Garbarsch C, Price PA, Graudal N. Increased serum YKL-40 in patients with pulmonary sarcoidosis--a potential marker of disease activity? Respir Med. 2005;99:396–402.
12. Long X, He X, Ohshimo S, Griese M, Sarria R, Guzman J, et al. Serum YKL-40 as predictor of outcome in hypersensitivity pneumonitis. Eur Respir J. 2017. https://doi.org/10.1183/13993003.01924-2015.
13. Harris M, Clark J, Coote N, Fletcher P, Harnden A, McKean M, et al. British Thoracic Society guidelines for the management of community acquired pneumonia in children: update 2011. Thorax. 2011;66:ii1–23.
14. Eccles S, Pincus C, Higgins B, Woodhead M. Guideline Development Group Diagnosis and management of community and hospital acquired pneumonia in adults: summary of NICE guidance. BMJ. 2014;349:g6722.
15. Abers MS, Musher DM. The yield of sputum culture in bacteremic pneumococcal pneumonia after initiation of antibiotics. Clin Infect Dis. 2014;58:1782–3.
16. Jiang W, Wu M, Zhou J, Wang Y, Hao C, Ji W, et al. Etiologic spectrum and occurrence of coinfections in children hospitalized with community-acquired pneumonia. BMC Infect Dis. 2017;17:787.
17. Scott JA, Wonodi C, Moïsi JC, Deloria-Knoll M, DeLuca AN, Karron RA, et al. The definition of pneumonia, the assessment of severity, and clinical standardization in the pneumonia etiology research for child health study. Clin Infect Dis. 2012;54:S109–16.
18. Bradley JS, Byington CL, Shah SS, Alverson B, Carter ER, Harrison C, et al. The management of community-acquired pneumonia in infants and children older than 3 months of age: clinical practice guidelines by the Pediatric Infectious Diseases Society and the Infectious Diseases Society of America. Clin Infect Dis. 2011;53:e25–76.
19. Marguet C, Dean TP, Warner JO. Soluble intercellular adhesion molecule-1 (sICAM-1) and interferon-gamma in bronchoalveolar lavage fluid from children with airway diseases. Am J Respir Crit Care Med. 2000;162:1016–22.
20. Specjalski K, Chelminska M, Jassem E. YKL-40 protein correlates with the phenotype of asthma. Lung. 2015;193:189–94.
21. Konradsen JR, James A, Nordlund B, Reinius LE, Söderhäll C, Melén E, et al. The chitinase-like protein YKL-40: a possible biomarker of inflammation and airway remodeling in severe pediatric asthma. J Allergy Clin Immunol. 2013; 132:328–35 e5.
22. Waldon EG, Lesser A, Weeden L, Messick E. The music attentiveness screening assessment, revised (MASA-R): a study of technical adequacy. J Music Ther. 2016;53:75–92.
23. García C, Soriano-Fallas A, Lozano J, Leos N, Gomez AM, Ramilo O, et al. Decreased innate immune cytokine responses correlate with disease severity in children with respiratory syncytial virus and human rhinovirus bronchiolitis. Pediatr Infect Dis J. 2012;31:86–9.
24. Mella C, Suarez-Arrabal MC, Lopez S, Stephens J, Fernandez S, Hall MW, et al. Innate immune dysfunction is associated with enhanced disease severity in infants with severe respiratory syncytial virus bronchiolitis. J Infect Dis. 2013;207:564–73.
25. Muszynski JA, Nofziger R, Greathouse K, Steele L, Hanson-Huber L, Nateri J, et al. Early adaptive immune suppression in children with septic shock: a prospective observational study. Crit Care. 2014;18:R145.
26. Gudmundsdottir S, Lieder R, Sigurjonsson OE, Petersen PH. Chitosan leads to downregulation of YKL-40 and inflammasome activation in human macrophages. J Biomed Mater Res A. 2015;103:2778–85.
27. Fantino E, Gangell CL, Hartl D, Sly PD, Airway ARESTCF. But not serum or urinary, levels of YKL-40 reflect inflammation in early cystic fibrosis lung disease. BMC Pulm Med. 2014;14:28.

23

Nebulised hypertonic saline (3 %) among children with mild to moderately severe bronchiolitis

Aayush Khanal[1*], Arun Sharma[1], Srijana Basnet[1], Pushpa Raj Sharma[1,2] and Fakir Chandra Gami[1]

Abstract

Background: To Assess the efficacy of nebulised hypertonic saline (HS) (3 %) among children with mild to moderately severe bronchiolitis.

Methods: Infants aged 6 weeks to 24 months, with a first episode of wheezing and Clinical Severity scores (Arch Dis Child 67:289-93, 1992) between 1 and 8, were enrolled over 4 months duration. Those with severe disease, co-morbidities, prior wheezing, recent bronchodilator and steroid use were excluded. Patients were randomized in a double-blind fashion, to receive two doses of nebulized 3 % HS (Group 1) or 0.9 % normal saline (Group 2) with 1.5 mg of L-Epineprine, delivered 30 min apart. Parents were contacted at 24 h and 7 days. The principal outcome measure was the mean change in clinical severity score at the end of 2 h of observation.

Results: A total of 100 infants (mean age 9.6 months, range 2–23 months; 61 % males) were enrolled. Patients in both groups had mild to moderately severe disease at presentation. On an intention-to-treat basis, the infants in the HS group had a significant reduction (3.57 ± 1.41) in the mean clinical severity score compared to those in the NS group (2.26 ± 1.15); [$p < 0.001$; CI: 0.78–1.82]. More children in the HS group ($n = 35/50$; 70.0 %) were eligible for ER/OPD discharge at the end of 2 h than those in the NS group ($n = 15/50$; 30 %; $p < 0.001$), and less likely to need a hospital re-visit ($n = 5/50$; 10.0 %) in the next 24 h as compared to the NS group ($n = 15/50$, 30.0 %; $p < 0.001$). The treatment was well tolerated, with no adverse effects.

Conclusions: Nebulized 3 % HS is effective, safe and superior to normal saline for outpatient management of infants with mild to moderately severe viral bronchiolitis in improving Clinical Severity Scores, facilitating early Out-Patient Department discharge and preventing hospital re-visits and admissions in the 24 h of presentation.

Keywords: Bronchiolitis, Clinical severity score, Epinephrine, Hypertonic saline

Background

Bronchiolitis is a common, occasionally severe viral infection of the lower respiratory tract responsible for significant morbidity and mortality in children under two years of age [1]. According to World Health Organization bulletin, an estimated 150 million new cases of clinical pneumonia (principally Pneumonia and Bronchiolitis) occur annually [2]; 11–20 million among them requiring hospital admission. Worldwide, 95 % of all cases occur in developing countries [2]. Epidemiologic data show that RSV accounts for about 65 % of hospitalizations due to Bronchiolitis [3].

Multiple studies [4–7] have documented variation in diagnostic testing, treatment modalities practiced and their outcomes in Bronchiolitis suggesting a lack of consensus for this common disorder. Likewise, despite the frequency of this condition, there is no unanimously accepted evidence driven treatment approach [8, 9]. Besides supplemental oxygen, fluids and supportive care, treatment

* Correspondence: aayush_khanal@iom.edu.np; aayush_khanal@yahoo.com
[1]Department of Pediatrics, Tribhuvan University Teaching Hospital, Institute of Medicine, Maharajgunj-44600, P.O. Box 1524, Kathmandu, Nepal
Full list of author information is available at the end of the article

options include, bronchodilators, epinephrine and corticosteroids [9]. Hypertonic saline (3 %) is a new agent that has been found to be promising in recent studies [10–20]. The proposed mechanism are by improving mucus rheology, reducing airway wall edema and causing sputum induction and cough [12]. A recent meta-analysis [10] also showed a consistent improvement in clinical severity scores and suggested HS may also decrease the length of hospital stay in Bronchiolitis. However, multiple other studies [8, 13, 21–25] have shown equivocal results with little or no clinical benefits with the use of hypertonic saline (3, 6 or 7 %). Similary, there is a paucity of data on comparison of important outcomes like readiness for discharge, need for repeat hospital visits and hospitalization rates, which are important reflectors of morbidity and economic burden [10]. In the paucity of rigorously controlled studies in developing countries using 3 % HS, lack of a consensus regarding management of bronchiolitis in our practice and an opportunity to improve care for this common disorder this study was conducted to assess the therapeutic efficacy of 3 % HS. We tried to study primarily the improvement in CS scores but also looked at parameters like readiness for discharge, need for hospital revisit rates and hospitalization which would reflect the morbidity and financial burden of disease.

Methods

Trial design

This study was a prospective, interventional, double-blind randomized controlled trial.

Ethical clearance

A written informed consent was obtained from the primary caretaker of the patients prior to the enrollment. The study was approved by the Department of Research, Institutional Review Board and Ethics Committee of Tribhuvan University Teaching Hospital.

Study participants

Subjects were recruited from previously healthy children visiting the Emergency Room (ER) and Out-Patient Department (OPD) of Kanti Children Hospital with the following inclusion criteria:

1. Age between 6 weeks and 2 years
2. First Episode of Wheezing
3. Meets Clinical Definition of Bronchiolitis
4. Clinical severity (CS) scores (Wang et al [26]) between 1 and 9 (Table 1).

Bronchiolitis was clinically defined as per the AAP consensus guidelines [4, 27] as the first episode of acute wheezing in children less than two years of age, starting as a viral upper respiratory infection (coryza, cough or fever).

Exclusion criteria

1. Any underlying disease (e.g., cystic fibrosis, bronchopulmonary dysplasia and cardiac or renal disease),
2. Prior history of wheezing,
3. Diagnosed case of asthma,
4. Oxygen saturation (SpO2) <85 % on room air,
5. CS score > 9,
6. Progressive respiratory distress requiring mechanical ventilation,
7. Previous treatment with bronchodilators within last 4 h, and
8. Any steroid therapy within 48 h

Study setting

The study was carried out in the ER, Observation room (OR) and OPD. Recruitment occurred at the peak of bronchiolitis season in between January 15th to April 15th for duration of 4 months.

Patient assessment

Patient enrollment occurred on weekdays between 08.00 and 17.00 h. The investigator assessed the children for eligibility and assigned a clinical severity (CS) score described by Wang et al. [26] (Table 1). Data were collected using standardized forms to document pertinent history and physical exam. Each children's weight, temperature, respiratory rate, SpO2 in room air (determined by pulse oximeter, Siemens), heart rate, CS Score and hydration status were recorded. The children were stabilized with antipyretics if necessary (temperature > 38.3°C) and/or nasal suction if the nose was blocked. Supplemental oxygen by face mask was provided to maintain SpO2 > 90 %.

Table 1 Wang et al. clinical severity score

Variables	Score			
	0	1	2	3
RR	< 30	31–45	46–60	> 60
Wheezing	None	Terminal expiration/only with stethoscope	Entire expiration or audible on exp. without stethoscope	Inspiration and expiration without stethoscope
Retraction	None	Intercostals	Tracheo-sternal	Severe with nasal flaring
General condition	Normal			Irritable, lethargic, poor feeding

Patients determined to be in life threatening condition were immediately managed for same and were not further considered for study.

Interventions

The study drugs were prepared by a pharmacist, administered by an ER/OPD nurse and compliance with medication administration was assured by the investigator's direct observation of each nebulization.

All eligible patients were randomly assigned to one of the two groups:

1. Group 1 ($n = 50$) received inhalation of L-Epinephrine 1.5 mg, diluted to 4 ml with 3 % Hypertonic 1 Saline (HS) solution;
2. Group 2 ($n = 50$) received inhalation of L-Epinephrine, 1.5 mg, diluted to 4 ml with 0.9 % Normal Saline solution.

The study drug was administered at 0 and 30 min by a Jet nebulizer using a face mask. The investigator assessed the children's general condition and recorded the CS score, SpO2, RR and HR prior to each drug administration and at 30, 60 and 120 min after the first nebulization.

The study design is shown in Fig. 1.

Adverse events were defined as heart rate > 200, tremor and worsening clinical status. Patients were excluded from the study if the two courses of nebulisation was not delivered, the drug delivery was delayed by 10 min or more (protocol deviation) or if clinical deterioration mandated escalation of therapy and/or support.

The investigator contacted the parents via telephone 24 h after their ED/OPD discharge to determine the need for any unscheduled hospital visit and hospitalization within the next 24 h of OPD/ ER visit: their readmission (relapse) rate. The register at the ER/OR was checked daily for any unscheduled visits by the caretakers. They were also contacted at the end of 1 week in order to record any unscheduled medical visits, missed working days of caregivers and persistence of cough. Patients were labeled as Lost-to-Follow up if there was failure to communicate for 3 consecutive attempts for 2 consecutive days at their 7th and 8th day of initial presentation to the OPD/ER.

Primary outcome

Compare the mean change in Clinical Severity score among patients with bronchiolitis treated with either L-Epinephrine- 3 % Hypertonic saline or L-Epinephrine-0.9 % saline.

Secondary outcomes

a. Assess the improvements in SpO2, respiratory rate and heart rate in both intervention groups.
b. Compare the discharge readiness and readmission rates in both intervention groups at the end of 2 h of observation and within 24 h following discharge respectively.
c. Describe the socioeconomic burden of illness.

Sample size

Sample size was determined by the following formula:

$$\mathbf{N} = [(\mathbf{z1} + \mathbf{z2})^2 (\mathbf{\acute{O}1}^2 + \mathbf{\acute{O}2}^2)] / \left(\mathbf{\hat{u}1} - \mathbf{\hat{u}2}\right)^2.$$

- N: Sample Size
- z1: The confidence level, for p value: 0.05, z1: 1.96.
- z2: 0.84 for Power of 80 %
  1.28 for Power of 90 %
  1.64 for Power of 95 %
- Ó1: Standard Deviation of the Outcome Variable (Clinical Severity Score) in the 1st intervention group (HS)
- Ó2: Standard deviation of the outcome variable (Clinical severity score) in the 2nd intervention group (NS)
- Û 1: Mean change in clinical severity score among 1st intervention group (HS)

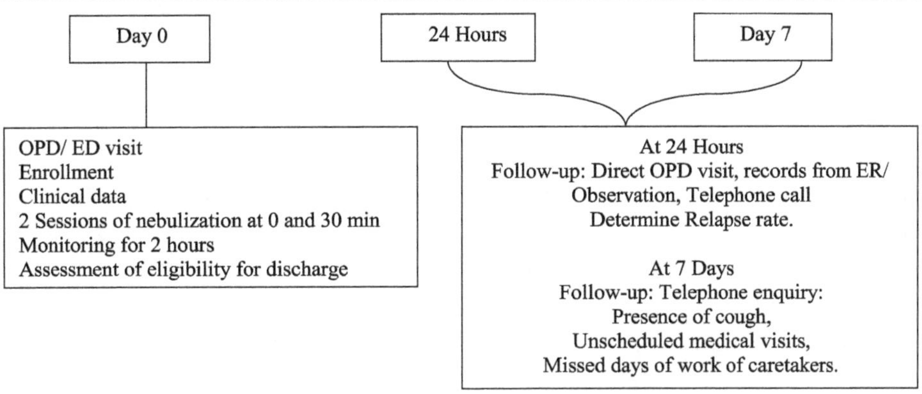

Fig. 1 The study design

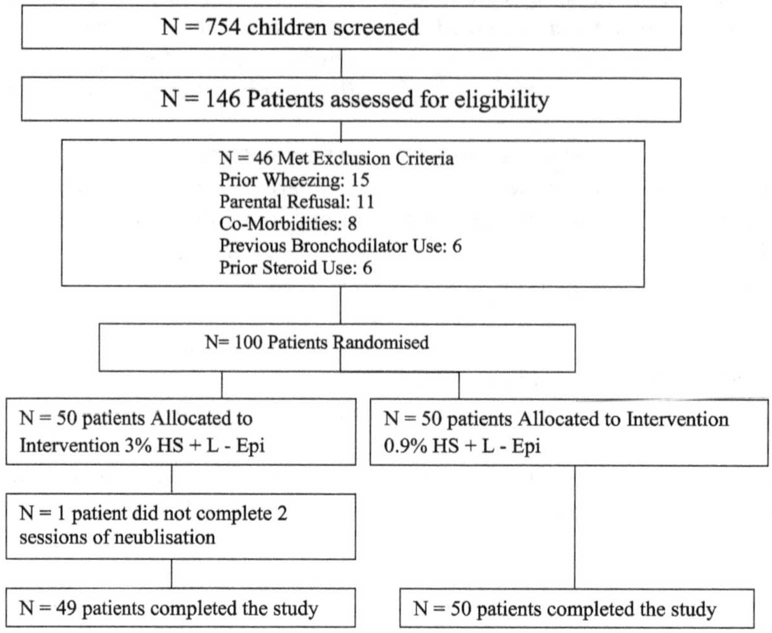

Fig. 2 The trial profile

- Û 2: Mean change in clinical severity score among 2nd intervention group (NS)
- Allowing a Type1 error of 5 % (α: 0.05), z1 score: 1.96.
- For a Power of 95 %, z2 = 1.64.

The standard deviation of the change in CS score is derived from previous studies [8] and taken as 1.3. We proposed that a difference of 1 point in the CS score between the two intervention groups will be considered clinically significant. To detect this mean difference of 1 unit in the CS score, with a power of 95 %, a sample size of 44 in each intervention group was required. This required a total of 88 patients to be enrolled in the study. Considering the drop out/lost to follow up to be approximately 10 %, 100 patients were enrolled, allowing 50 in each group.

Randomization

Sequence generation

A Random Allocation Software [28] generated by computer, identified patients by a triple digit mixed numeric code, was used by the study coordinator to allocate patients to treatment groups, and he was the only person with access to the randomization.

Type of randomization

Block Randomization method was used to stratify patients into blocks of 10 each, each comprising of 10 patients.

Allocation concealment

After preparation, the study solutions were labeled with the codes and wrapped in an envelope bearing the

Table 2 Baseline characteristics of 2 groups

Characteristics; mean(SD); (range)	Intervention L-Epi + 3 % HS (*n* = 50)	Intervention L-Epi + 0.9 % NS (*n* = 50)	*p* value
Age (months), mean (SD); (range)	9.82 (5.06); (2–23)	9.51 (4.28); (3–22)	0.74
Males, n(%)	27 (54.0 %)	21 (42.0 %)	0.40
Duration of illness (days), Mean ± SD	3.43 ± 1.02	3.33 ± 0.96	0.64
Mean (SD) respiratory rate (range)	49.1 (2.5) (46–60)	49.0 (2.0) (46–58)	0.79
Mean (SD) heart rate (range)	148.7 (7.5) (132–168)	149.7 (7.1) (132–166)	0.49
Mean (SD) Spo2 (range)	93.4 (0.8) (90–95)	93.5 (0.7) (90–94)	0.69
Mean (SD) clinical severity score (range)	5.3 (1.6) (3–9)	5.2 (1.1) (3–9)	0.57
Mean temperature (SD) temperature (*C) (range)	37.2 (−17.4) (36.7–38.0)	37.3 (−17.4) (36.6–38.0)	0.82
Urine specific gravity	1016	1022	0.001
ER enrollment, n (%)	2 (4 %)	2 (4 %)	1.00

Table 3 Distribution of risk factors proposed to contribute to prolonged disease course and, or severity in both intervention groups

Variables	3 % HS + L-Epi (*n* = 50)	0.9 % NS + L-Epi (*n* = 50)	*p*-value
Family history of asthma, n (%)	4 (8.0)	5 (10.0)	1.00
Parental smoking, n (%)	30 (60.0)	21 (42.0)	0.05
Exposure to biofuels, n (%)	14 (28.0)	8 (16.0)	0.11
Breastfeeding status, n (%)	48 (96.0)	48 (96.0)	0.75
Prematurity, n (%)	3 (6.0)	2 (4.0)	0.50
Atopic history, n (%)	7 (14.0)	3 (6.0)	0.15

respective codes. Study solutions were identical in appearance and odor. Their identity was blinded to all participants, care providers, and investigators and outcome assessor.

Implementation

Randomization was done by the study coordinator (not involved in the study), who was the only person to have access to the codes. The codes were a mixed 3 digit numeric code. The study solutions prepared by a pharmacist (not involved in the study) were stored in the non-freezer compartment (2–8*C) of the refrigerator and discarded if not used within 72 h of preparation. The investigator assessed the patients and allocated the treatment modalities to each one of them himself.

Blinding

The study was a Double Blind Randomized Controlled Trial with the investigator, the participants, the nurses who delivered the drug being blinded to the therapeutic option.

Statistical methods

Statistical analysis was performed using SPSS for Windows, Release 16.0 (SPSS Inc., Chicago, IL). Dichotomous events were analyzed by using the Chi-Square test. Continuous variables were compared by Student *t*-test. Statistical significance was defined as *p*-value < 0.05. This trial has been reported in accordance to the Consolidated Standards of Reporting Trials (CONSORT, 2010) guidelines [29].

Results and discussion

A total of 754 children were screened and 146 previously well children were assessed for eligibility in the study periodas shown in Fig. 2. Forty-Six children were

Table 4 Mean (± SD) for CS Score, respiratory rate, heart rate and SpO_2 for patients in each group at 0,30, 60 and 120 min of assessment

	Intervention 0.9 % NS + L-Epi (*n* = 50)	Intervention 3 % HS + L-Epi (*n* = 50)	*p* value	95 % confidence interval lower limits – upper limits (mean)
CS score, n, Mean ± S.D; range				
0 min	5.2 ± 1.1 (3–9)	5.3 ± 1.6; (3–9)	0.57	−0.73; 0.41 (−0.15)
30 min	4.9 ± 1.1; (3–8)	4.3 ± 2.0; (2–8)	0.10	−0.11; 1.21 (0.55)
60 min	3.2 ± 1.0; (1–6)	2.2 ± 1.2; (1–7)	0.001	0.52; 1.43 (0.97)
120 min	2.9 ± 0.8; (1–5)	1.7 ± 0.9; (1–7)	0.001	0.77; 1.52 (1.14)
Respiratory rate, breaths/minute, Mean ± S.D; range				
0 min	49.0 ± 2.0; (46–58)	49.1 ± 2.5; (46–60)	0.79	−1.01;0.81 (−0.12)
30 min	47.4 ± 1.7; (46–54)	46.6 ± 2.1; (42–56)	0.04	0.04; 1.61 (0.81)
60 min	45.3 ± 1.4; (42–50)	43.5 ± 2.0; (40–52)	0.001	1.13; 2.57 (1.85)
120 min	43.6 ± 2.6; (40–48)	40.7 ± 2.0; (38–49)	0.001	1.97; 3.86 (2.91)
Oxygen saturation,%, Mean ± S.D; range				
0 min	93.5 ± 0.7; (90–94)	93.4 ± 0.8 (90–95)	0.69	−0.22; 0.40 (0.09)
30 min	93.8 ± 0.8; (91–96)	94.2 ± 1.2; (90–96)	0.07	−0.79; 0.06 (−0.36)
60 min	94.9 ± 0.9; (92–97)	95.8 ± 1.1; (92–98)	0.001	−1.34; −0.48 (−0.97)
120 min	95.6 ± 1.0; (93–98)	97.0 ± 1.0; (93–99)	0.001	−1.77; −0.91 (−1.14)
Heart rate, beats/minute, Mean ± S.D; range				
0 min	149.7 ± 7.1; (132–166)	148.7 ± 7.5; (132–168)	0.49	−1.94; 3.98 (0.80)
30 min	149.7 ± 7.9; (130–164)	147.1 ± 9.1; (130–164)	0.13	−0.93; 6.04 (2.91)
60 min	145.2 ± 6.4; (130–156)	142.6 ± 7.2; (126–156)	0.06	−0.20; 5.30 (2.55)
120 min	141.8 ± 5.8; (126–154)	138.3 ± 6.6; (124–152)	0.006	1.02; 6.03 (3.53)

excluded and 99 patients completed the study. Data was analyzed on an intention to treat basis.

No significant differences were noted between the study groups with respect to baseline characteristics ($p > 0.05$) and risk factors for severity as shown in Table 2 and Table 3 respectively. Patients in both groups had moderately severe bronchiolitis with mean CS score above 5. There is gradual improvement in CS score with time in both the groups and the effect seemed to be more pronounced after the second session of nebulisation at 60 min. Patients who received nebulised HS had more significant improvement in the baseline CS scores (Group 1, a change of 3.57 ± 1.41; Group 2, a change of 2.26 ± 1.15; $p < 0.01$) at the end of 2 h of therapy as shown in Table 5. There was also significant difference in the mean change in CS scores, HR, RR and SpO2 between the two groups at the start of treatment and at the end of 2 h of therapy (p <0.001) as shown in Table 4 and Table 5. More infants who received HS were eligible for discharge at the end of 2 h as compared to NS [Group 1, $n = 35$(71.0 %); Group 2, $n = 15$(30.0 %); $p < 0.001$] as shown in Table 6.

In addition, in our trial the need for repeat medical visits and hospital admission within the next 24 h of initial hospital visit (Relapse rate) was 20 %, which was significantly lesser in the babies who received HS compared to those who received NS [Group 1, $n = 5$(10.0 %); Group 2, $n = 15$ (30.0 %); $p < 0.001$] as shown in Table 6. During the subsequent week, 78 out of 100 patients (Group 1, $n = 37$; Group 2, $n = 41$) were accessible. As shown in Table 7, a large number of patients in both groups had persistent cough at the end of 1 week (Group 1, $n = 31$; Group 2, $n = 37$; $p = 0.45$). Eighteen patients from HS Group and 23 patients from NS Group had at least 1 unscheduled medical visit within 1 week ($p = 0.58$; overall revisit rates 41/88; 46.5 %) and 3 parents from HS Group and 10 patients from NS Group reported at missing least 1 day of work ($p = 0.17$; total missed days of work 10/77; 12.9 %). No adverse events occurred in either treatment groups. No children were withdrawn from the trial due to side effects or clinical deterioration.

Table 5 Clinical outcomes in the two intervention groups at the end of 2 h of treatment

Variables (Mean ± SD)	Intervention 3 % HS + L-Epi	Intervention 0.9 % NS+ L-Epi	*p* value	95 % confidence interval (mean)
Change in CS Score	3.57 ± 1.41	2.26 ± 1.15	0.001	0.78; 1.82 (1.30)
Change in HR	10.38 ± 4.54	7.87 ± 3.63	0.003	0.86; 4.16 (2.50)
Change in RR	8.44 ± 2.15	5.40 ± 2.57	0.001	2.08; 3.99 (3.04)
Change in SpO_2	3.53 ± 0.84	2.12 ± 0.80	0.001	1.07; 1.73 (1.30)

Table 6 Secondary outcomes

	Intervention 3 % HS + L-Epi	Intervention 0.9 % + L-Epi	*p* value
Met criteria for ER/OPD discharge after 120 mins, n (%)	35 (70.0 %)	15 (30.0 %)	0.001
Relapse rate, n (%)	5 (10.0 %)	15 (30.0 %)	0.02
Need for intensive care	1 (2.0 %)	1 (2.0 %)	1.00

Ours is one of the few studies conducted in South-East Asia with a rigorously controlled design that has not only tried to look at the role of hypertonic saline in improving the CS scores but also studied its impact on early discharge eligibility and hospital revisit rates. In both treatment groups, change in CS was greater than 2 scores suggesting that both treatment combinations were effective. More infants with bronchiolitis were eligible for early discharge and less likely to need any hospital re-visit within the next 24 h ($p < 0.001$). This outcome seems to be particularly relevant in planning resource allocation and staffing in treatment of this common condition.

Similar findings were reported in a recent Cochrane review [10] by Zhang et al., where a total of 560 patients treated with nebulised 3 % saline had a significantly shorter mean length of hospital stay and significantly lower post-inhalation clinical score than the 0.9 % saline group in the first three days of treatment ($p < 0.001$). The effects of improving clinical score were observed in both outpatients and inpatients.

On the Contrary, in another double blind RCT, Wu et al. in 2014 [24] assessed the role of nebulised 3 % HS on change in RDAI scores, admission rates and length of stay in Bronchiolitis. They concluded that HS given to children in the ED decreases hospital admissions but did not produce any significant difference in Respiratory Distress Assessment Instrument score or length of stay as compared to NS.

Likewise, Florin et al. [22] conducted a RCT in ER setting and found that at 1 h after the intervention, the

Table 7 Burden placed on caretakers due to bronchiolitis

	Intervention 3 % HS + L-Epi	Intervention 0.9 % NS + L-Epi	*p* value
Need for unscheduled medical visits within 1 week, n (%)	18 (36.0 %)	23 (46.0 %)	0.58
Missed days of work	3 (6.0 %)	10 (20.0 %)	0.17
Persistence of cough at the end of 1 week, n (%)	31 (62.0 %)	37 (74.0 %)	0.37

HS group demonstrated significantly less improvement in the median RDAI Score compared with the NS group ($p < 0.001$) and hence concluded that nebulised 3 % Saline was not effective in improving RDAI scores in the ER setting.

Previously, Sarrell et al. [19] had shown that substituting hypertonic saline for normal saline solution (2 ml) in the inhalation mixture for delivering bronchodilator improved clinical scores and decreased hospitalization rates in ambulatory children. In hospitalized children with more severe bronchiolitis, nebulized 4 ml hypertonic saline solution with or without epinephrine was found to be more effective treatment. In our study all infants recovered in both the groups, there was no treatment failure or significant adverse events following nebulisation, as previously reported by Ralston et al. [30].

Our study was well designed to minimize the common bias and limitations associated with research. Sampling bias was addressed by block randomization of patients. Blinding was maintained throughout the study period. A single observer's assessments nullified the chances of inter-observer variability. Despite these measures, some amount of bias and attrition is inevitable. We could not clarify the additional benefits of supportive care alone in infants with bronchiolitis since we didn't have a placebo arm. Although we considered important outcomes such as hospital revisit and admission rates, we did not assess the impact of therapy on the length of hospital stay. Our study population consisted mainly of infants who presented earlier, had mostly mild symptoms and experienced significant benefits. We are unsure, if similar benefits could be reproduced in infants with a more severe disease presentation. Although, we had strict inclusion and exclusion criteria, and identified potential risk factors for asthma, we might have included infants with first episode of asthma. RSV testing was unavailable and hence not done. We are also unsure if co-infection worsens the outlook in our infants.

Our study was conducted at the largest tertiary level pediatric referral centre of our country with over 1000 ER visits per month and more than 10,000 OPD visits per month with seasonal variation. Our sampled population characteristics were truly representative of the general population visiting Kanti Children's Hospital. Strict inclusion and exclusion criteria were used to minimize possible confounding effects of uncharacterized and evolving wheezing phenotypes. A well defined objective, previously validated scoring system was used to assess the clinical response. Our adequate sample size, and double blinded design minimizes the common bias and limitations associated with research. Since our study only consisted of mild to moderate patients with Bronchiolitis, results may need caution while extrapolating to infants with severe disease.

Conclusion

Nebulised 3 % hypertonic saline in combination with epinephrine was effective in reducing the Clinical Severity scores, meeting the eligibility criteria for OPD/ER discharge and reducing the need for hospital admission among ambulatory children with bronchiolitis. We believe this simple, inexpensive, safe, and effective treatment intervention could minimize the morbidity of Bronchiolitis by generalizing its use in centers caring for pediatric patients. Similar study could be done in multicentric settings with a larger sample size, involving more severely affected patients, and with a placebo control design in order to confirm and extend our results.

Abbreviations

AAP: American Academy of Pediatrics; CI: 95 % confidence interval; CS: Clinical severity score; ER: Emergency room; HS: Hypertonic saline; OPD: Out-patient department; OR: Observation room; L-Epi: L-Epinephrine; Spo2: Oxygen saturation as measured by pulse oximeter; HR: Heart rate; RR: Respiratory rate.

Competing interests

The authors declare that they have no competing interests.

Authors' contributions

AK: Selected and designed the study, enrolled the patients and prepared the results. AS: Edited the Study Protcol including design, randomization and blinding techniques, made amendments where required, Performed critical Appraisal. SB: Revision of the Study Protocol and Performed Statistical analysis and Critical Appraisal. PS: Reviewed and Edited the Study Protocol and performed Critical Appraisal. FG: Reviewed and Edited the Study Protocol and performed Critical appraisal. All authors read and approved the final manuscript.

Author details

[1]Department of Pediatrics, Tribhuvan University Teaching Hospital, Institute of Medicine, Maharajgunj-44600, P.O. Box 1524, Kathmandu, Nepal. [2]Kathmandu Medical College Teaching Hospital, Sinamangal, Kathmandu, Nepal.

References

1. Chaudhary K, Sinert R. Is nebulized hypertonic saline solution an effective treatment for bronchiolitis in infants? Ann Emerg Med. 2010;55:120–2.
2. Igor R, Tomaskovic L, Boschi-Pinto C, Campbell H. Global estimate of the incidence of clinical pneumonia among children under 5 years of age. Bull World Health Organ. 2004;82:895–903.
3. Weber MW, Mulholland EK, Greenwood BM. Respiratory syncytial virus infection in tropical and developing countries. Trop Med Int Health. 1998;3(4):268–80.
4. Zorc JJ, Hall CB. Bronchiolitis: recent evidence on diagnosis and management. Pediatrics. 2010;125:342–9.
5. Behrendt CE, Decker MD, Burch DJ, Watson PH. International variation in the management of infants hospitalized with respiratory syncytial virus. International RSV Study Group. Eur J Pediatr. 1998;157(3):215–20.
6. Christakis DA, Cowan CA, Garrison MM, Molteni R, Marcuse E, Zerr DM. Variation in inpatient diagnostic testing and management of bronchiolitis. Pediatrics. 2005;115(4):878–84.
7. Willson DF, Horn SD, Hendley JO, Smout R, Gassaway J. Effect of practice variation on resource utilization in infants hospitalized for viral lower respiratory illness. Pediatrics. 2001;108(4):851–5.
8. Anil AB, Anil M, Saglam AB, Cetin N, Bal A, Aksu N. High volume normal saline alone is as effective as nebulized salbutamol-normal saline, epinephrine-normal saline, and 3 % saline in mild bronchiolitis. Pediatr Pulmonol. 2010;45:41–7.
9. Wainwright C. Acute Viral Bronchiolitis in children- a very common condition with few therapeutic options. Paediatr Respir Rev. 2010;11:39–45.

10. Zhang L, Mendoza-Sassi RA, Wainwright C, Klassen TP. Nebulised hypertonic saline solution for acute bronchiolitis in infants. Cochrane Database of Syst Rev. 2013, Issue 7. Art. No.: CD006458. doi:10.1002/14651858.CD006458.pub3.
11. Al-Ansari K, Sakran M, Davidson BL, El Sayyed R, Mahjoub H, Ibrahim K. Nebulised 5 or 3 or 0.9 % saline for treating acute bronchiolitis in infants. J Pediatr. 2010;157:630–4.
12. Mandelberg A, Amirav I. Hypertonic saline or high volume normal saline for viral bronchiolitis: mechanisms and rationale. Pediatr Pulmonol. 2010;45:36–40.
13. Giudice M, Saitta F, Leonardi S. Effectiveness of nebulized hypertonic saline and epinephrine in hospitalized infants with bronchiolitis. Int J Immunopathol Pharmacol. 2012;25(2):485–91.
14. Kuzik BA, Al Qadhi SA, Kent S. Nebulised hypertonic saline in the treatment of viral bronchiolitis 1 in infants. J Pediatr. 2007;151:266–70.
15. Luo Z, Fu Z, Liu E. A randomized controlled trial of nebulised hypertonic saline treatment in hospitalized children with moderate to severe viral bronchiolitis. J Clin Microbiol Inf. 2011;17(12):1829–33.
16. Luo Z, Liu E, Luo J, Li S, Zeng F, Yang X, et al. Nebulized hypertonic saline/ salbutamol solution treatment in hospitalized children with mild to moderate bronchiolitis. Pediatr Int. 2010;52(2):199–202.
17. Mandelberg A, Tal G, Witzling M, Someck E, Houri S, Balin A, et al. Nebulised 3 % hypertonic saline solution treatment for hospitalized infants with bronchiolitis. Chest. 2003;123:483–7.
18. Sarrell EM, Tal G, Witzling M, Someck E, Houri S, Cohen HA, et al. Nebulised 3 % hypertonic saline solution for treatment of ambulatory children with viral bronchiolitis decreases symptoms. Chest. 2002;122:2015–20.
19. Tal G, Cesar K, Oron A. Hypertonic saline/ epinephrine treatment in hospitalized infants with viral bronchiolitis reduces hospitalization stay: 2 years experience. IMAJ. 2006;8:169–73.
20. Ipek IO, Yalchin EU, Sezer RG, Bozaykut A. The efficacy of nebulized salbutamol, hypertonic saline and salbutamol/hypertonic saline combination in moderate bronchiolitis. Pulm Pharmacol Ther. 2011;24(6):633–7.
21. Grewal S, Ali S, McConnell DW, Vandermeer B, Klassen TP. A randomized trial of nebulised 3 % hypertonic saline with epinephrine in the treatment of acute bronchiolitis in the emergency department. Arch Pediatr Adolesc Med. 2009;163(11):1007–12.
22. Florin TA, Shaw KN, Kittick M, Yaskscoe S, Zorc JJ. Nebulized hypertonic saline for bronchiolitis in the emergency department: a randomized clinical trial. 1. JAMA Pediatr. 2014;168(7):664–702.
23. Teunissen J, Hochs AH, Vaessen-Verberne A, Boehmer AL, Smeets CC, Brackel H, et al. The effect of 3 and 6 % hypertonic saline in viral bronchiolitis: a randomised controlled trial. Eur Respir J. 2014;44(4):913–21.
24. Wu S, Baker C, Lang ME. Nebulized hypertonic saline for bronchiolitis: a randomized controlled trial. JAMA Pediatr. 2014;168(7):657–63.
25. Jacobs J, Foster M, Wan J, Pershad J. 7 % hypertonic saline in acute bronchiolitis: a randomized controlled trial. Pediatrics. 2014;133:e8.
26. Wang EE, Milner R, Allen U, Maj H. Bronchodilators for treatment of mild bronchiolitis: a factorial randomised trial. Arch Dis Child. 1992;67:289–93.
27. Subcommittee on Diagnosis and Management of Bronchiolitis. Diagnosis and management of bronchiolitis. Pediatrics. 2006;118:1774–93.
28. Saghaei M. Random allocation software for parallel group randomised trials. BMC Med Res Methodol. 2004;4:26.
29. Schultz KF, Altman DG, Moher D. CONSORT 2010 Statement: updated guidelines for reporting parallel group randomized trials. BMJ. 2010;340:c332.
30. Ralston S, Hill V, Martinez M. Nebulised hypertonic saline without adjunctive bronchodilators for children with bronchiolitis. Pediatrics. 2010;126:e520–5.

24

Predictors of treatment failure for non-severe childhood pneumonia in developing countries: systematic literature review and expert survey – the first step towards a community focused mHealth risk-assessment tool?

Eric D. McCollum[1,2*], Carina King[2], Robert Hollowell[3], Janet Zhou[4], Tim Colbourn[2], Bejoy Nambiar[2], David Mukanga[4] and Deborah C. Hay Burgess[4]

Abstract

Background: Improved referral algorithms for children with non-severe pneumonia at the community level are desirable. We sought to identify predictors of oral antibiotic failure in children who fulfill the case definition of World Health Organization (WHO) non-severe pneumonia. Predictors of greatest interest were those not currently utilized in referral algorithms and feasible to obtain at the community level.

Methods: We systematically reviewed prospective studies reporting independent predictors of oral antibiotic failure for children 2–59 months of age in resource-limited settings with WHO non-severe pneumonia (either fast breathing for age and/or lower chest wall indrawing without danger signs), with an emphasis on predictors not currently utilized for referral and reasonable for community health workers. We searched PubMed, Cochrane, and Embase and qualitatively analyzed publications from 1997–2014. To supplement the limited published evidence in this subject area we also surveyed respiratory experts.

Results: Nine studies met criteria, seven of which were performed in south Asia. One eligible study occurred exclusively at the community level. Overall, oral antibiotic failure rates ranged between 7.8-22.9 %. Six studies found excess age-adjusted respiratory rate (either WHO-defined very fast breathing for age or 10–15 breaths/min faster than normal WHO age-adjusted thresholds) and four reported young age as predictive for oral antibiotic failure. Of the seven predictors identified by the expert panel, abnormal oxygen saturation and malnutrition were most highly favored per the panel's rankings and comments.

Conclusions: This review identified several candidate predictors of oral antibiotic failure not currently utilized in childhood pneumonia referral algorithms; excess age-specific respiratory rate, young age, abnormal oxygen saturation, and moderate malnutrition. However, the data was limited and there are clear evidence gaps; research in rural, low-resource settings with community health workers is needed.

Keywords: integrated Community Case Management (iCCM), Community health workers, Childhood pneumonia, Pediatrics, Developing countries, Predictors, Treatment failure, mHealth

* Correspondence: Eric.D.McCollum@gmail.com
[1]Department of Pediatrics, Division of Pulmonology, Johns Hopkins School of Medicine, Baltimore, USA
[2]Institute for Global Health, University College London, London, UK
Full list of author information is available at the end of the article

Background

Healthcare providers in resource-limited countries use practical, standardized case management guidelines to diagnose pneumonia [1]. Although mortality reductions of 36 % have been attributed to standardized management, pneumonia remains the second leading cause of childhood death globally with nearly one million deaths annually [2]. Three-quarters of all deaths occur in Africa and Asia, and it is estimated that a majority of all childhood pneumonia deaths occur outside of the hospital [3, 4]. Incomplete antibiotic coverage and care-seeking delays negatively influence pneumonia outcomes in low-resource settings and improvements have been inconsistent and difficult to sustain [4].

The World Health Organization (WHO) recommends expansion of basic healthcare beyond traditional facilities to community health workers (CHWs). This strategy, called 'integrated Community Case Management' (iCCM), includes childhood pneumonia care [5]. iCCM can address gaps in antibiotic access and care seeking delays by providing antibiotics earlier in a pneumonia illness when the disease is more responsive to treatment [5, 6]. Likewise, iCCM can permit earlier referral if treatment fails - defined as disease persistence or progression despite antibiotics. Evidence from Zambia and Pakistan has demonstrated improved childhood pneumonia antibiotic coverage and reduced treatment failure with iCCM [7–9]. As a result, iCCM expansion is a key strategy against childhood pneumonia [5, 6].

Despite iCCM's potential there are challenges, such as sustaining quality of care. CHWs receive limited training and are difficult to supervise in remote areas [5, 6]; consistent supervision and retraining is likely important for successful iCCM pneumonia management to ensure standardized recording of subjective clinical danger signs [10]. Strengthening CHW decision-making and identification of higher-risk patients, including those that do not meet current referral criteria, could reduce incorrect pneumonia diagnosis, antibiotic prescription, and referrals. Mobile health, or *mHealth*, may help to address these weaknesses [11]. mHealth utilizes user-friendly software compatible with mobile phones for healthcare delivery and capitalizes on mobile networks with wide coverage and usage in developing countries [11]. New mHealth applications that provide an array of performance support for CHWs are in development [12, 13].

An iCCM mHealth mobile phone application could assist CHWs to identify two groups of children with pneumonia; (1) those who meet current referral criteria but are mis-classified, and (2) those who do not meet current referral criteria but are still at greater risk for treatment failure based upon their initial clinical assessment. Both groups of children could then be referred for more appropriate treatment or be flagged for closer community-based monitoring. An improved referral mHealth tool could provide the result as a simple audio recommendation translated into the preferred local language, allowing both the CHW and caregiver to hear the recommendation. Facilitating objective decision-making by CHWs with a mHealth tool could complement existing guidelines to expand appropriate, timely antibiotic coverage and further reduce life-threatening treatment delays.

This systematic review and expert opinion survey aimed to identify predictors of WHO non-severe pneumonia treatment failure that are not currently used in referral algorithms and are also realistic for CHWs. The ultimate aim of a prediction algorithm would be to facilitate improved referral pathways originating from the community level, leading both to improved antibiotic stewardship and decreased morbidity and mortality.

Methods

Systematic review

We conducted a systematic review in accordance with PRIMSA (see Additional file 1) [14]. All studies from January 1, 1997 - June 25, 2014 listed in PubMed, Cochrane Central Register of Controlled Trials, and Embase were eligible. The following search terms were used: pneumonia; predictors or risk factors or prognostic; treatment failure or death; and Africa or Asia or developing country. These were combined with the following search filters: clinical trial, humans, and infant or preschool ages. No language restrictions were applied. We conducted the search on June 25, 2014. We also conducted a supplementary, non-systematic search that did not filter for geographical region. Please see Additional file 2 for these findings.

Titles and abstracts were reviewed twice and those which both reviewers agreed were relevant underwent full text review. Reference lists of reviewed manuscripts were screened for additional studies. Eligibility criteria included: 1) Study design: Prospective observational studies and clinical trials. 2) Participants: Aged 2–59 months treated with *oral* antibiotics for WHO-defined non-severe pneumonia per the 2013 revised WHO guidelines (Fig. 1) [15]. 3) Data collection dates: 1997 or more recent. The current WHO guidelines were formally disseminated in 1997 [1]. 4) Geographic regions: Africa and/or Asia, representing the highest burden of disease. 5) Outcome: *A priori* defined treatment failure, with statistical analysis for independent baseline clinical predictors of treatment failure.

We used a structured data extraction tool to describe key data from the eligible studies including: region, study design, primary outcome, data collection dates, enrollment criteria, treatment failure definition, sample size, age range of participants, treatment failure rate, and independent predictors of treatment failure. The Cochrane

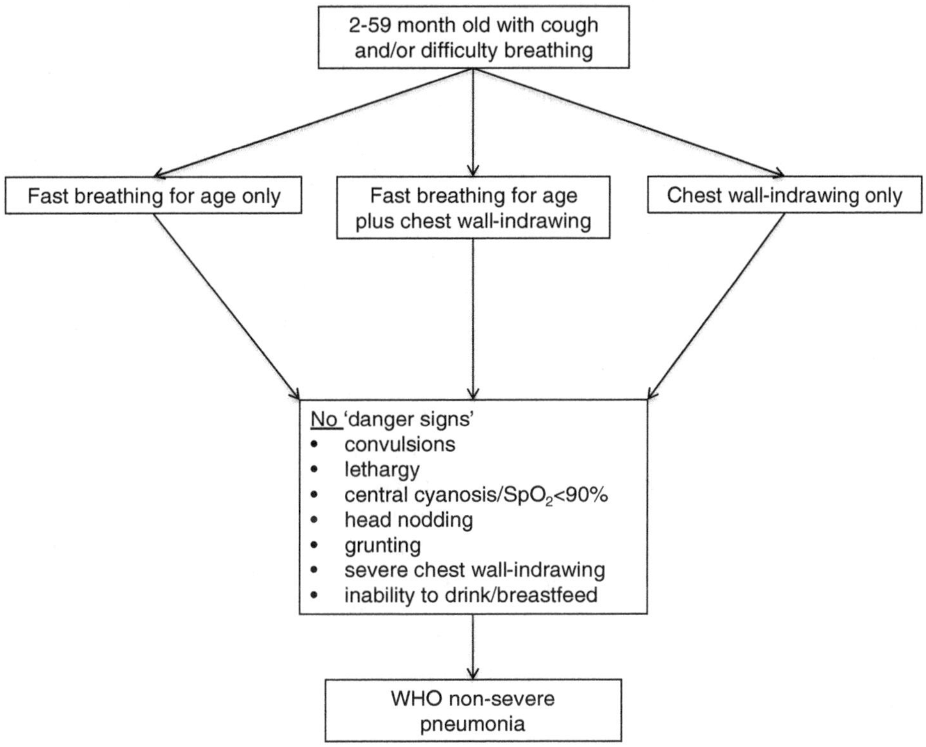

Fig. 1 2013 World Health Organization non-severe pneumonia case definition

Risk of Bias tool was used to qualitatively assess the risk of bias in individual studies [16].

Expert opinion

We complemented the systematic literature review by surveying childhood pneumonia experts. The experts were all healthcare professionals experienced in childhood pneumonia in the African or Asian region across hospital and community care settings, many with research experience [17]. We used a modified Delphi consensus process, administering two separate structured phone interviews and a final electronic survey to 13 experts, concluding when a general consensus was reached (see Additional file 3 for interview materials). Participants were asked to assess the potential role for a pneumonia treatment prognostic, including where in the health system (the home, a community health clinic, or the hospital) a prognostic would be best utilized.

The literature search provided the initial prognostic indicators to test with interviewees, using WHO definitions [15]. The panel was allowed to adjust these indicators, as well as the definitions of them and we encouraged the panel to use their own knowledge and experience. Fever was modified to an axillary temperature >38.0 °C, high blood lactate levels to >2 mmol/l, and low weight for age as a standardized z score < −2. The definition of 'human immunodeficiency virus (HIV)-affected' included HIV-exposed children (i.e. born to an HIV-infected mother but not HIV tested *or* previously tested HIV-negative with ongoing breastfeeding) or HIV-infected per standard guidelines [18].

The experts qualitatively and quantitatively estimated each predictor's potential value. Qualitative estimates of each prognostic indicator's value were allocated using an ordinal scale (0 = unfavorable, 1 = minimally favorable, 2 = favorable, 3 = highly favorable), along with any comments regarding each indicator's likely performance and feasibility. Panel members provided quantitative estimates by assigning a childhood pneumonia mortality rate to community oral *or* parenteral hospital antibiotic treatment.

An anonymous summary of panel answers were provided to interviewees after the first interview and each expert was encouraged to revise their answers after considering the panel's overall results. For the final survey, the expert opinion results were rephrased into binary yes/no questions to determine a final consensus. This research was approved by the Johns Hopkins Institutional Review Board (IRB00047406) and written consent was obtained from survey participants.

Results

Systematic review

Our search yielded 7,649 studies; of these, 59 manuscripts were retrieved for full text review. Nine studies met all eligibility criteria, including quality control, and were qualitatively analyzed (Fig. 2). We found no publications that included children with fast breathing *and* lower chest indrawing (LCI)-defined pneumonia together, probably because the WHO guidelines were only recently revised and disseminated in 2013.

Table 1 summarizes the six studies reporting predictors of oral antibiotic failure in fast breathing non-severe pneumonia [19–24]. All studies were from developing countries in south Asia. Five of the six studies included amoxicillin treatment and only one included community clinics. Five studies defined treatment failure as either a persistence of fast breathing after 3–5 days or disease progression (development of LCI or danger signs) between 1–5 days after antibiotic initiation. One study included peripheral oxygen saturation (SpO_2) less than 90 % in the definition of treatment failure. The proportion of children that failed oral antibiotic treatment ranged from 7.8 % to 22.9 %. Three studies identified baseline excess age-specific respiratory rate, and two studies found history of difficulty breathing, age, and illness duration of ≥3 days as independent predictors of oral antibiotic failure.

Table 2 summarizes the three studies reporting independent predictors of oral antibiotic failure in LCI non-severe pneumonia [25–27]. Two studies were multi-country with sites in Africa. In two of the three studies, treatment failure was assigned on day six after antibiotic initiation. Treatment failure rates for the three studies ranged from 8.1 % to 19.3 %. All studies found young age and very fast breathing at baseline to be independent predictors of treatment failure. One study collected SpO_2 measurements and found low baseline SpO_2 to predictive; another study found malnutrition to be predictive of treatment failure.

Expert opinion

Of the 13 experts interviewed, eight reported experience in Africa, four in Asia, and one in both. All interviewees agreed that the development of a pneumonia treatment prognostic could significantly advance childhood pneumonia care and that the community-level was the most attractive setting for implementation.

The panel qualitatively evaluated seven prognostic indicators for performance and feasibility at the community level (Table 3). Abnormal SpO_2 and malnutrition were ranked highest while fever and high blood lactate

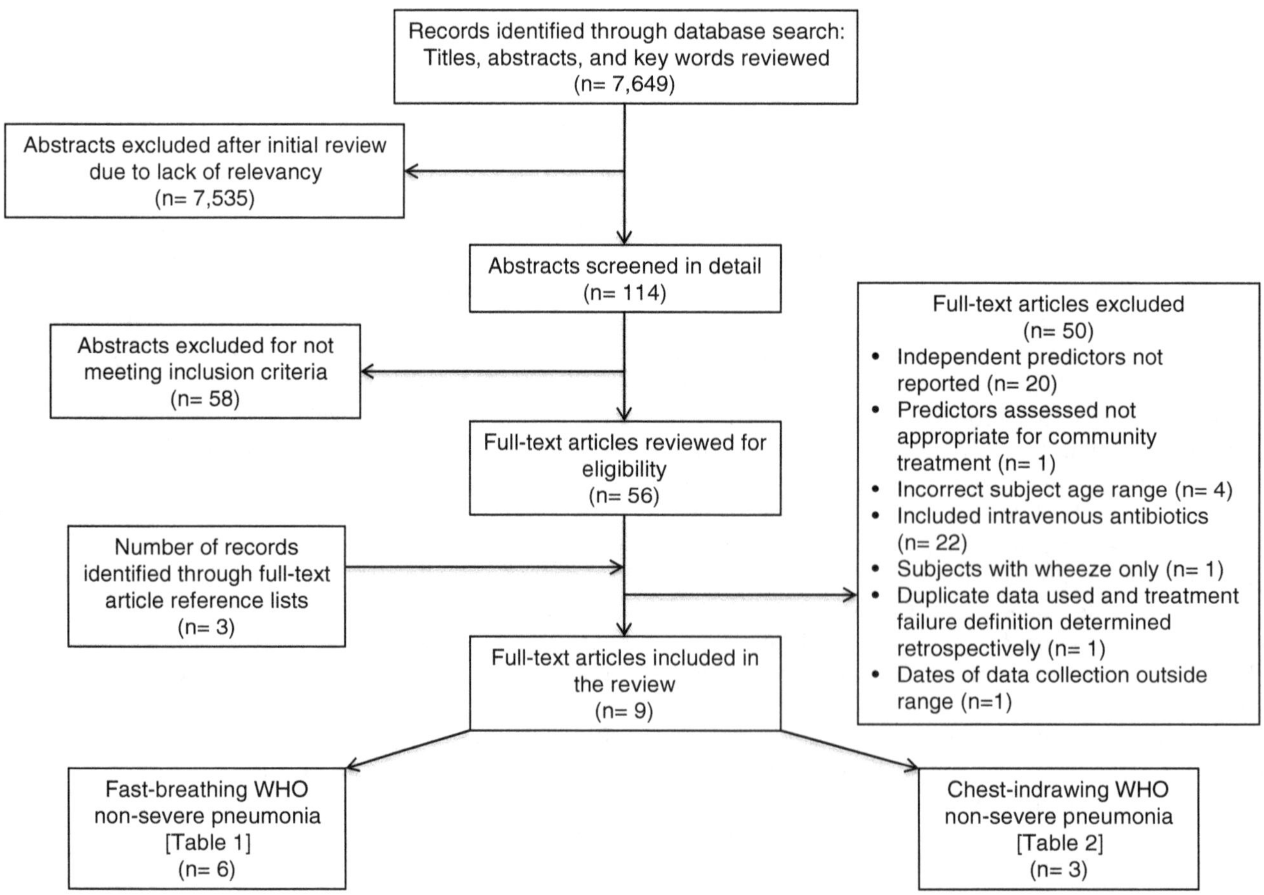

Fig. 2 Flow diagram of study identification and selection

Table 1 Independent predictors of oral antibiotic failure in fast breathing WHO non-severe childhood pneumonia[a]

Study overview	Awasthi S et al.	CATCH UP	MASCOT	Agarwal G et al.	Noorani QA et al.	Hazir T et al.
Region (country)	Asia (India)	Asia (Pakistan)	Asia (Pakistan)	Asia (India)	Asia (Pakistan)	Asia (Pakistan)
Data collection dates	2004–2006	1998–1999	1999–2001	2000–2002	2000–2001	2005–2008
Enrollment criteria	2–59 months old	2–59 months old	2–59 months of age	2–59 months of age	2–59 months of age	2–59 months of age
Study design	Cluster randomized study	Randomized multicenter equivalency study	Randomized multicenter equivalency study	Randomized multicenter equivalency study	Multicenter observational study	Randomized multicenter equivalency study
Intervention arm	Oral amoxicillin 31–51 mg/kg/day for 3 days	Oral amoxicillin 50 mg/kg/day for 5 days	Oral amoxicillin 45 mg/kg/day for 3 days	Oral amoxicillin 31–54 mg/kg/day for 3 days	-	Placebo for 3 days
Control arm (or standard of care)	Oral trimethoprim (7–11 mg/kg/day)-sulfamethoxazole for 5 days	Oral trimethoprim (8 mg/kg/day)-sulfamethoxazole for 5 days	Oral amoxicillin 45 mg/kg/day for 5 days	Oral amoxicillin 31–54 mg/kg/day for 5 days	Oral trimethoprim (8 mg/kg/day)-sulfamethoxazole for 5 days	Oral amoxicillin 45 mg/kg/day for 3 days
Blinding	No	Yes	Yes	Yes	-	Yes
Study site types	Health centers	Tertiary care and secondary-level hospitals, and health center	Tertiary care and secondary-level hospitals	Tertiary care hospitals	Health centers	Tertiary care hospitals
Number of sites	14	8	7	7	14	4
Primary outcome	Treatment failure	Equivalency	Equivalency	Equivalency	Treatment failure	Equivalency
Treatment failure definition						
Day of assignment	Day 3 (intervention); Day 5 (control)	Days 3 to 5	Day 5	Days 3 to 5	Day 5	Day 3
Respiratory rate[a]	Yes, elevated for age (days 3–5)	Yes, +/−5 breaths/min or higher versus enrollment (days 3–5)	Yes, elevated for age (days 3–5)	Yes, elevated for age (days 3–5)	Yes, +/−5 breaths/min or higher versus enrollment (days 3–5)	No
Fever >38 °C *and* LCI	No	No	No	No	No	No
Fever >38 °C	Yes (days 3–5)	No	No	No	No	No
LCI	Yes (days 1–5)	Yes (days 3–5)	Yes (days 1–5)	Yes (days 1–5)	Yes (days 1–5)	Yes (days 1–3)
Convulsions	Yes (days 1–5)	Yes (days 3–5)	Not specified	Yes (days 1–5)	Not specified	Yes (days 1–3)
Abnormally sleepy	Yes (days 1–5)	Yes (days 3–5)	Not specified	Yes (days 1–5)	Not specified	Yes (days 1–3)
Inability to drink	Yes (days 1–5)	Yes (days 3–5)	Not specified	Yes (days 1–5)	Not specified	Yes (days 1–3)
Stridor in calm child	Yes (days 1–5)	Yes (days 3–5)	No	No	No	Yes (days 1–3)
Malnutrition	No	Yes (days 3–5)	No	No	No	Yes (days 1–3)
Cyanosis	Yes (days 1–5)	No	Yes	No	Yes	No
SpO_2	No	No	No	Yes, <90 % (on day 3 only)	No	No
Antibiotic change	No	Yes (days 3–5)	Yes (days 1–5)	No	Yes (days 1–5)	No
Hospitalization	No	Yes (days 1–5)	No	No	No	No
Lost to follow-up	Yes (days 3–5)	Yes (days 3–5)	No	Yes (days 1–5)	Yes (days 5–11)	No

Table 1 Independent predictors of oral antibiotic failure in fast breathing WHO non-severe childhood pneumonia[a] *(Continued)*

Study withdrawal	Yes (days 1–5)	No	No	Yes (days 1–5)	No	No
Death	Yes (days 1–14)	Yes (days 1–5)	Yes (days 1–5)	Yes (days 1–5)	Yes (days 1–5)	Yes (days 1–5)
Study participants and description						
Sample size[b]	2009	1459	1953	2188	944	873
Age 2–11 months	594/2009 (29.6 %)	732/1459 (50.2 %)	1051/1953 (53.8 %)	954/2188 (43.6 %)	334/944 (35.4 %)	573/873 (65.6 %)
Age 12–59 months	1415/2009 (70.4 %)	727/1459 (49.8 %)	902/1953 (46.2 %)	1234/2188 (56.4 %)	610/944 (64.6 %)	300/873 (34.4 %)
Treatment failure rate[b]	234/2009 (11.6 %)	256/1459 (17.5 %)	364/1953 (22.9 %)	225/2188 (10.3 %)	110/944 (11.6 %)	68/873 (7.8 %)
Independent predictors of treatment failure OR (95 % CI)[c,d]	Diarrhea, 1.65 (1.24–2.19)	History of difficulty breathing, 1.61 (1.13–2.15)	Excess respiratory rate >10 breaths/min for age[a], 1.4 (1.1–1.9)	Excess respiratory rate >10 breaths/min for age[a], 2.89 (1.83–4.55)	Excess respiratory rate ≥15 breaths/min for age[a], 2.0 (1.2–3.4)	History of difficulty breathing, 2.86 (1.29–7.23)
		Age 12–59 months, 1.5 (1.12–1.91)	Antibiotic non-adherence, 4.5 (95 % CI 2.9–7.0)	Antibiotic non-adherence, 11.57 (7.4–18.0	Wheeze on examination, 1.7 (1.1–2.6)	Temperature >37.5 °C at enrollment, 1.99 (1.37–2.90)
		Illness >3 days, 1.4 (1.03–1.8)	Illness ≥3 days, 1.7 (1.3–2.1)	RSV, 1.95 (1.0–3.8)		
			Age 2–11 months, 1.7 (1.1–2.1)			
			Persistent vomiting, 1.4 (1.0–2.0)			

Serious adverse event or drug reaction, and new comorbid condition were not considered in the treatment failure definitions for any of the studies. WHO: World Health Organization; LCI: lower chest wall indrawing; SpO_2: peripheral oxygen saturation; OR: odds ratio; CI: confidence interval; RSV: human respiratory syncytial virus

[a]Respiratory rate norms: <50 breaths/min for ages 2–11 months; <40 breaths/min for ages 12–59 months

[b]If primary outcome of trial was equivalency or no difference was found then intervention and control arm data was combined

[c]Multivariate logistic regression modeling was performed to determine independent predictors of treatment failure in all included studies. CATCHUP trial modeled age, history of difficulty breathing, duration of illness, and respiratory rate. The models were not reported for the MASCOT trial, Agarwal G et al., Noorani QA et al., Awasthi S et al., and Hazir T et al

[d]For Hazir T et al. multivariate logistic regression modeling was performed on cumulative treatment failure data from day 5 although primary outcome data was analyzed from day 3 treatment failure data

levels were lowest. Abnormal SpO_2 was judged to be objective, although the panel identified the need for a robust, precise, low-cost pulse oximeter for young children. Malnutrition was also valued by the experts as it is likely to have a high positive predictive value and the feasibility of reliable malnutrition screening was attractive, with tools such as tapes and scales being simple, accurate, and relatively inexpensive.

The panel's quantitative performance estimates for each prognostic indicator are presented in Table 4. Regardless of setting, children that are malnourished, HIV-affected or have an abnormal SpO_2, were estimated to be at the highest mortality risk by the panel. Estimated median mortality rates of community treatment with amoxicillin for children with abnormal SpO_2, malnutrition, or an HIV-affected status ranged from 15.5–20 %.

Discussion

WHO guidelines standardize pneumonia management in low-resource settings and stratify pneumonia severity according to the presence of severe clinical features [1, 15]. Currently, these guidelines do not further categorize non-severe pneumonia patients according to their treatment failure risk even though some children with non-severe disease have failure rates as high as 23 % [20]. Given the increased decentralization of pneumonia care to CHWs, improving baseline risk stratification with objective clinical measures may be an important next step for reducing pneumonia morbidity. To assist in algorithm development, we performed a systematic review and surveyed experts to identify predictors of oral antibiotic failure in children that fit the WHO case definition for non-severe pneumonia (2013 guidelines) [15]. We placed the greatest emphasis on predictors not currently incorporated into referral algorithms and those that were also measureable by CHWs. From the literature and expert review, we found some agreement for excess age-specific respiratory rate, abnormal baseline SpO_2 and moderate malnutrition as important predictors of treatment failure. However, the literature was limited and highlighted several key evidence gaps, and there were notable differences between those predictors

Table 2 Independent predictors of oral antibiotic failure in chest indrawing WHO non-severe childhood pneumonia

Study overview	Addo-Yobo E, Chisaka N et al.	Hazir T, Fox LM et al.	Addo-Yobo E, Anh DD et al.
Region (countries)	Africa (Ghana, South Africa, Zambia) Asia (India, Pakistan, Vietnam) South America (Columbia, Mexico)	Pakistan (Asia)	Africa (Egypt, Ghana) Asia (Bangladesh, Vietnam)
Data collection dates	1999–2002	2005–2006	2005–2008
Enrollment criteria	3–59 months	3–59 months	3–59 months
Study design	Randomized multicenter equivalency study	Randomized multicenter equivalency study	Multicenter observational study
Intervention arm	Oral amoxicillin 45 mg/kg/day for 5 days	Oral amoxicillin 80–90 mg/kg/day for 5 days	-
Control arm (or standard of care)	Intravenous 200,000 IU penicillin G for 2 days then oral amoxicillin 45 mg/kg/day for 3 days (total 5 days)	Intravenous ampicillin 100 mg/kg/day for 2 days then oral amoxicillin for 3 days (total 5 days)	Amoxicillin 80–90 mg/kg/day for 5 days
Blinding	No	No	-
Study site type(s)	Pediatric department of tertiary care hospitals	Pediatric department of tertiary care hospitals	Pediatric department of tertiary care and second-level hospitals, health centers
Number of study sites	9	7	5
Primary outcome	Equivalence	Equivalence	Treatment failure
Treatment failure definition			
Day of assignment	Day 3	Day 6	Day 6
Respiratory rate[a]	No	No	No
Fever >38 °C *and* LCI	No	Yes (days 3–6)	Yes (day 3)
Fever >38 °C	No	Yes (day 6)	Yes (day 6)
LCI	Yes (day 3)	Yes (day 6)	Yes (day 6)
Convulsions	Yes (days 1–3)	Yes (days 1–6)	Yes (days 1–6)
Abnormally sleepy	Yes (days 1–3)	Yes (days 1–6)	Yes (days 1–6)
Inability to drink	Yes (days 1–3)	Yes (days 1–6)	Yes (days 1–6)
Stridor in calm child	No	No	No
Malnutrition	No	No	No
Cyanosis	Yes (days 1–3)	Yes (days 1–6)	Yes (days 1–6)
SpO_2	<80 % at sea-level or <75 % below sea-level (days 1–3)	No	No
Antibiotic change	Yes (days 1–3)	No	Yes (days 1–6)
Hospitalization	No	Yes, if related to pneumonia (days 1–6)	No
Serious drug reaction	Yes (days 1–3)	No	Yes (days 1–6)
Serious adverse event	No	Yes (days 1–6)	No
	Yes (days 1–3)	Yes, if required antibiotic (days 1–6)	Yes (days 1–6)

Table 2 Independent predictors of oral antibiotic failure in chest indrawing WHO non-severe childhood pneumonia *(Continued)*

New comorbid condition			
Lost to follow-up	Yes (days 1–3)	Yes (days 1–6)	Yes (day 6)
Study withdrawal	Yes (days 1–3)	Yes (days 1–6)	No
Death	Yes (days 1–3)	Yes (days 1–14)	Yes (days 1–6)
Study participants and description			
Sample size[b]	1702	2037	823
Age: 3–11 months	1045/1669 (62.6 %)	1311/2037 (64.4 %)	562/873 (64.4 %)
12–59 months	624/1669 (37.4 %)	726/2037 (35.6 %)	310/873 (35.5 %)
Treatment failure rate[c]	328/1702 (19.3 %)	164/2037 (8.1 %)	76/823 (9.2 %)
Independent predictors of treatment failure[c] OR/RR (95 % CI)	Age 3–11 months, 2.72 OR (95 % CI 1.95–3.79)	Age 3–5 months, 3.22 OR, (95 % CI 1.87–5.52)	Age 3–5 months, 1.96 RR (95 % CI 1.09–3.51)
	Very fast breathing, 1.94 OR (95 % CI 1.42–2.65)[d]	Very fast breathing, 1.65 OR (95 % CI 1.07–2.57)[d]	Very fast breathing, 12.5 RR (95 % CI 1.74–89.1)[d]
	$SpO_2 < 90$ %, 2.11 OR (95 % CI 1.6–2.78)	Weight for age z score <−2, 1.79 OR (95 % CI 1.23–2.60)	

WHO: World Health Organization; *IU*: International Units; *LCI*: lower chest wall indrawing; *SpO_2*: peripheral oxygen saturation; *OR*: odds ratio; *RR*: relative risk; *CI*, confidence interval

[a]Respiratory rate norms: <50 breaths/min for ages 2–11 months; <40 breaths/min for ages 12–59 months

[b]If primary outcome of trial was equivalency then intervention and control arm data was combined

[c]Multivariate logistic regression modeling was used by Addo-Yobo E, Chisaka N et al. and Hazir T while log-linear regression modeling was used by Fox LM et al. Addo-Yobo E, Chisaka N et al. modeled age, very fast breathing, hypoxemia, and amoxicillin. Hazir T, Fox LM et al. modeled sex, age, breastfeeding, weight-for-age z score <−2, very fast breathing, and treatment group (home vs hospital). Addo-Yobo E, Anh DD et al. modeled sex, age, and respiratory rate

[d]Very fast breathing defined as ≥70 breaths/min for ages 3–11 months and ≥60 breaths/min for ages 12–59 months

supported by the literature and those favored by the experts.

Our systematic review and expert survey yielded several interesting comparisons. The panel strongly favored abnormal SpO_2 as a predictor, however, SpO_2 was evaluated in only two studies [21, 25], none of which examined SpO_2 at community clinics or assessed less severe, but still abnormal SpO_2 ranges (90–94 %). Similarly, malnutrition was highlighted by the panel but was only found to be predictive for oral antibiotic failure in one study conducted at tertiary hospital clinics [26]. Milder degrees of malnutrition were not evaluated, and the experts defined malnutrition in the moderate range. Although young age was found to be predictive in multiple studies [20, 25–27], the experts did not recommend young age as a candidate predictor. *Haemophilus influenzae* type B (HiB) vaccine or pneumococcal conjugate vaccine (PCV) status were not examined as predictors in our systematic review since most studies were performed before introduction of these vaccines, but it was also not recommended by the panel. These differences between the published literature and expert panel may in part reflect the panel's emphasis on personal experience to guide their answers and the overall lack of publications meeting eligibility criteria. In addition, a majority of the panel worked in Africa while in contrast the published literature was heavily represented by Asia.

The systematic review suggested that fast breathing and LCI pneumonia may be distinct groups with different drivers and predictors of failure. Our review of the literature consistently found excess age-specific respiratory rate as an important predictor in both LCI- and fast breathing non-severe pneumonia [20–22, 25–27], but abnormal baseline SpO_2 and young age were clearer predictors of treatment failure in children solely with LCI [25–27]. In those studies looking at fast-breathing defined pneumonia, the independent predictors were less consistent and included persistent vomiting, diarrhea, wheeze, human respiratory syncytial virus infection and history of difficult breathing; these may suggest a primarily viral cause of illness. Other studies support the notion that a low proportion of fast breathing pneumonia cases may be due to bacterial pneumonia. Hazir and colleagues reported that only 1.7 % of Pakistani children with fast breathing pneumonia had a radiographic consolidation consistent with a bacterial etiology [28], and the same group also published findings of equivalency when fast breathing cases were treated with either

Table 3 Expert panel qualitative assessments of potential prognostic indicators

Prognostic indicator	Overall favorability	Selected performance comments	Selected feasibility comments
Fever	Unfavorable	Low specificity for identifying children who will not fail treatment	High feasibility since already implemented and measurement tools simple
Rapid breathing	Minimally favorable	Normal range highly variable	Measurement tools inaccurate
		Low sensitivity for hypoxemic children	Low feasibility with respect to sequential monitoring of respiratory rates over time
		Performance profile improves with sequential monitoring of respiratory rates over time	
Lower chest wall indrawing	Favorable	Low specificity for identifying children who will not fail treatment	Subjective sign with variable inter-provider agreement levels
Abnormal oxygen saturation	Highly favorable	High specificity for identifying children who will not fail treatment	Objective measurement but inter-provider agreement levels unknown
		Later indicator decreases sensitivity for identifying children who will fail treatment at the community-level	Robust, precise, low-cost point-of-care instrument needed
			Likely costly to implement and sustain
High blood lactate levels	Unfavorable	Low specificity for identifying children who will not fail treatment	Point-of-care tool appropriate for community use not available, likely costly
		Very late indicator decreases sensitivity for identifying children who will fail treatment at the community-level	
Moderate malnutrition	Highly favorable	Mid-range sensitivity and specificity which likely improves greatly in combination with other indicators	High feasibility since measurement tools simple and accurate
		High positive predictive value	
HIV-affected	Minimally favorable	Geographically limited in relevancy (e.g. primarily in eastern and southern Africa)	Low feasibility since difficult to obtain HIV status at community-level (e.g. stigma)
		High positive predictive value	

HIV: Human Immunodeficiency Virus

placebo or amoxicillin [23]. At this time listening for wheeze with a stethoscope or testing for respiratory syncytial virus are not feasible for routine CHW care. The results from this systematic review should be interpreted within this context; LCI and fast breathing pneumonia may differ etiologically and the published literature on this subject has primarily focused on fast breathing pneumonia (only three studies meeting eligibility criteria for this work included LCI pneumonia).

Our systematic review found an overall paucity of community-level data, potentially limited by publication bias. However, we also found other important evidence gaps. Firstly, it is likely that predictors will differ between African and Asian populations, in part because HIV is endemic in southern Africa and a key driver of treatment unresponsive pneumonia [29]. However, our systematic review demonstrated that African data is limited, with only two studies including data from African countries. These studies did not explore region as a predictor of treatment failure, and did not report adjusting for region in their multivariate models. The experts also did not address this evidence gap since they did not explicitly factor regional differences into their responses, although the majority of experts worked in Africa and this is likely to have influenced their answers. The development of a sound prognostic algorithm for the southern African region that

Table 4 Expert panel quantitative assessments of potential prognostic indicators

Identified prognostic indicator[a]	Mortality rate according to location of care received if prognostic indictor positive	
	Community treatment with oral amoxicillin	Hospital treatment with parenteral antibiotics
Fever	0.5 % (0.5–1.0)	0.1 % (0.1–0.2)
Rapid breathing	1.0 % (1.0–2.0)	0.2 % (0.1–0.5)
Lower chest indrawing	5.8 % (5.1–7.4)	1.0 % (0.6–1.0)
Abnormal SpO_2	15.5 % (11.3–23.0)	6.3 % (5.0–7.5)
Moderate malnutrition	20.0 % (18.5–25.0)	10.5 % (5.0–12.8)
HIV-infected or HIV-exposed status	16.5 % (15.0–20.0)	7.5 % (6.1–8.6)

IQR: interquartile range; *SpO_2*: peripheral oxygen saturation
[a]Lactate not assessed quantitatively

accounts for HIV status may be challenging since HIV stigma persists, particularly in more rural, intimate community settings where anonymous testing is difficult to achieve [30]. Second, it is likely that pneumonia epidemiology, and thus treatment failure predictors, will shift after HiB vaccine and PCV introduction. However, data from developing countries after full vaccine introduction is only more recently becoming available [31]. Due to these limitations in the literature, the findings from the literature review need to be interpreted cautiously.

Although validated prognostic models that identify higher risk pneumonia patients exist, only two studies (both secondary analyses from the Amoxicillin Penicillin Pneumonia International Study (APPIS) [25]) present predictive models for children who fulfill the LCI non-severe pneumonia case definition [32, 33]. Mamtani et al. validated a clinical tool for predicting oral amoxicillin failure in children with LCI pneumonia and no danger signs, using the child's age and excess age-specific respiratory rate after 24 h of treatment to stratify patients' risk [32]. Fu et al. predicted the risk of oral amoxicillin treatment failure after 48 h, with the best performing model including a second clinical evaluation after 12 h of treatment and SpO_2 [33]. However both studies likely reflect different pneumonia epidemiology due to increasing HiB and PCV availability and current treatment failure definitions have been simplified [26, 27]. The feasibility of using models that rely on a single patient observation for an extended period or multiple clinical observations will need careful assessment at the CHW level.

At this time more evidence is needed to demonstrate effective use of pulse oximetry by CHWs, whether milder degrees of altitude-adjusted hypoxemia (90–94 %) are predictive of treatment failure, and if pulse oximetry can be cost-effective at the community level in low-resource countries where equipment maintenance can be challenging. Several low-cost respiratory rate counters, pulse oximeters and combination devices have recently been developed or are in development for low-resource settings [34–36]; there is an on-going evaluation of the clinical performance, usability, and acceptability of these devices currently underway by Malaria Consortium (D. Hay Burgess, personal communication).

Conclusion

In conclusion, we found that young age, excess age-specific respiratory rate, abnormal baseline SpO_2 and moderate malnutrition should be carefully considered for an automated mHealth iCCM tool for predicting oral antibiotic failure in children with pneumonia. However, the evidence is currently limited. Additional formative research to identify antibiotic failure predictors is needed at the community-level, in HIV and non-HIV endemic regions, with and without malaria, and that have introduced the HiB vaccine and PCV. Modeling patient and health system-level consequences of a prognostic, along with a cost analysis of device scale-up, are important next steps.

Abbreviations

WHO: World Health Organization; iCCM: integrated Community Case Management; CHW: Community health worker; mHealth: Mobile health; HIV: Human immunodeficiency virus; LCI: Lower chest indrawing; SpO_2: Peripheral oxygen saturation; HiB: *Haemophilus influenzae* type B; PCV: Pneumococcal conjugate vaccine.

Competing interests

The authors declare that they have no competing interests.

Authors' contributions

Conceived and designed the experiments: EDM, CK, RH, JZ, DM, DCHB. Performed the literature review and expert review: EDM, RH, JZ, DCHB. Analyzed the data: EDM, CK, RH, JZ, TC, BN. Wrote first draft of paper: EDM. Edited paper for content: EDM, CK, RH, JZ, TC, BN, DM, DCHB. All authors read and approved the final manuscript. EDM is the guarantor of the paper.

Acknowledgements

We would like to thank Saul S. Morris for his contributions to this research. EDM was supported by the Fogarty International Center of the National Institutes of Health under Award Number K01TW009988 for the research reported in this publication. The content is solely the responsibility of the authors and does not necessarily represent the official views of the National Institutes of Health.

Author details

[1]Department of Pediatrics, Division of Pulmonology, Johns Hopkins School of Medicine, Baltimore, USA. [2]Institute for Global Health, University College London, London, UK. [3]The Boston Consulting Group, Boston, USA. [4]Bill & Melinda Gates Foundation, Seattle, USA.

References

1. Handbook IMCI. Integrated management of childhood illness. World Health Organization. 2005. http://whqlibdoc.who.int/publications/2005/9241546441.pdf. Accessed 28 August 2014.
2. Sazawal S, Black RE. Effect of pneumonia case management on mortality in neonates, infants, and preschool children: a meta-analysis of community-based trials. Lancet Infect Dis. 2003;3(9):547–56.
3. Liu L, Oza S, Hogan D, Perin J, Rudan I, Lawn JE, et al. Global, regional, and national causes of child mortality in 2000–13, with projections to inform post-2015 priorities: an updated systematic analysis. Lancet. 2014;385(9966):430–40.
4. Pneumonia: the forgotten killer of children. United Nations Children's Fund. 2006. http://www.unicef.org/publications/files/Pneumonia_The_Forgotten_Killer_of_Children.pdf. Accessed 28 Aug 2014.
5. Management of pneumonia in community settings. United Nations Children's Fund/World Health Organization. 2006. http://whqlibdoc.who.int/hq/2004/WHO_FCH_CAH_04.06.pdf?ua=1. Accessed 28 Aug 2014.
6. Integrated Community Case Management (iCCM). World Health Organization/United Nations Children's Fund. 2012. http://www.unicef.org/health/files/iCCM_Joint_Statement_2012.pdf. Accessed 28 Aug 2014.

7. Yeboah-Antwi K, Pilingana P, Macleod WB, Semrau K, Siazeele K, Kalesha P, et al. Community case management of fever Due to malaria and pneumonia in children under five in Zambia: a cluster randomized controlled trial. PLoS Med. 2010;7(9):e1000340.
8. Bari A, Sadruddin S, Khan A, Khan I, Khan A, Lehri IA, et al. Community case management of severe pneumonia with oral amoxicillin in children aged 2–59 months in Haripur district, Pakistan: a cluster randomised trial. Lancet. 2011;378(9805):1796–803.
9. Soofi S, Ahmed S, Fox MP, MacLeod WB, Thea DM, Qazi SA, et al. Effectiveness of community case management of severe pneumonia with oral amoxicillin in children aged 2–59 months in Matiari district, rural Pakistan: a cluster-randomised controlled trial. Lancet. 2012;379(9817):729–37.
10. Kahigwa E, Schellenberg D, Schellenberg JA, Aponte JJ, Alonso PL, Menendez C. Inter-observer variation in the assessment of clinical signs in sick Tanzanian children. Trans R Soc Trop Med Hyg. 2002;96(2):162–6.
11. Mobile technologies and empowerment: enhancing human development through participation and innovation. United Nations Development Programme. 2012. http://www.undp.org/content/dam/undp/library/Democratic%20Governance/Access%20to%20Information%20and%20E-governance/Mobile%20Technologies%20and%20Empowerment_EN.pdf. Accessed 28 Aug 2014.
12. Mechael PN. The case for mHealth in developing countries. Innovations: Technology, Governance, Globalization. 2009;4:103–18.
13. Kallander K, Tibenderana JK, Akpogheneta OJ, Strachan DL, Hill Z, ten Asbroek AH, et al. Mobile health (mHealth) approaches and lessons for increased performance and retention of community health workers in low- and middle-income countries: a review. J Med Internet Res. 2013;15(1):e17.
14. Moher D, Liberati A, Tetzlaff J, Altman DG. Preferred reporting items for systematic reviews and meta-analyses: the PRISMA statement. PLoS Med. 2009;6(7):e1000097.
15. Pocket book of hospital care for children: guidelines for the management of common illnesses with limited resources. World Health Organization. 2013. http://apps.who.int/iris/bitstream/10665/81170/1/9789241548373_eng.pdf?ua=1. Accessed 28 Aug 2014.
16. Cochrane handbook for systematic reviews of interventions. The Cochrane Collaboration. 2011. http://handbook.cochrane.org. Accessed 3 June 2014.
17. Powell C. The Delphi technique: myths and realities. J Adv Nurs. 2003;41(4):376–82.
18. WHO recommendations on the diagnosis of HIV infection in infants and children. World Health Organization. 2010. http://whqlibdoc.who.int/publications/2010/9789241599085_eng.pdf?ua=1. Accessed 28 Aug 2014.
19. CATCH UP study group. Clinical efficacy of co-trimoxazole versus amoxicillin twice daily for treatment of pneumonia: a randomised controlled clinical trial in Pakistan. Arch Dis Child. 2002;86(2):113–8.
20. MASCOT pneumonia study group. Clinical efficacy of 3 days versus 5 days of oral amoxicillin for treatment of childhood pneumonia: a multicentre double-blind trial. Lancet. 2002;360(9336):835–41.
21. Agarwal G, Awasthi S, Kabra SK, Kaul A, Singhi S, Walter SD. Three day versus five day treatment with amoxicillin for non-severe pneumonia in young children: a multicentre randomised controlled trial. BMJ (Clin Res Ed). 2004;328(7443):791.
22. Noorani QA, Qazi SA, Rasmussen ZA, Rehman GN, Khan SS, Muhammadullah I, et al. Response to cotrimoxazole in the management of childhood pneumonia in first-level health care facilities. Int J Tuberc Lung Dis Off J Int Union Tuberc Lung Dis. 2006;10(8):932–8.
23. Hazir T, Nisar YB, Abbasi S, Ashraf YP, Khurshid J, Tariq P, et al. Comparison of oral amoxicillin with placebo for the treatment of world health organization-defined nonsevere pneumonia in children aged 2–59 months: a multicenter, double-blind, randomized, placebo-controlled trial in pakistan. Clin Infect Dis Off Publ Infect Dis Soc Am. 2011;52(3):293–300.
24. Awasthi S, Agarwal G, Singh JV, Kabra SK, Pillai RM, Singhi S, et al. Effectiveness of 3-day amoxycillin vs. 5-day co-trimoxazole in the treatment of non-severe pneumonia in children aged 2–59 months of age: a multi-centric open labeled trial. J Trop Pediatr. 2008;54(6):382–9.
25. Addo-Yobo E, Chisaka N, Hassan M, Hibberd P, Lozano JM, Jeena P, et al. Oral amoxicillin versus injectable penicillin for severe pneumonia in children aged 3 to 59 months: a randomised multicentre equivalency study. Lancet. 2004;364(9440):1141–8.
26. Hazir T, Fox LM, Nisar YB, Fox MP, Ashraf YP, MacLeod WB, et al. Ambulatory short-course high-dose oral amoxicillin for treatment of severe pneumonia in children: a randomised equivalency trial. Lancet. 2008;371(9606):49–56.
27. Addo-Yobo E, Anh DD, El-Sayed HF, Fox LM, Fox MP, MacLeod W, et al. Outpatient treatment of children with severe pneumonia with oral amoxicillin in four countries: the MASS study. Trop Med Int Health. 2011;16(8):995–1006.
28. Hazir T, Nisar YB, Qazi SA, Khan SF, Raza M, Zameer S, et al. Chest radiography in children aged 2–59 months diagnosed with non-severe pneumonia as defined by World Health Organization: descriptive multicentre study in Pakistan. BMJ (Clin Res Ed). 2006;333(7569):629.
29. McNally LM, Jeena PM, Gajee K, Thula SA, Sturm AW, Cassol S, et al. Effect of age, polymicrobial disease, and maternal HIV status on treatment response and cause of severe pneumonia in South African children: a prospective descriptive study. Lancet. 2007;369(9571):1440–51.
30. Goodson JL, Finkbeiner T, Davis NL, Lyimo D, Rwebembera A, Swartzendruber AL, et al. Evaluation of using routine infant immunization visits to identify and follow-up HIV-exposed infants and their mothers in Tanzania. J Acquir Immune Defic Syndr (1999). 2013;63(1):e9–15.
31. Levine OS, O'Brien KL, Deloria-Knoll M, Murdoch DR, Feikin DR, DeLuca AN, et al. The pneumonia etiology research for child health project: a 21st century childhood pneumonia etiology study. Clin Infect Dis Off Publ Infect Dis Soc Am. 2012;54 Suppl 2:S93–101.
32. Mamtani M, Patel A, Hibberd PL, Tuan TA, Jeena P, Chisaka N, et al. A clinical tool to predict failed response to therapy in children with severe pneumonia. Pediatr Pulmonol. 2009;44(4):379–86.
33. Fu LY, Ruthazer R, Wilson I, Patel A, Fox LM, Tuan TA, et al. Brief hospitalization and pulse oximetry for predicting amoxicillin treatment failure in children with severe pneumonia. Pediatrics. 2006;118(6):e1822–30.
34. Hudson J, Nguku SM, Sleiman J, Karlen W, Dumont GA, Petersen CL, et al. Usability testing of a prototype phone oximeter with healthcare providers in high- and low-medical resource environments. Anaesthesia. 2012;67(9):957–67.
35. Karlen W, Gan H, Chiu M, Dunsmuir D, Zhou G, Dumont GA, et al. Improving the accuracy and efficiency of respiratory rate measurements in children using mobile devices. PLoS One. 2014;9(6):e99266.
36. Petersen CL, Chen TP, Ansermino JM, Dumont GA. Design and evaluation of a low-cost smartphone pulse oximeter. Sensors (Basel, Switzerland). 2013;13(12):16882–93.

25

Lung ultrasound: a useful tool in diagnosis and management of bronchiolitis

Vincenzo Basile[1], Antonio Di Mauro[2], Egisto Scalini[1], Paolo Comes[3], Ignazio Lofù[1], Michael Mostert[4], Silvio Tafuri[5] and Mariano M. Manzionna[1*]

Abstract

Background: Clinical assessment is the gold standard for diagnosis of bronchiolitis. To date, only one study found LUS (Lung Ultrasound) to be a valuable tool in the diagnosis of bronchiolitis. Aim of this study is to evaluate the accuracy of lung ultrasonography in the diagnosis and management of bronchiolitis in infants.

Methods: This was an observational cohort study of infants admitted to our Pediatric Unit with suspected bronchiolitis. A physical examination and lung ultrasound scans were performed on each patient. Diagnosis and grading of bronchiolitis was assessed according to a clinical and a ultrasound score. An exploratory analysis was used to assess correspondence between the lung ultrasound findings and the clinical evaluation and to evaluate the inter-observer concordance between the two different sonographs.

Results: One hundred six infants were studied (average age 71 days). According to our clinical score, 74 infants had mild bronchiolitis, 30 had moderate bronchiolitis and two had severe bronchiolitis. 25 infants composed the control group. Agreement between the clinical and sonographic diagnosis was good (90.6 %) with a statistically significant inter-observer ultrasound diagnosis concordance (89.6 %).
Lung ultrasound permits the identification of infants who are in need of supplementary oxygen with a specificity of 98.7 %, a sensitivity of 96.6 %, a positive predictive value of 96.6 % and a negative predictive value of 98.7 %. An aberrant ultrasound lung pattern in posterior chest area was collected in 86 % of infants with bronchiolitis. In all patients clinical improvement at discharge was associated with disappearance of the previous LUS findings. Subpleural lung consolidation of 1 cm or more in the posterior area scan and a quantitative classification of interstitial syndrome based on intercostal spaces involved bilaterally, good correlate with bronchiolitis severity and oxygen use.

Conclusions: The lung ultrasound findings strictly correlate with the clinical evaluations in infants with bronchiolitis and permit the identification of infants who are in need of supplementary oxygen with high specificity. Scans of the posterior area are more indicative in ascertaining the severity of bronchiolitis.

Keywords: Chest ultrasound, Sonographic interstitial syndrome, Bronchiolitis

* Correspondence: mariano.manzionna@alice.it
[1]Pediatric Unit, Maternal and Child Health Department, "S. Giacomo" Hospital, ASL BA, Largo Simone Veneziani, 21, Monopoli (Bari), Italy
Full list of author information is available at the end of the article

Background

Bronchiolitis is the most common lower respiratory tract illness that affects infants and children <2 years of age. It is usually caused by a viral infection with a peak of incidence and morbidity among infants of 1–3 months of age [1].

The diagnosis of bronchiolitis should be made on the basis of medical history and a clinical examination. Up to date, there are no serological or radiological signs included in the diagnostic work-up [2].

The pathophysiology of bronchiolitis is characterized by edema, an increased production of mucus and necrosis of the infected epithelial cells of the small airways that cause a heterogeneous obstruction of the distal bronchioles.

This process leads to a reduction in the air content in the lung with impaired diffusion across the blood-gas membrane and ventilation-perfusion inconsistency [3].

Lung ultrasound (LUS) is performed in adult and pediatric care for the evaluation of several cardiopulmonary conditions and with respect to the use of X-rays offers advantages as concerns the employment of ionizing radiation [4–7].

A healthy, normally-aerated lung reflects ultrasound beams due to its high acoustic impedance and shows only an anatomic indication of a hyper-reflective pleural line that slides, with breathing, towards the interface between tissue and air. A normal lung also reveals horizontal artifacts below the pleural line, called A lines, due to reverberations of ultrasound beam [8].

The gradual passage from a dry to a wet lung allows the reflection of the ultrasound beam and leads to the formation of vertical artifacts called B-lines [9]. An increasing concentration of vertical artifacts corresponds with the increasing extent of lung congestion and permits a quantification of pulmonary interstitial syndrome [10, 11].

The areas of lung dysventilation with an absence of alveolar air are visualized in the form of consolidations adjacent to the pleural line [12].

To date, only one study by Caiulo et al. found LUS to be a valuable tool in the diagnosis of bronchiolitis and at present LUS is not recommended for its management [13].

This study aims to compare the agreement between lung ultrasonography and clinical score in the diagnosis of infants with suspected bronchiolitis. In addition the present study explores the potential of ultrasound in bronchiolitis management in predict need for oxygen supplementation.

Methods

This is an observational cohort study, performed at the Pediatric Unit of S. Giacomo Hospital of Monopoli (Bari, Italy) in association with the Radiology Department.

The local Ethics Committee and the Institutional Review Board of the S. Giacomo Hospital in Monopoli (Bari, Italy) approved the protocol. Written informed parental consent was obtained.

All patients were admitted from January 2010 to December 2013 with history, signs and symptoms of suspected bronchiolitis, according to the American Academy of Pediatrics [1, 2]. They all then underwent a routine clinical evaluation and a Rapid Test for Syncytial Respiratory Virus (SRV) (BinaxNOW®SRV). Infants admitted for routine hip and kidney echography composed the control group.

The attending physician assessed the overall clinical impression on the basis of a modified previously published protocol for bronchiolitis [14] (Table 1).

Tachypnea, signs of dyspnea, use of accessory respiratory muscle and aberrant auscultation are thought to be the best clinical signs of bronchiolitis.

According to our clinical score, the diagnosis and grading of bronchiolitis was:

A. Mild bronchiolitis: score 1–4
B. Moderate bronchiolitis: score 5–8
C. Severe bronchiolitis: score 9–12
D. Healthy infant: score 0

To complete and widen the clinical evaluation, chest ultrasound scans were acquired by a pediatrician (VB) and a radiologist (PC) with a 10–12 MHZ linear transducer (LOGIQ P5 portable ultrasound system). All sonographers were equally skilled in chest scans and were unaware of the clinical score. The unavailability of a sonographer in the pediatric and radiology unit was considered exclusion criteria. We excluded patients with other major pathologies or previous chest-radiographs confirming pneumonia. In case of preterm intants, we excluded patients affected by bronchopulmonary dysplasia whose ultrasound pattern could be similar to bronchiolitis ultrasound appearance.

Ultrasonography examinations were performed following the methodology previously described by Copetti, Cattarossi et al. [15–17]. Both longitudinal and transversal sections were collected on the anterior, lateral, and posterior chest wall.

Data were classified according to the study protocol, on the basis of a proposed echographic score (Table 2). We decided to adopt this echographic score with the aim of answering a few simple queries about some bronchiolitis ultrasound findings that emerged from previous evaluations, such as a characteristic pattern of viral infections [18]; a presence of lung sliding with B-lines, confluent B-lines and sub pleural consolidations (Fig. 1) which were thought to be the best ultrasound signs of bronchiolitis [19].

Table 1 Clinical score

Clinical score	0	1	2	3
Respiratory rate	<50	50 - 60	61-69	>70
Dyspnea	Normal feeding	Difficulty feeding	2 of the following: difficulty feeding, pallor, perioral cyanosis OR agitation.	2 of the following: cyanosis, stopped feeding OR drowsiness.
Use of accessory respiratory muscles	None	Subcostal or intercostal retractions	2 of the following: subcostal, intercostal, substernal retractions OR nasal flaring	3 of the following: subcostal, intercostal, substernal, suprasternal, supraclavicular retractions OR nasal flaring
Auscultation	Normal breathing	End-expiratory wheeze only OR crackles.	Expiratory wheeze and/or crackles	Inspiratory and expiratory wheeze OR diminished breath sounds OR both

An accurate scanning of the posterior and paravertebral areas of the thorax was performed to increase the accuracy of the US examination [20].

A quantitative classification of echographic interstitial syndrome was proposed, based on the extent of lung involvement, using the bilaterally involved posterior intercostal spaces as coordinates (Fig. 2).

According to the ultrasound findings, diagnosis and severity of bronchiolitis were assessed as follows:

A. Mild bronchiolitis: score 1–3
B. Moderate bronchiolitis: score 4–6
C. Severe bronchiolitis: score 7–8
D. Normal lung ultrasound pattern: score 0

Reference diagnosis made by sonographers, who independently reviewed the ultrasound findings, was collected and inter-observer concordance was assessed. Furthermore, the ultrasound score was correlated with the clinical data to estimate the agreement between clinical and echographic diagnosis.

The attending physician was unaware of the LUS score and was responsible for treatment decisions. Hypoxia due to ventilation/perfusion incongruity was evaluated by way of arterialized capillary blood gas determinations. Normal values for capillary blood oxygen tension were assumed to be >45 mmHg in air. Pulse oximetry (PM-7000, Masimo SET®) was used for monitoring trends in oxygenation. In accordance with local protocols, the infants were treated with oxygen supplementation when supplementary O_2 was needed to keep saturation at >94 % (<90 if asleep) or capillary blood oxygen tension at <45 mmHg.

All patients underwent an echographical follow-up in order to obtain data on the disappearance of ultrasound pulmonary abnormalities during the course of the disease. At discharge, the US Score was recalculated. Clinical and ultrasonographical evaluation was performed even on infants without signs of bronchiolitis, admitted for routine hip and kidney echography (control group).

Statistical analysis

Cohen's kappa coefficient was calculated to assess agreement on diagnosis between the attending physician and the pediatric sonographer. The sonographer inter-observer concordance was also assessed.

According to recent literature[2], 25 % of infants hospitalized for bronchiolitis need oxygen supplementation. With an α level of 0.05 and a power of 90 % a sample size of 19 infants was needed.

We calculated the specificity, sensitivity, positive predictive value and negative predictive value of the

Table 2 Bronchiolitis ultrasound score

US score		0	1	2
Anterolateral data		Normal lung sliding with horizontal artifacts (A-lines). Vertical artifacts (B-lines) in limited number or absent.	Diffuse and dishomogeneous interstitial syndrome with confluent, multiple B lines and spared areas.	Diffuse and dishomogeneous interstitial syndrome and/or subpleural lung consolidations.
Paravertebral/ posterior data	Interstitial syndrome	Individual B line or absent	Focal, multiple B-lines	Confluent, multiple B lines
	Extension on interstitial syndrome	0-6 bilaterally involved intercostal spaces	6-12bilaterally involved intercostal spaces	>12 bilaterally involved intercostal spaces
	Presence of subpleural lung consolidation	Absent	Subcentimeter-subpleural lung consolidation	Subpleural lung consolidation of 1 cm or more

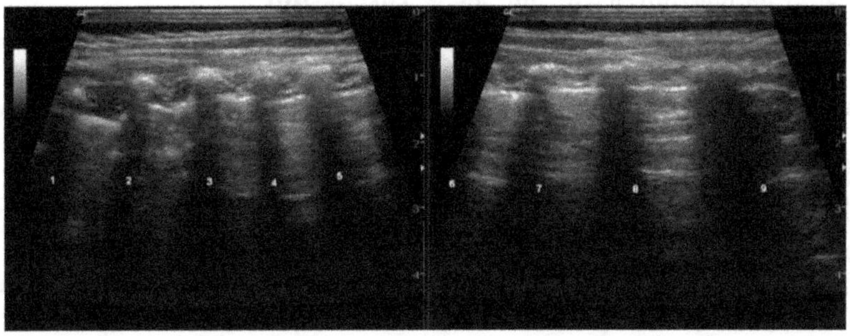

Fig. 1 Quantitative classification of echographic interstitial syndrome

sonographic profile to predict the need for supplementary oxygen also when during acquiring the scan, saturation was more than 94 % or capillary blood oxygen tension was more than 45 mmHg. We defined true positive (TP) as US score >3 indicating that supplementary O_2 was required. We defined true negative (TN) as US score <3 indicating that supplementary O_2 was not required. False positive (FP) as US score >3 indicating that supplementary O_2 was not required and false negative (FN) as US score <3 indicating that supplementary O_2 was required.

The categorical data were expressed as counts and percentages. As regards the ultrasound findings, the x^2 test was used to compare the percentages between different groups: mild bronchiolitis vs. moderate-severe bronchiolitis; infants in need of oxygen supplementation vs infants not in need of oxygen supplementation; SRV positive bronchiolitis vs SRV negative bronchiolitis.

For all tests, $P<0.05$ was considered significant.

Results

One hundred eighteen infants were eligible for the study. Six were excluded for unavailability of sonographer, three for chest X-ray- diagnosed pneumonia, two for other concomitant pathologies.

One hundred six infants, aged from 9 to 239 days of life (median 71, mean: 87.4 ± 59.3) were enrolled.

Seventy three were positive for SRV. Seven infants were preterm newborns.

The characteristics of the infants at the time of enrollment are described in Table 3.

The control group was composed by 25 infants (11 males, 14 females). Ages ranged from 32 to 160 days of life. No one of the control group was positive for SRV. Only one was preterm newborns.

According to our clinical score performed by the attending physician: 76 infants had mild bronchiolitis, 27 had moderate bronchiolitis, and three had severe bronchiolitis.

According to our US score performed by the pediatric sonographer: 68 infants had mild bronchiolitis, 26 had moderate bronchiolitis, three had severe bronchiolitis and nine had a normal ultrasound pattern.

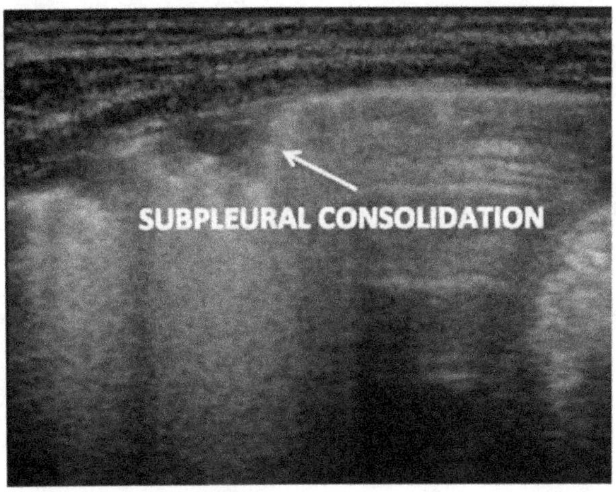

Fig. 2 Subpleural consolidation

Table 3 Study population

Mode of delivery					
	Vaginal	64 (60 %)	Age		
	Cesarean	42 (40 %)		<3 month	40 (38 %)
Gender				>3 month	66 (62 %)
	Male	59 (56 %)	Use of drugs before enrollment		
	Female	47 (44 %)		Yes	46 (43 %)
				No	60 (57 %)
Feeding					
	Bottlefed	43 (41 %)	VRS		
	Breastfed	63 (59 %)		Yes	73 (69 %)
Gestational age				No	33 (31 %)
	Preterm	7 (7 %)	Auscultation of lung		
	Term	99 (93 %)		Normal	10 (9 %)
Family history of atopy				Wheeze	36 (34 %)
	Yes	25 (24 %)		Crackles	41 (39 %)
	No	81 (76 %)		Both	19 (18 %)

Agreement between the attending physician and the pediatric sonographer on the severity of bronchiolitis was high (agreement: 90.6 %; expected agreement: 52.3 %; K = 0.8; Std error = 0.0765; z = 10.19; $p = 0.000$).

According to our US score performed by the radiologist sonographer: 65 infants had mild bronchiolitis, 26 had moderate bronchiolitis, three had severe bronchiolitis and 12 had a normal pattern. Three of these 12 infants scanned by radiologist was considered with a mild bronchiolitis by pediatric sonographer.

Inter-observer concordance on the basis of the US findings between the two different sonographers was excellent (Cohen's kappa coefficient: agreement = 89.6 %; expected agreement 46.4 %; K = 0.8; Std error = 0.07; z = 11.33; $p = 0.000$).

On the basis of our protocol on bronchiolitis, 29 (27 %) infants were in need of oxygen supplementation. LUS permits the identification of those infants that are in need of supplementary oxygen with a specificity of 98.7 % (95 % CI: 93 % to 99.8 %), a sensitivity of 96.6 % (95 % CI: 82.2 % to 99.4 %), a positive predictive value of 96.6 % (95 % CI: 82.2 % to 99.4 %) and a negative predictive value of 98.7 % (95 % CI: 92.95 % to 99.8 %).

In all patients with clinical sign of bronchiolitis, 56/106 (58 %) scans revealed alterations only in the posterior and paravertebral areas against 6/106 (6 %) only in the anterior areas. 35/106 (33 %) infants revealed alterations in both the posterior and anterior areas. 9/106 (8 %) scans revealed no alteration in either the posterior or anterior areas.

The distribution of LUS findings and scan position between the different groups are presented, expressed as counts and percentages, in Tables 4, 5 and 6.

In all patients (100 %) the clinical improvement at discharge was associated with the disappearance of the previous LUS findings and a lower US score.

Ultrasound findings in the control group were all compatible as a normal pattern: subpleural lung consolidations or compact B-lines were observed in 0/25 (0 %) infants, an Individual B line without any pathological significance was observed in 5/25 (20 %) infants.

Discussion

Traditionally, the evaluation of the chest is considered possible only through exposure to radiation. Not long ago, the text *"Harrison's principles of internal medicine"* considered the lung unsuitable for ultrasonographic examination [21]. Nevertheless, lung ultrasound has recently been applied to the diagnosis and management of several diseases and many authors have conducted several studies with promising results, all analyzed in the recent *"International evidence-based recommendations for point-of-care lung ultrasound"* [22].

We demonstrated that sonographers were able to accurately identify bronchiolitis using LUS with a good agreement on its severity between clinical and ultrasound evaluations. Our study confirms LUS as a valuable tool in the diagnosis and management of bronchiolitis and upholds previous conclusions made by Caiullo et al. that recently showed how the use of ultrasound can drastically reduce the need for chest X-ray [10].

Differently from Caiulo et al. [11] who reported data from a single operator, we used different ultrasound operators to evaluate diagnostic accuracy and reproducibility. It is important that every ultrasound examination is carried out in a standard manner and that the same anatomical or artifactual signs can be collected from one patient to another. We identified an echographic score with the aim of elaborating a unified and reproducible approach to LUS by different sonographers which permits consistency when different physicians scan one patient. Our calculated Cohen's Kappa was 0.8, which means that the inter-observer agreement between the pediatric operator's interpretation and that of the blinded radiologist operator was excellent. The evidence of an excellent inter-observer agreement between two operators suggests that lung ultrasound is not only easy to perform but also easy to read. Pediatric and radiologist diagnosis differs only in 3/12 cases where a normal US pattern according to radiologist was considered a mild bronchiolitis US pattern by pediatric sonographer. All these 12 infants did not need oxygen supplementation in the next hours, despite clinically diagnosed as

Table 4 Quantitative classification of echographic interstitial syndrome between the different groups: clinically mild bronchiolitis vs. moderate-severe bronchiolitis; infants in need of oxygen supplementation vs infants in no need of oxygen supplementation

LUS data	Mild	Moderate Severe	χ^2 test	p	Oxygen No	Oxygen Yes	χ^2 test	P
Less than 6 bilaterally involved intercostal spaces in the posterior and paravertebral area of the lung	61/76 (80 %)	3/30 (10 %)	44.3	0.00	61/77 (79 %)	3/29 (10 %)	41.7	0.00
6 to 12 bilaterally involved intercostal spaces in the posterior and paravertebral area of the lung	15/76 (20 %)	18/30 (60 %)	16.2	0.00	16/77 (21 %)	17/29 (59 %)	14	0.00
Up to 12 bilaterally involved intercostal spaces, in the posterior and paravertebral area of the lung	0/76 (0 %)	9/30 (30 %)	24.9	0.00	0/77 (0 %)	9/29 (31 %)	26.1	0.00

Table 5 Subpleural lung consolidation in the posterior area of the lung between the different groups: clinically mild bronchiolitis vs. moderate-severe bronchiolitis; infants in need of oxygen supplementation vs infants in no need of oxygen supplementation

LUS data	Mild	Moderate Severe	x^2 test	p	Oxygen No	Oxygen Yes	x^2 test	P
No presence of subpleural lung consolidations in the posterior and paravertebral area of the lung	53/76 (70 %)	5/30 (17 %)	24.4	0.00	53/77 (69 %)	5/29 (18 %)	22.6	0.00
Subcentimetersubpleural lung consolidations in the posterior and paravertebral area of the lung	20/76 (26 %)	12/30 (40 %)	1.9	0.16	20/77 (26 %)	12/29 (41 %)	2.3	0.1
Subpleural lung consolidation of 1 cm or more in the posterior and paravertebral area of the lung	3/76 (4 %)	13/30 (43 %)	26.4	0.00	4/77 (5 %)	12/29 (41 %)	21.5	0.00

Table 6 LUS findings between SRV positive bronchiolitis vs SRV negative bronchiolitis

LUS data	SRV neg	SRV pos	x^2 test	P
Normal lung sliding with horizontal artifacts (A-lines), and vertical artifacts (B-lines) in limited number or absent in the anterolateral area of the lung	27/33 (82 %)	37/73 (51 %)	9.21	0.00
Diffused and dishomogeneous interstitial syndrome with confluent, multiple B lines and spared areas in the anterolateral area of the lung	5/33 (15 %)	30/73 (41 %)	6.92	0.00
Diffused and dishomogeneous interstitial syndrome and/or subpleural lung consolidations in the anterolateral area of the lung	1/33 (3 %)	6/73 (8 %)	0.9	0.31
Less than 6 bilaterally involved intercostal spaces in the posterior and paravertebral area of the lung	22/33 (67 %)	42/73 (58 %)	0.7	0.3
6 to 12 bilaterally involved intercostal spaces in the posterior and paravertebral area of the lung	9/33 (27 %)	24/73 (33 %)	0.3	0.5
Up to 12 bilaterally involved intercostal spaces, in the posterior and paravertebral area of the lung	2/33 (6 %)	7/73 (9 %)	0.3	0.5
No presence of subpleural lung consolidations in the posterior and paravertebral area of the lung	22/33 (67 %)	36/73 (49 %)	2.7	0.09
Subcentimetersubpleural lung consolidations in the posterior and paravertebral area of the lung	7/33 (21 %)	25/73 (34 %)	1.8	0.17
Subpleural lung consolidation of 1 cm or more in the posterior and paravertebral area of the lung	4/33 (12 %)	12/73 (17 %)	0.3	0.5
No interstitial syndrome ultrasound signs in the posterior and paravertebral area of the lung	8/33 (24 %)	14/73 (19 %)	0.3	0.5
Focal, multiple B-lines in the posterior and paravertebral area of the lung	20/33 (61 %)	37/73 (51 %)	0.9	0.3
Confluent, multiple B lines in the posterior and paravertebral area of the lung	5/33 (15 %)	22/73 (30 %)	2.6	0.1
Only posterior area	23/33 (70 %)	33/73 (45 %)	5.4	0.01
Only anterior area	3/33 (9 %)	3/73 (4 %)	1.06	0.3
Both anterior and posterior area	3/33 (9 %)	32/72 (44 %)	12.7	0.00
No alteration	4/33 (12 %)	5/72 (7 %)	0.8	0.3

affected by mild bronchiolitis and hospitalized. We speculate that pediatric sonographer over-diagnosed US data, influenced by clinical signs because could not avoid observing the patients. Based on our data, clinicians were able to detect infants that will be in need of supplementary oxygen using ultrasonography with high specificity and sensitivity. It means that we can claim a possible prognostic use of LUS in discriminate patients in need of hospitalization and oxygen supplementation, when saturation is more than 94 % and capillary blood oxygen tension was >45 mmHg in air. The use of LUS as a rapid and efficient screening tool to grant respiratory assistance in a timely fashion was already demonstrated in neonatal respiratory distress by Raimondi et al. [23].

A great percentage of our infants with bronchiolitis presented ultrasound anomalies on posterior and paravertebral scans. This data can be explained because the posterior area is more involved in bronchiolitis pathophysiology due to the gravity of obligate supine newborns and infants. Up to date, to our knowledge, it is the first time that the ultrasound involvement of paravertebral areas is described.

Our quantitative classification of echographic interstitial syndrome (Fig. 1) based on posterior bilaterally involved intercostal spaces correlates well with the need for oxygen supplementation and the severity of the bronchiolitis (Table 4).

Particular importance has to be given to infants with a subpleural lung consolidation of 1 cm or more in the posterior area scan (Fig. 2) as a great percentage of these are in need of oxygen supplementation (Table 5).

Our LUS data showed a great percentage of both posterior and anterior areas involved in patients positive for SRV and a great percentage of no alteration in LUS data in patients negative for SRV. Nevertheless, we couldn't find any particular US findings related to SRV infections and, according to previous data published by Tsung et al. [18], it is unknown if different viruses have specific LUS patterns (Table 6).

We acknowledge some limitations of our study. Firstly, we had only three infants diagnosed with severe bronchiolitis. Secondly, our study population age span is considerably wide and is mainly represented by term infants and not by pre-terms who are at a higher risk of developing more serious illnesses. Further research into an intensive care setting and into a wider population are required in order to improve our findings. Thirdly, in this study, experienced physicians in LUS performed the ultrasound evaluations, and the results might not be extrapolated to all pediatricians. However, other authors have reported that physicians without previous knowledge of LUS can acquire the basic skills following a short intensive training period [24–26].

Up to date, LUS has to be considered as a rapidly expanding field and its use in pediatric care has to be implemented, in order to minimize the use of ionizing radiation and the risk of cancer.

At present, LUS is not included in the management of bronchiolitis but if our results are further upholded in larger, multicentric studies, the use of LUS could be routinely recommended in infants with clinical signs and symptoms of suspected bronchiolitis.

Conclusions

The diagnosis of bronchiolitis is mainly based on clinical signs and symptoms but lung ultrasound (LUS), given the absence of radiation, may offer a non-invasive, rapid, reproducible, and relatively inexpensive diagnostic tool that could be of exceptional help in the clinical management of bronchiolitis. Thinner chest walls and smaller lung mass make infants and neonates ideal candidates for ultrasound scans, without exposing them to the greater cancer risk of ionizing radiation relative to adults [27, 28].

In pediatric patients with bronchiolitis, LUS reflects the clinical respiratory status and can be used as a rapid and reproducible screening technique to help the physician in the unequivocal identification of infants in need of hospitalization and oxygen supplementation.

In-patient health care costs of bronchiolitis are high [29, 30]. Despite clinical assessment continues to be the gold standard for diagnosis of bronchiolitis, use of LUS for safely reducing hospitalization, might have a great impact on socioeconomic aspect of this disease thereby decreasing health care costs.

In summary, this pilot study demonstrates that the use of LUS in bronchiolitis can be considered as an extension of the clinical evaluation and could be incorporated into clinical algorithms to aid decision-making. Our promising data needs to be confirmed in larger cohort studies also involving critical patients.

Abbreviations

LUS: Lung ultrasound; SRV: Syncytial respiratory virus.

Competing interests

The authors declare that they have no competing interests.

Authors' contributions

VB and PC conceptualized and designed the study. ADM drafted the manuscript. ES and ST carried out the statistical analyses. MM and IL critically reviewed the manuscript. MMM was responsible for the concept, design and writing of the final version of the manuscript, which was seen and finally approved by all authors.

Acknowledgements

We would like to acknowledge all the families for their participation and the "S. Giacomo" Hospital staff for assistance. We are grateful to all paediatric colleagues who examined these children and whose work underpinned this study.

The authors would also like to thank Prof. Nicola Laforgia, (University of Bari), to had approved Dr Di Mauro's support for this research project; and Prof. Paolo Manzoni (Sant'Anna Hospital, Turin), whose "International Conference on Clinical Neonatology" inspired this work. The authors declare no funding source for the study.

Author details
[1]Pediatric Unit, Maternal and Child Health Department, "S. Giacomo" Hospital, ASL BA, Largo Simone Veneziani, 21, Monopoli (Bari), Italy. [2]Neonatology and Neonatal Intensive Care Unit, Department of Biomedical Science and Human Oncology, University of Bari "Aldo Moro", Bari, Italy. [3]Radiodiagnostic Unit, "S. Giacomo" Hospital, ASL BA, Largo Simone Veneziani, 21, Monopoli (Bari), Italy. [4]Pediatric Unit University of Turin, Turin, Italy. [5]Section of Hygiene, Department of Biomedical Sciences and Human Oncology, University of Bari "Aldo Moro", Bari, Italy.

References

1. Subcommittee on Diagnosis and Management of Bronchiolitis. Diagnosis and management of bronchiolitis. Pediatrics. 2006;118:1774–92.
2. Ralston SL, Lieberthal AS, Meissner HC, Alverson BK, Baley JE, Gadomski AM, et al. Clinical practice guideline: the diagnosis, management, and prevention of bronchiolitis. Pediatrics. 2014;134(5):e1474–502.
3. Wagner T. Bronchiolitis. Pediatr Rev. 2009;30:386–95.
4. Cattarossi L. Lung utrasound: its role in neonatology and pediatrics. Early Hum Dev. 2013;89 Suppl 1:S17–9.
5. Smargiassi A, Inchingolo R, Soldati G, Copetti R, Marchetti G, Zanforlin A, et al. The role of chest ultrasonography in the management of respiratory diseases: document II. MultidiscipRespir Med. 2013;8(1):55.
6. Mong A, Epelman M, Darge K. Ultrasound of the pediatric chest. PediatrRadiol. 2012;42(11):1287–97.
7. Raimondi F, Cattarossi L, Copetti R. Point of care chest ultrasound in the neonatal intensive care unit; an Italian perspective. NeoReviews. 2014;1:e1–5.
8. Zanforlin A, Giannuzzi R, Nardini S, Testa A, Soldati G, Copetti R, et al. The role of chest ultrasonography in the management of respiratory diseases: document I. MultidiscipRespir Med. 2013;8(1):54.
9. Lichtenstein D, Mézière G, Biderman P, Gepner A, Barré O. The comet-tail artifact. An ultrasound sign of alveolar-interstitial syndrome. Am J RespirCrit Care Med. 1997;156(5):1640–6.
10. Soldati G, Giunta V, Sher S, Melosi F, Dini C. "Synthetic" comets: a new look at lung sonography. UltrasoundMedBiol. 2011;37(11):1762–70.
11. Volpicelli G, Melniker LA, Cardinale L, Lamorte A, Frascisco MF. Lung ultrasound in diagnosing and monitoring pulmonary interstital fluid. Radiol Med. 2013;118(2):196–205.
12. Yang PC, Luh KT, Chang DB, Yu CJ, Kuo SH, Wu HD. Ultrasonographic evaluation of pulmonary consolidation. Am Rev Respir Dis. 1992;146(3):757–62.
13. Caiulo VA, Gargani L, Caiulo S, Fisicaro A, Moramarco F, Latini G, et al. Lung ultrasound in bronchiolitis: comparison with chest X-ray. Eur J Pediatr. 2011;170(11):1427–33.
14. Liu L, Gallaher M, Davis R, Rutter CM, Lewis TC, Marcuse EK. Use of respiratory clinical score among different providers. Pediatr Pulmonol. 2004;37:243–8.
15. Copetti R, Cattarossi L. Ultrasound diagnosis of pneumonia in children. Radiol Med. 2008;113(2):190–8.
16. Copetti R, Cattarossi L, Macagno F, Violino M, Furlan R. Lung ultrasound in respiratory distress syndrome: a useful tool for early diagnosis. Neonatology. 2008;94(1):52–9.
17. Copetti R, Cattarossi L. The 'double lung point': an ultrasound sign diagnostic of transient tachypnea of the newborn. Neonatology. 2007;91(3):203–9.
18. Scalini E, Basile IV, Lofù I, De Bellis T, Fortunato M, Laforgia F, et al. Correlation between clinical and chest ultrasound findings in infants with bronchiolitis: A preliminary study. Early Hum Dev. 2011;87S:S96.
19. Lichtenstein DA, Meziere GA. Relevance of lung ultrasound in the diagnosis of acute respiratory failure: the BLUE protocol. Chest. 2008;134(1):1140–7.
20. Tsung JW, Kessler DO, Shah VP. Prospective application of clinician-performed lung ultrasonography during the 2009 H1N1 influenza A pandemic:distinguishing viral from bacterial pneumonia. Crit Ultrasound J. 2012;4(1):16.
21. Kasper DL, Braunwald E, Fauci AS, Hauser SL, Longo DL, Jameson JL, et al. Harrison's principles of internal medicine. 17th ed. New York: McGraw-Hill Medical Publishing Division; 2008.
22. Volpicelli G, Elbarbary M, Blaivas M, Lichtenstein DA, Mathis G, Kirkpatrick AW, et al. International evidence-based recommendations for point-of-care lung ultrasound. Intensive Care Med. 2012;38(4):577–91.
23. Raimondi F, Migliaro F, Sodano A, Umbaldo A, Romano A, Vallone G, et al. Can neonatal lung ultrasound monitor fluid clearance and predict the need of respiratory support? Crit Care. 2012;16(6):R220.
24. Chalumeau-Lemoine L, Baudel JL, Das V, Arrive L, Noblinski B, Guidet B, et al. Results of short-term training of naive physicians in focused general ultrasonography in an intensive-care unit. Intensive Care Med. 2009;35:1767–71.
25. Shah VP, Tunik MG, Tsung JW. Prospective evaluation of point-of-care ultrasonography for the diagnosis of pneumonia in children and young adults. JAMA Pediatr. 2013;167(2):119–25.
26. Bedetti G, Gargani L, Corbisiero A, Frassi F, Poggianti E, Mottola G. Evaluation of ultrasound lung comets by hand-held echocardiography. Cardiovasc Ultrasound. 2006;4:34.
27. Shu XO, Jin F, Linet MS, Zheng W, Clemens J, Mills J, et al. Diagnostic X-ray and ultrasound exposure and risk of childhood cancer. Br J Cancer. 1994;70:531–6.
28. Hall EJ, Brenner DJ. Cancer risks from diagnostic radiology. Br J Radiol. 2008;81(965):362–78.
29. Stang P, Brandenburg N, Carter B. The economic burden of respiratory syncytial virus associated bronchiolitis hospitalization. Arch Pediatric Asolesc Ned. 2001;155:95–6.
30. Pelletier AJ, Mansbach JM, Camargo CA. Direct medical costs of bronchiolitis hospitalizations in the United States. Pediatrics. 2006;118:2418.

26

Neonatal respiratory distress syndrome revealing a cervical bronchogenic cyst

Penelope Thaller[1], Catherine Blanchet[2], Maliha Badr[1], Renaud Mesnage[1], Nicolas Leboucq[3], Michel Mondain[2] and Gilles Cambonie[1*]

Abstract

Background: Bronchogenic cyst is a congenital malformation, rarely located in the cervical region and almost never involved in a neonate with acute respiratory distress in the delivery room.

Case presentation: A female newborn with respiratory distress syndrome caused by a large left cervical mass. Intubation was difficult due to tracheal deviation. Magnetic resonance imaging confirmed a left cervical cyst displacing the trachea and esophagus laterally. Surgical excision was performed via a cervical approach on the 5th day, and pathological examination revealed a bronchogenic cyst. The patient's course was complicated by left vocal cord paralysis and necrotic lesions in the glottic and subglottic regions; she required a tracheostomy on the 13th day. Inflammatory stenosis in the subglottic region required balloon dilation once, 20 days later. Proximal esophageal stenosis induced transient upper airway obstruction with salivary stasis. Decannulation was performed at 2 months and the patient was discharged 10 days later.

Conclusion: A bronchogenic cyst can exceptionally obstruct the airways in the neonatal period. Surgical excision is necessary, but postoperative complications may occur if the cyst is in close contact with the trachea and esophagus, including necrotic and stenotic lesions of the upper aerodigestive tract. In those situations, tracheostomy may be necessary for mechanical ventilation weaning and the initiation of oral feeding.

Keywords: Cervical bronchogenic cyst, Neonatal respiratory distress syndrome, Tracheostomy

Background

Bronchogenic cyst is a congenital malformation of the tracheobronchial tree. It is usually located in the mediastinum or lung parenchyma, though rarely can be seen in extrathoracic locations such as the neck. In 2004, Mehta et al. reported a series of 4 cases of cervical bronchogenic cysts over a 22-year period, with the age of discovery ranging from 3 weeks to 6 years [1]. In 2008, Teissier et al. reported 8 cases over a period of 13 years [2]. The signs and symptoms are variable, but usually consistent with a neck mass associated with chronic cough or stridor [3]. Some cases are not diagnosed until adulthood, when an isolated laterocervical mass is discovered incidentally [4]. We report an exceptional case of cervical bronchogenic cyst revealed by acute respiratory distress in the neonatal period.

* Correspondence: g-cambonie@chu-montpellier.fr
[1]Department of Neonatology and Pediatric Intensive Care Unit, Hôpital Arnaud de Villeneuve, 371 Avenue du Doyen Gaston Giraud, 34295 Montpellier Cedex 5, France
Full list of author information is available at the end of the article

Case presentation

The patient's mother received prenatal care during pregnancy, with 3 antenatal US exams showing normal fetal development. Labor was induced at 41^{+4} gestational weeks in a type 2a maternity ward and delivery was by cesarean section because of abnormal fetal heart rate. The newborn was female with a birth weight of 3045 g. The newborn showed ineffective ventilation from the first postnatal minute, and positive pressure ventilation with a bag and mask was immediately started. A left cervical swelling was also observed. Respiratory distress, with suprasternal tugging and stridor, occurred at every attempt to withdraw ventilatory support. Furthermore, FiO_2 of 90 % was required to maintain SpO_2 above 90 %. Two attempts of orotracheal intubation failed because the larynx could not be visualized. A more experienced pediatrician was called for help. Standard direct laryngoscopy found a right laryngeal deviation with a restricted laryngeal orifice. After sedation with midazolam (0.1 mg/kg intravenous, 2 doses 10 min apart), tracheal intubation was achieved at the 3rd attempt, with a 2.5-mm endotracheal tube, at 1 h 30 min after birth. The newborn was then transferred to a type 3 neonatal unit.

On admission, the newborn was ventilated in assist-control pressure mode with FiO_2 set at 21 %. Clinical examination confirmed a noninflammatory cervical swelling that was soft on palpation. Chest x-ray revealed the endotracheal tube deflected to the right with respect to the spinal axis. Cervical US showed a thin-walled cystic mass measuring 24 × 28 × 37 mm displacing the trachea and the left thyroid lobe medially and forward, and the carotid and jugular vessels laterally and posteriorly. MRI identified a large cystic mass with well-defined walls that laterally displaced the aerodigestive tract (Fig. 1).

In the first 48 h of management, peak inspiratory pressures > 25 cm H_2O were necessary to observe chest expansion and hear vesicular breath sounds at auscultation. Volume mode was tested, but it also generated high inspiratory pressures, between 25 and 30 cm H_2O, despite the selection of a minimal tidal volume (5 ml/kg) and the use of permissive hypercapnia (PCO_2 allowed to rise as high as 60 mmHg). On the assumption that the cyst might be squeezing the endotracheal tube, we performed fine needle aspiration of the cyst in the operating room, under general anesthesia, on postnatal day 3. Twenty milliliters of clear liquid was removed for cytological analysis, which revealed both respiratory-type epithelium and squamous epithelium. Rigid bronchoscopy performed at the same time confirmed tracheal compression and no laryngeal fistula. A 3-mm endotracheal tube was put into place to secure the airway. On day 5, surgery using a cervical approach isolated a unilocular cystic structure measuring 25 × 23 × 6 mm in close contact with the trachea and esophagus. Dissection was not possible from the trachea or the esophagus, and limited resection of trachea and esophagus was therefore mandatory, resulting in an opening of both structures. Both were then sutured. Histological examination showed that the cyst wall was composed of fibrous and smooth fibromuscular tissue, with some seromucinous bronchial gland cells. The wall was lined by a layer of respiratory-type ciliated cells. These findings suggested the diagnosis of bronchogenic cyst.

After the first attempt at extubation on the day after surgery, the infant had respiratory distress due to laryngotracheal edema and left vocal fold paresis that was refractory to treatment with nebulized epinephrine and corticosteroids and required reintubation. The second attempt at 8 days postsurgery was equally unsuccessful. The upper respiratory tract was explored under general anesthesia at a postnatal age of 13 days. We observed edema of the left laryngeal ventricle and the anterior third of the glottis, associated with the necrotic appearance of the mucosa in the left lateral subglottis (Fig. 2). Such lesions in a newborn who could not be weaned from mechanical ventilatory support prompted immediate tracheostomy.

Sedation was gradually reduced over 48 h postsurgery, and mechanical ventilation was ended 2 weeks later with the infant ventilating effectively with the tracheal cannula.

Laryngotracheobronchoscopy under general anesthesia on day 33 revealed a subglottic stenosis treated with a 6-mm diameter balloon dilation. Proximal esophageal stenosis was also observed and not treated. Videographic exploration of swallowing confirmed the images of a very proximal partial esophageal stenosis, from C3 to C4.

After a final endoscopic assessment at 2 months showing the absence of airway stenosis, the cannula was withdrawn. The infant was then discharged 10 days later. She was exclusively breastfed and weight and height

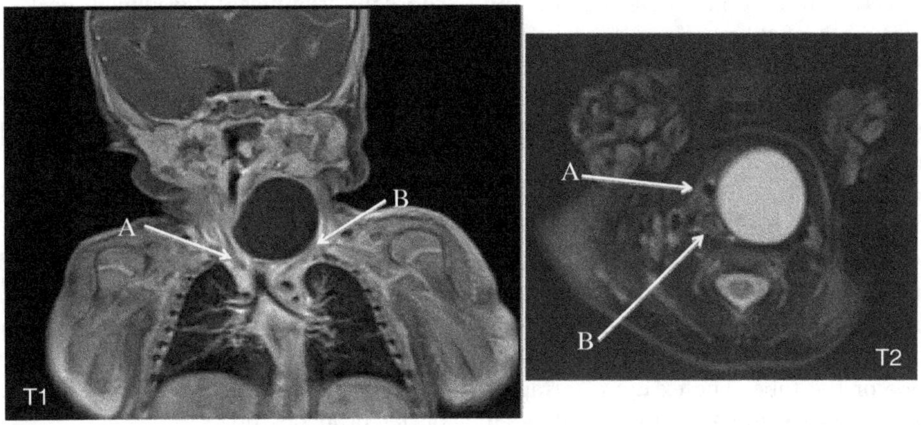

Fig. 1 Cervical thoracic MRI. Coronal T1-weighted sequence showing a voluminous left laterocervical mass displacing the trachea (**a**) and carotid-jugular axis (**b**). Axial T2-weighted sequence showing tracheal compression (**a**) and esophageal compression (**b**) by the cyst

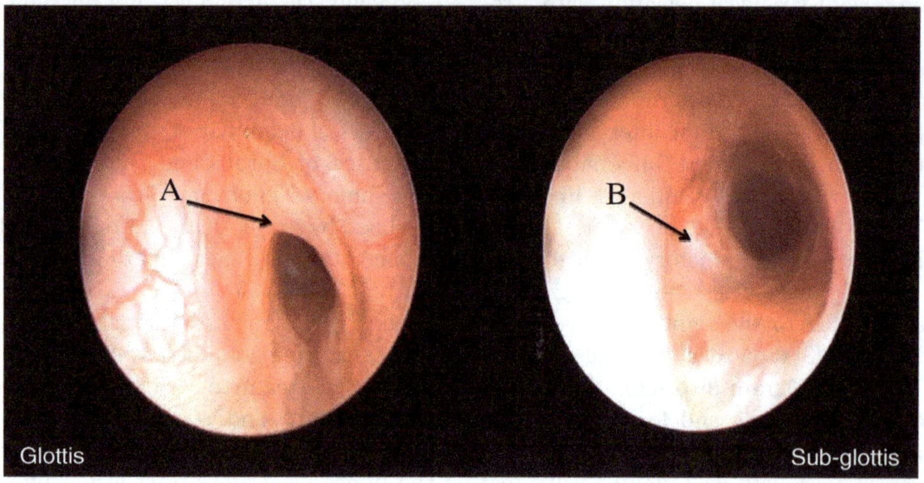

Fig. 2 Postoperative endoscopy. Glottic region: anterior synechia (**a**) causing luminal stenosis of 50 %. Subglottic region: sutured tracheal wound (**b**) and inflammatory alterations causing grade 1 stenosis

gains were satisfactory, with respective gains of 915 g and 7 cm since birth, with absence of swallowing difficulty in relation to the partial esophageal stenosis.

Discussion

The respiratory bud develops from the ventral side of the primitive foregut from the 4th week of development. Cervical bronchogenic cyst may result from an abnormal division of the bud and migration to an ectopic localization in the neck region [1,5,6]. Other extrathoracic localizations have been described, including subcutaneous [7] and even abdominal [8] sites.

Antenatal discovery of a bronchogenic cyst is rare and localization is generally intrathoracic [9,10]. One case has been reported of a cervico-mediastinal bronchogenic cyst detected by a cervical mass on prenatal US [11]. Undetected cervical bronchogenic cyst may also cause polyhydramnios by esophageal compression [12]. In both this case and ours, an abnormal fetal heart rate precipitated delivery by cesarean section. Nevertheless, the direct and indirect impact of this malformation on disturbances in fetal monitoring is difficult to establish.

The immediate neonatal respiratory distress of our patient was explained by direct compression of the trachea, causing major difficulties for intubation because the larynx could not be visualized. The use of a video-laryngoscope for intubation can improve the viewing conditions of the upper airways, making it easier to identify the laryngeal inlet. Rigid bronchoscopy or a flexometallic tube can also relieve glottic-subglottic compression, although great caution is required while advancing the scope or the tube. The ex utero intrapartum treatment (EXIT) procedure can also be done if prenatal diagnosis suggests fetal airway obstruction by a neck mass. Its use in this context has mainly been reported for cervical lymphatic malformations and cervical teratomas [13,14].

The main differential diagnosis is cystic hygroma, which is more likely in the setting of a multilocular cyst, and more unlikely in the setting of a unilocular cyst. Other differential diagnoses include thymic cyst, branchial cyst and thyroglossal duct cyst, but they are rarely responsible for neonatal respiratory distress. Only histological examination of the resected specimen confirms the diagnosis.

MRI is essential before surgery, as it provides the surgeon with precise information on the anatomical relationships with adjacent organs [15]. Rigid bronchoscopy assesses the degree of cyst-trachea contact and the need for tracheal surgery [12]. Needle aspiration of the cyst usually has low diagnostic value [16]. It was performed in our patient to temporarily reduce the tracheal compression. However, neither cyst aspiration nor the larger caliber endotracheal tube introduced following bronchoscopy significantly reduced peak inspiratory pressures, which remained high until surgery.

The only treatment is surgical excision, even for an asymptomatic cyst, given the risks of infection, hemorrhage and, rarely, malignant transformation [17]. The paralysis of the left vocal cord may have resulted from direct injury to the laryngeal nerve during surgery. Paralysis was reported in two other cases [2,12], but in one of these cases this condition had already been observed during the preoperative bronchoscopy, suggesting direct mechanical interference between the cyst and the ipsilateral laryngeal nerve [2]. Evaluation of vocal cord mobility before surgery was not possible in our case because of the depth of sedation during bronchoscopy.

Several factors probably contributed to the alterations in the glottic and subglottic regions observed after the intervention, including intubation and the repeated attempts to intubate, the inflammation associated with laryngeal surgery, and the prolonged mechanical ventilation. In a newborn, edemic and necrotic lesions further narrow an already physiologically narrow larynx, which is an additional motivation to perform tracheostomy.

In addition to the vocal cord paralysis, persistent airway obstruction after laryngeal surgery should always raise the suspicion of a local cause, such as stenosis. In our patient, a proximal esophageal stenosis was also present after surgery. The damage to the esophageal mucosa was probably caused by the surgery, secondary to cyst resection and the suturing of borders. This stenosis, however, had only transient and moderate clinical consequences and did not preclude satisfactory breastfeeding, even with the tracheal cannula.

Conclusion

Cervical bronchogenic cyst is rare and diagnosis is most often made in childhood. However, it should be systematically considered in all cases of neonatal cervical tumor, especially if respiratory distress is present. Prenatal diagnosis may be guided by an unexplained polyhydramnios and/or direct visualization of a cyst, in which case delivery should be performed in a maternity hospital with a type 3 neonatal unit. The EXIT procedure, with a multidisciplinary team approach, should also be planned for fetuses with evidence of airway obstruction on prenatal images.

Abbreviations

US: Ultrasound; FiO_2: Fraction of inspired oxygen; SpO_2: Oxygen saturation by pulse oximetry; MRI: Magnetic resonance imaging; cm H_2O: centimeter of water (0.7355 mmHg); PCO_2: Partial pressure of carbon dioxide measured on capillary blood gas sampling (mmHg); C3: 3rd cervical vertebra; C4: 4th cervical vertebra.

Competing interests

The authors declare that they have no competing interests.

Authors' contributions

PT reviewed the literature and prepared the manuscript, CB helped to draft the manuscript, MB and RM made a critical reading of the manuscript and participated to revisions, NL helped to draft the manuscript, MM helped to draft the manuscript and participated to revisions, GC reviewed the literature, prepared the manuscript and is the corresponding author. All authors read and approved the final version of the manuscript.

Acknowledgement

The authors thank Mrs C Stott-Carmeni for reviewing the manuscript and for editorial assistance.
This case study is from the Neonatal Intensive Care Unit, Arnaud de Villeneuve Hospital, Montpellier University Hospital Center.

Author details

[1]Department of Neonatology and Pediatric Intensive Care Unit, Hôpital Arnaud de Villeneuve, 371 Avenue du Doyen Gaston Giraud, 34295 Montpellier Cedex 5, France. [2]Department of Pediatric Otorhinolaryngology, Hôpital Arnaud de Villeneuve, 371 Avenue du Doyen Gaston Giraud, 34295 Montpellier Cedex 5, France. [3]Department of Neuroradiology, CHU Montpellier, F-34000 Montpellier, France.

References

1. Mehta RP, Faquin WC, Cunningham MJ. Cervical bronchogenic cysts: a consideration in the differential diagnosis of pediatric cervical cystic masses. Int J Pediatr Otorhinolaryngol. 2004;68:563–8.
2. Teissier N, Elmaleh-Bergès M, Ferkdadji L, François M, Van den Abbeele T. Cervical bronchogenic cysts: usual and unusual clinical presentations. Arch Otolaryngol Head Neck Surg. 2008;134:1165–9.
3. Goswamy J, de Kruijf S, Humphrey G, Rothera MP, Bruce IA. Bronchogenic cysts as a cause of infantile stridor: case report and literature review. J Laryngol Otol. 2011;125:1094–7.
4. Bocciolini C, Dall'olio D, Cunsolo E, Latini G, Gradoni P, Laudadio P. Cervical bronchogenic cyst: asymptomatic neck mass in an adult male. Acta Otolaryngol. 2006;126:553–6.
5. Marks C, Marks P. The embryologic basis of tracheobroncho-pulmonary maldevelopment. Int Surg. 1987;72:109–14.
6. Joshi R, Cobb AR, Wilson P, Bailey BM. Lingual cyst lined by respiratory and gastric epithelium in a neonate. Br J Oral Maxillofac Surg. 2013;51:173–5.
7. Gaikwad P, Muthusami JC, Raj JP, Rajinikanth J, John GM. Subcutaneous bronchogenic cyst. Otolaryngol Head Neck Surg. 2006;135:951–2.
8. El Youssef R, Fleseriu M, Sheppard BC. Adrenal and pancreatic presentation of subdiaphragmatic retroperitoneal bronchogenic cysts. Arch Surg. 2010;145:302–4.
9. Levine D, Jennings R, Barnewolt C, Mehta T, Wilson J, Wong G. Progressive fetal bronchial obstruction caused by a bronchogenic cyst diagnosed using prenatal MR imaging. AJR Am J Roentgenol. 2001;176:49–52.
10. Bernasconi A, Yoo SJ, Golding F, Langer JC, Jaeggi ET. Etiology and outcome of prenatally detected paracardial cystic lesions: a case series and review of the literature. Ultrasound Obstet Gynecol. 2007;29:388–94.
11. Kaji T, Takamatsu H, Noguchi H, Tahara H, Fukushige T, Mukai M, et al. Cervico-mediastinal bronchogenic cyst occurring in the prenatal period: report of a case. Surg Today. 2000;30:1016–8.
12. Cavel O, Kokta V, Reveret M, L'Allier M, Froehlich P, Lapointe A. Subglottic bronchogenic cyst presenting as neonatal asphyxia. Case report and literature review. Int J Pediatr Otorhinolaryngol Extra. 2013;8:92–6.
13. Liechty KW. Ex-utero intrapartum therapy. Semin Fetal Neonatal Med. 2010;15:34–9.
14. Laje P, Peranteau WH, Hedrick HL, Flake AW, Johnson MP, Moldenhauer JS, et al. Ex utero intrapartum treatment (EXIT) in the management of cervical lymphatic malformation. J Pediatr Surg. 2015;50:311–4.
15. Kieran SM, Robson CD, Nosé V, Rahbar R. Foregut duplication cysts in the head and neck: presentation, diagnosis, and management. Arch Otolaryngol Head Neck Surg. 2010;136:778–82.
16. Sumiyoshi K, Shimizu S, Enjoji M, Iwashita A, Kawakami K. Bronchogenic cyst in the abdomen. Virchows Arch A Pathol Anat Histopathol. 1985;408:93–8.14.
17. Ashizawa K, Okimoto T, Shirafuji T, Kusano H, Ayabe H, Hayashi K. Anterior mediastinal bronchogenic cyst: demonstration of complicating malignancy by CT and MRI. Br J Radiol. 2001;74:959–61.

Permissions

All chapters in this book were first published in PEDIATRICS, by BioMed Central; hereby published with permission under the Creative Commons Attribution License or equivalent. Every chapter published in this book has been scrutinized by our experts. Their significance has been extensively debated. The topics covered herein carry significant findings which will fuel the growth of the discipline. They may even be implemented as practical applications or may be referred to as a beginning point for another development.

The contributors of this book come from diverse backgrounds, making this book a truly international effort. This book will bring forth new frontiers with its revolutionizing research information and detailed analysis of the nascent developments around the world.

We would like to thank all the contributing authors for lending their expertise to make the book truly unique. They have played a crucial role in the development of this book. Without their invaluable contributions this book wouldn't have been possible. They have made vital efforts to compile up to date information on the varied aspects of this subject to make this book a valuable addition to the collection of many professionals and students.

This book was conceptualized with the vision of imparting up-to-date information and advanced data in this field. To ensure the same, a matchless editorial board was set up. Every individual on the board went through rigorous rounds of assessment to prove their worth. After which they invested a large part of their time researching and compiling the most relevant data for our readers.

The editorial board has been involved in producing this book since its inception. They have spent rigorous hours researching and exploring the diverse topics which have resulted in the successful publishing of this book. They have passed on their knowledge of decades through this book. To expedite this challenging task, the publisher supported the team at every step. A small team of assistant editors was also appointed to further simplify the editing procedure and attain best results for the readers.

Apart from the editorial board, the designing team has also invested a significant amount of their time in understanding the subject and creating the most relevant covers. They scrutinized every image to scout for the most suitable representation of the subject and create an appropriate cover for the book.

The publishing team has been an ardent support to the editorial, designing and production team. Their endless efforts to recruit the best for this project, has resulted in the accomplishment of this book. They are a veteran in the field of academics and their pool of knowledge is as vast as their experience in printing. Their expertise and guidance has proved useful at every step. Their uncompromising quality standards have made this book an exceptional effort. Their encouragement from time to time has been an inspiration for everyone.

The publisher and the editorial board hope that this book will prove to be a valuable piece of knowledge for researchers, students, practitioners and scholars across the globe.

List of Contributors

Kohei Tsukahara, Emily Knaup, Kumiko Hayashi and Yoshihito Ujike
Advanced Emergency and Critical Care Medical Center, Okayama University Hospital, Okayama, Japan

Nobuyuki Nosaka
Department of Pediatrics, Okayama University Graduate School of Medicine, Dentistry and Pharmaceutical Sciences, Okayama, Japan
Advanced Emergency and Critical Care Medical Center, Okayama University Hospital, Okayama, Japan

Shingo Ichiba
Department of Community and Emergency Medicine, Okayama University Graduate School of Medicine, Dentistry and Pharmaceutical Sciences, Okayama, Japan
Advanced Emergency and Critical Care Medical Center, Okayama University Hospital, Okayama, Japan

Shingo Kasahara
Department of Cardiovascular Surgery, Okayama University Graduate School of Medicine, Dentistry and Pharmaceutical Sciences, Okayama, Japan

Yoshinori Kobayashi, Makio Oka, Katsuhiro Kobayashi and Harumi Yoshinaga
Department of Child Neurology, Okayama University Graduate School of Medicine, Dentistry and Pharmaceutical Sciences, Okayama, Japan

Rei-Cheng Yang, Jong-Hau Hsu, Jiunn-Ren Wu and Zen-Kong Dai
Department of Respiratory Therapy, College of Medicine, Kaohsiung Medical University, Kaohsiung, Taiwan
School of Medicine, College of Medicine, Kaohsiung Medical University, Kaohsiung, Taiwan
Department of Pediatrics, Kaohsiung Medical University Hospital, No.100, Tzyou 1st RoadSan Ming District, Kaohsiung 807, Taiwan

Hsiu-Lin Chen, Wei-Te Lee and Pei-Lun Lee
Department of Pediatrics, Kaohsiung Medical University Hospital, No.100, Tzyou 1st RoadSan Ming District, Kaohsiung 807, Taiwan
Department of Respiratory Therapy, College of Medicine, Kaohsiung Medical University, Kaohsiung, Taiwan

Ali Arabkhazaeli, Susanne J. H. Vijverberg, Jan A. M. Raaijmakers and Anke H. Maitland van der Zee
Division of Pharmacoepidemiology & Clinical Pharmacology, Utrecht Institute for Pharmaceutical Sciences (UIPS), Faculty of Science, Utrecht University, David de Wied Building, Universiteitsweg 99, Utrecht 3508 TB, The Netherlands

Francine C. van Erp and Cornelis K. van der Ent
Department of Pediatric Respiratory Medicine, Wilhelmina Children's Hospital, University Medical Centre Utrecht, Lundlaan 6, Utrecht 3584 EA, The Netherlands

Sa'ed H. Zyoud
Poison Control and Drug Information Center (PCDIC), College of Medicine and Health Sciences, An-Najah National University, Nablus 44839, Palestine
Department of Clinical and Community Pharmacy, College of Medicine and Health Sciences, An-Najah National University, Nablus 44839, Palestine
WHO Collaborating Centre for Drug Information, National Poison Centre, Universiti Sains Malaysia (USM), Penang 11800, Malaysia

Samah W. Al-Jabi
Department of Clinical and Community Pharmacy, College of Medicine and Health Sciences, An-Najah National University, Nablus 44839, Palestine

Rahmat Awang
WHO Collaborating Centre for Drug Information, National Poison Centre, Universiti Sains Malaysia (USM), Penang 11800, Malaysia

Adham Abu Taha, Ansam F. Sawalha and Waleed M. Sweileh
Department of Pharmacology and Toxicology, College of Medicine and Health Sciences, An-Najah National University, Nablus 44839, Palestine

Khulood F. Araj and Islam A. Abahri
PharmD Program, College of Medicine and Health Sciences, An-Najah National University, Nablus, Palestine

Archana B. Patel and Leena Dhande
Lata Medical Research Foundation and Indira Gandhi Government Medical College, Nagpur, India

Akash Bang
Mahatma Gandhi Institute of Medical Sciences, Sewagram, Maharashtra, India

Meenu Singh
Post Graduate Institute of Medical Sciences, Chandigarh, India

Luke Ravi Chelliah
Institute of Child Health, Chennai, India

Ashraf Malik
Jawaharlal Nehru Medical College, Aligarh Muslim University, Aligarh, India

Sandhya Khadse
B.J. Medical College, Pune, India

Lene Lochte and Poul Erik Petersen
Department of Odontology, University of Copenhagen, Copenhagen 1014, Denmark

Kim G. Nielsen
Department of Pediatrics and Adolescent Medicine, Copenhagen University Hospital, Rigshospitalet, Copenhagen 2100, Denmark

Thomas A. E. Platts-Mills
Department of Medicine, Division of Allergy and Clinical Immunology, University of Virginia, Charlottesville 22908, VA, USA

Amanda C. Nascimento-Carvalhos
Bahiana School of Medicine, Bahiana Foundation for Science Development, Salvador, Bahia, Brazil

Olli Ruuskanen
Department of Paediatrics, Turku University and University Hospital, Turku, Finland

Cristiana M. Nascimento-Carvalho
Department of Paediatrics, Federal University of Bahia School of Medicine, Salvador, Bahia, Brazil

Xiaoling Wang and Libo Zhao
Department of Pharmacy, Beijing Children's Hospital, Capital Medical University, Beijing 100045, China

Zhenwei Xie
School of Pharmaceutical Science, Peking University, Beijing 100191, China
Department of Pharmacy, Beijing Children's Hospital, Capital Medical University, Beijing 100045, China

Lin Sun and Adong Shen
Key Laboratory of Pediatric Respiratory Infection Diseases, Beijing Pediatric Research Institute, Beijing Children's Hospital, Capital Medical University, Beijing 100045, China

Jun Liu, Yan Guo and Baoping Xu
Department of Respiratory, Beijing Children's Hospital, Capital Medical University, Beijing 100045, China

Wenjing Gu, Wujun Jiang, Xinxing Zhang, Zhengrong Chen, Yongdong Yan, Li Huang, Meijuan Wang, Shuhui Wang and Wei Ji
Department of Respiration, Children's Hospital of Soochow University, Suzhou 215003, China

Xuejun Shao
Department of Clinical laboratory, Children's Hospital, Children's Hospital of Soochow University, Suzhou 215003, China

H. Turnham
Bristol Royal Hospital for Children, University Hospitals Bristol NHS Foundation Trust, Bristol, United Kingdom

S. Agbeko
Great North Children's Hospital, The Newcastle upon Tyne Hospitals NHS Foundation Trust, Newcastle University, Newcastle upon Tyne, UK
Institute of Cellular Medicine, Newcastle University, Newcastle upon Tyne, UK

J. Furness
Country Durham and Darlington NHS Foundation trust, Darlington, UK

J. Pappachan
Southampton Children's Hospital, Southampton, UK

A. G. Sutcliffe
Institute of Child Health, University College London, GAP unit, Institute of Child Health, 30 Guilford Street, London WC1N 1EH, UK

P. Ramnarayan
Children's Acute Transport Service, Great Ormond Street Hospital NHS Foundation Trust, London, UK

Magdeldin Elgizouli and Alexandra Nieters
Center for Chronic Immunodeficiency, Medical Center - University of Freiburg, Faculty of Medicine, University of Freiburg, Breisacherstr. 115 4, Freiburg D-79106, Germany

Chad Logan and Dietrich Rothenbacher
Institute of Epidemiology and Medical Biometry, Ulm University, Ulm, Germany

Ruth Grychtol and Andrea Heinzmann
Department of Pediatrics and Adolescent Medicine, Medical Center - University of Freiburg, Faculty of Medicine, University of Freiburg, Freiburg, Germany

Chia-Chin Li
Departments of Laboratory Medicine, Kaohsiung Chang Gung Memorial Hospital, Kaohsiung, Taiwan

Huey-Ling You
Department of Medical Laboratory Sciences and Biotechnology, Fooyin University, Kaohsiung, Taiwan
Departments of Laboratory Medicine, Kaohsiung Chang Gung Memorial Hospital, Kaohsiung, Taiwan

Shun-Jen Chang
Department of Kinesiology, Health and Leisure Studies, National University of Kaohsiung, Kaohsiung, Taiwan

Hong-Ren Yu
Department of Pediatrics, Kaohsiung Chang Gung Memorial Hospital and Chang Gung University College of Medicine, Kaohsiung, Taiwan

Chang-Han Chen
Institute for Translational Research in Biomedicine, Kaohsiung Chang Gung Memorial Hospital, Kaohsiung, Taiwan
Institute for Translational Research in Biomedicine, Kaohsiung Chang Gung Memorial Hospital, Kaohsiung, Taiwan
Department of Applied Chemistry, and Graduate Institute of Biomedicine and Biomedical Technology, National Chi Nan University, Nanto, Taiwan

Wei-Ting Liao
Department of Biotechnology, College of Life Science, Kaohsiung Medical University, No. 100 Shih-Chuan 1st Road, Kaohsiung 807, Taiwan
Department of Biological Sciences, National Sun Yat-Sen University, Kaohsiung, Taiwan

Hye-Rim Kim, Chang Won Choi and Beyong Il Kim
Department of Pediatrics, Bundang CHA Medical Center, CHA University, Seongnam, Republic of Korea
Department of Pediatrics, Seoul National University College of Medicine, Seoul, Republic of Korea
Department of Pediatrics, Seoul National University Bundang Hospital, 82 Gumi-ro 173 Beon-gil, Bundang-gu, Seongnam 13620, Republic of Korea

Ji Young Kim and Bo La Yun
Department of Radiology, Seoul National University Bundang Hospital, Seongnam, Republic of Korea

Byoungkook Lee
Department of Pediatrics, Wonju Severance Christian Hospital, Wonju, Republic of Korea

Yuan-Jian Sheng, Xue-Jing Li, Jin-Ling Liu, Xi-Ling Wu and Xue-Feng Xu
Department of Respiratory Medicine, The Children's Hospital, Zhejiang University School of Medicine, Hangzhou 310052, China

Shan-Shan Xu
Department of Neonatology, The Children's Hospital, Zhejiang University School of Medicine, Hangzhou 310052, People's Republic of China

V. Oktaria, C. D. Satria, J. Atthobari, H. Nirwati and Y. Soenarto
Pediatrics Research Office, Child Health Department, Faculty of Medicine, Universitas Gadjah Mada/ DR Sardjito Hospital, Yogyakarta, Indonesia

V. Oktaria, K. J. Lee, J. E. Bines and M. H. Danchin
Department of Pediatrics, Faculty of Medicine, Dentistry and Health Sciences, The University of Melbourne, Melbourne, Australia

V. Oktaria, K. J. Lee, J. E. Bines, E. Watts M. H. Danchin
Murdoch Childrens Research Institute (MCRI), The Royal Children Hospital, Melbourne, Australia

J. Atthobari
Department of Pharmacology & Therapy, Faculty of Medicine, Universitas Gadjah Mada, Yogyakarta, Indonesia

H. Nirwati
Department of Microbiology, Faculty of Medicine, Universitas Gadjah Mada, Yogyakarta, Indonesia

C. D. Kirkwood
Bill and Melinda Gates Foundation, Seattle, USA
Murdoch Childrens Research Institute (MCRI), The Royal Children Hospital, Melbourne, Australia

Virginia Mirra, Silvia Montella and Francesca Santamaria
Department of Translational Medical Sciences, Federico II University, Via Sergio Pansini 5, 80131 Naples, Italy

Hiroki Miura, Fumihiko Hattori, Hidetoshi Uchida, Kazuko Kudo and Tetsushi Yoshikawa
Department of Pediatrics, Fujita Health University School of Medicine, 1-98, Dengakugakubo, Kutsukake-cho, Toyoake, Aichi 470-1192, Japan

Tadayoshi Hata
Graduate School of Health Sciences, Fujita Health University, Toyoake, Aichi, Japan

Masatoki Sato
Department of Pediatrics, School of Medicine, Fukushima Medical University, Fukushima, Japan

Kaia Skromme and Maria Vollsæter
Department of Pediatrics, Haukeland University Hospital, N-5021 Bergen, Norway

Maria Vollsæter and Trond Markestad
Department of Clinical Science, Faculty of Medicine and Dentistry, University of Bergen, Bergen, Norway

Thomas Halvorsen
Department of Pediatrics, Haukeland University Hospital, N-5021 Bergen, Norway
Department of Clinical Science, Faculty of Medicine and Dentistry, University of Bergen, Bergen, Norway

Knut Øymar
Department of Clinical Science, Faculty of Medicine and Dentistry, University of Bergen, Bergen, Norway
Department of Pediatrics, Stavanger University Hospital, Stavanger, Norway

Chiyoe Shirota, Takahisa Tainaka, Yujiro Tanaka, Akinari Hinoki, Wataru Sumida, Naruhiko Murase, Kazuo Oshima, Kosuke Chiba, Ryo Shirotsuki and Hiroo Uchida
Department of Pediatric Surgery, Nagoya University Graduate School of Medicine, 65 Tsurumai-cho, Showa-ku, Nagoya 466-8550, Japan

Toshiki Nakane
Department of Radiology, Nagoya University Graduate School of Medicine, Nagoya, Japan

Yosra Azizpour
Department of Clinical Epidemiology, Student Research Committee, Ilam University of Medical Sciences, Ilam, Iran

Ali Delpisheh
Department of Clinical Epidemiology, Psychosocial Injuries Research Center, Ilam University of Medical Sciences, Ilam, Iran

Zahra Montazeri
School of Epidemiology, Public Health and Preventive Medicine, Faculty of Medicine, University of Ottawa, Ottawa, Canada

Kourosh Sayehmiri
Department of Biostatistics, Psychosocial Injuries Research Center, Ilam University of Medical Sciences, Ilam, Iran

Behzad Darabi
Department of Pediatrics, Faculty of Medicine, Ilam University of Medical Sciences, Ilam, Iran

Tao Zhou, Tianli Zheng, Lingxu Zhou, Chunping Jiang and Xiaofang Pei
Department of Public Health Laboratory Sciences, West China School of Public Health (No.4 West China Teaching Hospital), Sichuan University, 16#, Section 3, Renmin Road South, Chengdu 610041, Sichuan, People's Republic of Chinas

Jiayi Chen
Research Center for Occupational Respiratory Diseases, West China School of Public Health (No.4 West China Teaching Hospital), Sichuan University, 16#, Section 3, Renmin Road South, Chengdu 610041, Sichuan, China
Department of Public Health Laboratory Sciences, West China School of Public Health (No.4 West China Teaching Hospital), Sichuan University, 16#, Section 3, Renmin Road South, Chengdu 610041, Sichuan, People's Republic of Chinas

Pengwei Hu
Shenzhen Nanshan Center for Disease Control and Prevention, 95#, Nanshang Road, Shenzhen 518054, Guangdong, China
Department of Public Health Laboratory Sciences, West China School of Public Health (No.4 West China Teaching Hospital), Sichuan University, 16#, Section 3, Renmin Road South, Chengdu 610041, Sichuan, People's Republic of Chinas

Lingxu Zhou
Chongqing Yuzhong District Center for Disease Control and Prevention, 254#, Heping Road, Yuzhong District, Chongqing 400010, China

Xingge Yang and Guangyao Sheng
Pediatrics, the First Affiliated Hospital of Zhengzhou University, No. 1 East Jianshe Road, Zhengzhou 450052, Henan, China

Aayush Khanal, Arun Sharma, Srijana Basnet, Pushpa Raj Sharma and Fakir Chandra Gami
Department of Pediatrics, Tribhuvan University Teaching Hospital, Institute of Medicine, Maharajgunj-44600, Kathmandu, Nepal

Pushpa Raj Sharma
Kathmandu Medical College Teaching Hospital, Sinamangal, Kathmandu, Nepal

Eric D. McCollum
Department of Pediatrics, Division of Pulmonology, Johns Hopkins School of Medicine, Baltimore, USA
Institute for Global Health, University College London, London, UK

Carina King, Tim Colbourn and Bejoy Nambiar
Institute for Global Health, University College London, London, UK

Robert Hollowell
The Boston Consulting Group, Boston, USA

Janet Zhou, David Mukanga and Deborah C. Hay Burgess
Bill & Melinda Gates Foundation, Seattle, USA

Vincenzo Basile, Egisto Scalini, Ignazio Lofù and Mariano M. Manzionna
Pediatric Unit, Maternal and Child Health Department, "S. Giacomo" Hospital, ASL BA, Largo Simone Veneziani, 21, Monopoli (Bari), Italy

Antonio Di Mauro
Neonatology and Neonatal Intensive Care Unit, Department of Biomedical Science and Human Oncology, University of Bari "Aldo Moro", Bari, Italy

Paolo Comes
Radiodiagnostic Unit, "S. Giacomo" Hospital, ASL BA, Largo Simone Veneziani, 21, Monopoli (Bari), Italy

Michael Mostert
Pediatric Unit University of Turin, Turin, Italy

Silvio Tafuri
Section of Hygiene, Department of Biomedical Sciences and Human Oncology, University of Bari "Aldo Moro", Bari, Italy

Penelope Thaller, Maliha Badr, Renaud Mesnage and Gilles Cambonie
Department of Neonatology and Pediatric Intensive Care Unit, Hôpital Arnaud de Villeneuve, 371 Avenue du Doyen Gaston Giraud, 34295 Montpellier Cedex 5, France

Catherine Blanchet and Michel Mondain
Department of Pediatric Otorhinolaryngology, Hôpital Arnaud de Villeneuve, 371 Avenue du Doyen Gaston Giraud, 34295 Montpellier Cedex 5, France

Nicolas Leboucq
Department of Neuroradiology, CHU Montpellier, F-34000 Montpellier, France

Index

www.ingramcontent.com/pod-product-compliance
Lightning Source LLC
LaVergne TN
LVHW080704210926
848485LV00003B/414